ANTIEPILEPTIC DRUGS:
QUANTITATIVE ANALYSIS AND INTERPRETATION

Antiepileptic Drugs: Quantitative Analysis and Interpretation

Editors

C. E. Pippenger, Ph.D.
Assistant Professor of Neuropharmacology (Neurology)
Columbia University College of Physicians and Surgeons
New York, New York 10032

J. Kiffin Penry, M.D.
Chief, Epilepsy Branch
Neurological Disorders Program
National Institute of Neurological and Communicative Disorders and Stroke
National Institutes of Health
Bethesda, Maryland 20014

Henn Kutt, M.D.
Associate Professor of Neurology and Pharmacology
Cornell University Medical College
New York, New York 10021

Raven Press ▪ New York

Raven Press, 1140 Avenue of the Americas, New York, New York 10036

Made in the United States of America

Library of Congress Cataloging in Publication Data

Main entry under title:

Antiepileptic drugs.

Includes bibliographical references and index.
1. Epilepsy—Chemotherapy. 2. Anticonvulsants—Analysis. I. Pippenger, C. E. II. Penry, J. Kiffin, 1929– III. Kutt, Henn. [DNLM: 1. Anticonvulsants. 2. Epilepsy—Drug therapy. 3. Monitoring systems. 4. Quality control. QV85 A629]
RC374.C48A59 615′.784 76–58055
ISBN 0–89004–197–0

Preface

During the past ten years, the value of routine monitoring of serum antiepileptic drug levels as an adjunct to the provision of better patient care has been repeatedly demonstrated. Clinical studies have shown a strong correlation betwen serum antiepileptic drug concentrations and seizure control, and it has been suggested that nearly 80% of all epileptic patients could become seizure-free with the currently available antiepileptic drugs if their serum drug concentrations were accurately and routinely monitored. The demand for services for the quantitation of antiepileptic drugs has increased as physicians have recognized the value of serum monitoring. This demand has stimulated many laboratories without extensive experience in drug monitoring techniques to establish routine testing procedures for the various antiepileptic drugs.

The establishment of a large number of laboratories engaged in routine antiepileptic drug analysis, particularly those without previous experience in drug monitoring, has resulted in a great deal of confusion with respect to accuracy of results, analytical methodology, and the clinical application of drug concentrations determined in the laboratory. In 1974, a blind survey of laboratories in the United States that routinely analyze antiepileptic drugs revealed that more than half were reporting unacceptable results. Inaccurate reports of serum antiepileptic drug levels could lead to inappropriate adjustment of a patient's medication regimen and could cause the physician to conclude that quantitation of serum drug levels is of no clinical value. Failure to monitor serum antiepileptic drug levels denies the physician a valuable means of enhancing the management of patients with epilepsy and deprives the patient of optimum care.

As a result of the blind survey, a voluntary Antiepileptic Drug Levels Quality Control program was instituted under the auspices of the Epilepsy Foundation of America. One of the recurrent requests from the participants in this program was for a national workshop to discuss the analytical methodology employed in the quantitative analysis of antiepileptic drugs and the clinical applications of therapeutic monitoring. Consequently, in November 1976, a symposium on the Reliable Quantitation of Antiepileptic Drugs was held in Kansas City, Missouri, under the sponsorship of the National Institute of Neurological and Communicative Disorders and Stroke and the Epilepsy Foundation of America. Many of the symposium participants expressed a desire for a definitive source of current knowledge on the therapeutic monitoring of antiepileptic drugs. This volume was developed in response to that identified need.

The volume treats essentially three aspects of the subject: (1) general overviews of the various analytical techniques employed in the quantitation of antiepileptic drugs, (2) reviews of the fundamental principles of clinical pharmacology and the application of these principles to the clinical management of the epilepsies for each of the commonly prescribed antiepileptic drugs, and (3) detailed instructions for the quantitation of antiepileptic drugs by proven methodologies, and a detailed summary of the chemical and pharmacological properties of the currently marketed antiepileptic drugs. The information contained in this volume provides a concise reference source for laboratories engaged in the quantitative analysis of antiepileptic drugs and for physicians who treat patients with epilepsy. The importance of reliable antiepileptic drug level determinations and their rational clinical application to the successful management of the epilepsies cannot be overemphasized.

The Editors

Acknowledgments

This work could not have been presented without the contributions and cooperation of the authors, and we are grateful for their efforts. We also wish to express our special gratitude to Bettie Jean Hessie for her editorial efforts in the creation of this volume.

Contents

Special Analytical Techniques

Antiepileptic Drug Quality Control

Clinical Applications of Antiepileptic Drug Concentrations

Contributors

William H. Barr, Pharm. D., Ph.D.
Professor and Chairman, Department of Pharmacy and Pharmaceutics
Medical College of Virginia
Virginia Commonwealth University
Richmond, Virginia 23298

H. Bryan Bente, Ph.D.
Applications Chemist
Hewlett-Packard Company
Avondale Division
Avondale, Pennsylvania 19311

Daniel L. Bius, B.S.
Research Analyst, Epilepsy and Anticonvulsant Drug Research Laboratory
Department of Pharmacology
University of North Carolina School of Medicine
Chapel Hill, North Carolina 27514

Harold E. Booker, M.D.
Professor of Neurology
University of Wisconsin Center for Health Sciences
Madison, Wisconsin 53704

Larry W. Boyles, M.D.
Assistant Professor of Neurology and Assistant Director, Epilepsy and Anticonvulsant Drug Research Laboratory
University of North Carolina School of Medicine
Chapel Hill, North Carolina 27514

Thomas C. Butler, M.D.
Professor of Pharmacology
University of North Carolina School of Medicine
Chapel Hill, North Carolina 27514

C. E. Cook, Ph.D.
Director for Life Sciences and Bioorganic Chemistry
Research Triangle Institute
Research Triangle Park, North Carolina 27709

David D. Daly, M.D.
Professor of Neurology
University of Texas Southwestern Medical School
Dallas, Texas 75235

Barbara A. Darcey, B.S.
Research Assistant, Department of Neurology
University of Wisconsin Center for Health Sciences
Madison, Wisconsin 53704

J. Arthur F. de Silva, Ph.D.
Research Section Head
Bioanalytical Methods Development
Department of Biochemistry and Drug Metabolism
Hoffmann–La Roche Inc.
Nutley, New Jersey 07110

Kenneth H. Dudley, Ph.D.
Associate Professor of Pharmacology and Director, Epilepsy and Anticonvulsant Drug Research Laboratory
University of North Carolina School of Medicine
Chapel Hill, North Carolina 27514

Richard W. Fincham, M.D.
Professor of Neurology
University of Iowa College of Medicine
University Hospitals
Iowa City, Iowa 52242

Edward Fingl, Ph.D.
Professor of Pharmacology
University of Utah College of Medicine
Salt Lake City, Utah 84132

Louis C. Franconi, B.A.
Manager, International Applications
Waters Associates, Inc.
Milford, Maine 01757

Patrick N. Friel
Research Technologist, Department of Neurological Surgery
University of Washington School of Medicine
Seattle, Washington 98195

Erich L. Gibbs, Ph.D.
Director, Gibbs Laboratory
Evanston, Illinois 60201

Trudy J. Gibbs, M.S.
Director, Gibbs Laboratory
Evanston, Illinois 60201

Horace E. Hamilton, M.S.
Instructor, Department of Pathology
The University of Texas Health Science Center at San Antonio
San Antonio, Texas 78284

Christine D. Harvey, M.Sc.
Senior Technician, Neuropharmacology Laboratory
Montreal Neurological Institute
Montreal H3A 2B4, Quebec, Canada

Gerald L. Hawk, Ph.D.
Technical Manager, Life Science Division
Waters Associates, Inc.
Milford, Maine 01757

Betsy L. Kraus, B.S.
Research Technician, Epilepsy and Anticonvulsant Drug Research Laboratory
Department of Pharmacology
University of North Carolina School of Medicine
Chapel Hill, North Carolina 27514

Harvey J. Kupferberg, Ph.D.
Pharmacologist, Epilepsy Branch
Neurological Disorders Program
National Institute of Neurological and Communicative Disorders and Stroke
National Institutes of Health
Bethesda, Maryland 20014

Henn Kutt, M.D.
Associate Professor of Neurology and Pharmacology
Cornell University Medical College
New York, New York 10021

H. Paris-Kutt, M.D.
Staff Associate in Neurology
Columbia University College of Physicians and Surgeons
New York, New York 10032

J. Kiffin Penry, M.D.
Chief, Epilepsy Branch
Neurological Disorders Program
National Institute of Neurological and Communicative Disorders and Stroke
National Institutes of Health
Bethesda, Maryland 20014

Robert J. Perchalski, M.S.
Research Chemist
Veterans Administration Hospital
Gainesville, Florida 32602

C. E. Pippenger, Ph.D.
Assistant Professor of Neuropharmacology (Neurology)
Columbia University College of Physicians and Surgeons
New York, New York 10032

Dorothy D. Schottelius, Ph.D.
Assistant Professor of Neurology
University of Iowa College of Medicine
University Hospitals
Iowa City, Iowa 52242

Allan L. Sherwin, M.D., Ph.D.
Associate Professor of Neurology
McGill University Faculty of Medicine
Montreal H3A 2B4, Quebec, Canada

Donald W. Sichler, B.S.
Research Associate, Department of Neurology
Columbia University College of Physicians and Surgeons
New York, New York 10032

Elizabeth B. Solow, M.S.
Associate Professor in Neurological Surgery Research
Indiana University School of Medicine
Indianapolis, Indiana 46202

Allan S. Troupin, M.D.
Assistant Professor of Neurosurgery
University of Washington School of Medicine
Seattle, Washington 98195

Jack E. Wallace, Ph.D.
Associate Professor of Pathology
The University of Texas Health Science Center at San Antonio
San Antonio, Texas 78284

B. Joe Wilder, M.D.
Chief, Neurology Service
Veterans Administration Hospital
Gainesville, Florida 32602

Robert A. Williamson
Senior Technician, Department of Neurology
Cornell University Medical College
New York, New York 10021

Antiepileptic Drugs: Quantitative Analysis and Interpretation, edited by C. E. Pippenger, J. K. Penry, and H. Kutt, Raven Press, New York, © 1978.

Chapter 1
Reliability of Serum Antiepileptic Drug Concentrations and Patient Management

J. Kiffin Penry

The clinical management of epilepsy has improved dramatically in the past decade through the determination of serum antiepileptic drug concentrations (1). Sherwin (Chapter 25) has clearly demonstrated over a period of 5 years that the number of patients with completely controlled absence seizures can be increased by improving compliance and adjusting the prescribed dosage based on the measurement of serum ethosuximide concentrations. Similar results were obtained by Lund (2), who monitored serum phenytoin concentrations in patients suffering primarily from generalized tonic-clonic and complex partial seizures. In both studies, reliable determinations of serum antiepileptic drug concentrations were available to the investigators.

Not infrequently, however, serum antiepileptic drug concentrations are not readily available to physicians treating patients with epilepsy, or they are unreliable when available. Pippenger and colleagues (3) found that only 54 of 109 laboratories reported serum phenytoin concentrations within a range of $\pm$ 1 standard deviation of the mean of five reference laboratories. In other words, half of the laboratories reported unreliable and misleading phenytoin concentrations. The reported results were no better for phenobarbital and much worse for primidone and ethosuximide. The magnitude of the error ranged from 0.1 μg/ml to more than 100 μg/ml. How does the magnitude of the error affect patient management? Is it the same for all antiepileptic drugs?

Each antiepileptic drug in each class of compounds has unique physical and chemical properties that are further amplified by specific phamacologic and pharmacokinetic characteristics. This is illustrated by a superficial comparison and contrast of phenytoin (Dilantin®) and ethosuximide (Zarontin®). Phenytoin is a five-membered heterocyclic compound with two nitrogens in the heterocycle and phenyl radicals. It is almost insoluble in water. With a pK_a of 9.2, it is far more basic than the gastric pH and even more basic than the normal serum and intercellular pH. The peak absorption is highly variable and often delayed. Serum protein binds 88 to 90% of the molecules in the blood, leaving only 10% free to enter CSF and tissues. The biologic half-life is 24 to 30 hr, but highly variable. Biotransformation, principally to hydroxyphenylphenylhydantoin, occurs largely in the liver where competitive drug interactions and enzyme inductions occur. Most responsive patients will benefit throughout a narrow range of 10 to 20 μg/ml at a steady-state serum concentration of phenytoin. Most patients will exhibit fine nystagmus on lateral gaze with a serum phenytoin concentration above 20 μg/ml.

Ethosuximide is also a heterocyclic compound, but the five-membered heterocycle contains only one nitrogen. The radicals are the short, straight-chained hydrocarbons, ethyl and methyl. It is highly soluble in acidic water at pH 3 to 7.9. Ethosuximide is more rapidly absorbed than phenytoin but it is not bound to serum proteins, so that the CSF concentration equals that of the serum. It is biotransformed in the liver through hydroxylation and subsequent oxidation. However, there appears to be little competitive drug interaction or enzyme induction in man. The biologic half-life is 24 to 30 hr in children and about 60 hr in adults. As much as 12 to 20% of the ethosuximide is excreted unchanged in the urine. Most responsive patients will benefit throughout a wide range of 40 to 100 μg/ml at a steady-state serum ethosuximide concentration. Occasionally, complete seizure control can be achieved with an even higher ethosuximide level without eliciting toxic side effects. In contrast to phenytoin, there is no single level where the majority of patients will experience toxic side effects; they appear over a wide range from 80 to 120 μg/ml. However, when toxic side effects appear, slight lowering of the level often relieves the symptoms, revealing the dose dependency of the side effect.

When antiepileptic drug concentrations are used as a guide to dosage adjustment for achieving effectiveness or controlling toxic side effects, the impact of error in the concentration reported from the laboratory will differ for each antiepileptic drug and in relation to the actual value of the concentration. Table 1 describes the impact of error in reported phenytoin concentrations when the error is 0.5, 2, 5, and 30 μg/ml and when the actual phenytoin concentration is 0, 5, 10, 20, 40, and 100 μg/ml. It is worthwhile to consider each of these examples in the context of patient management. Consider, first, the patient who is on 100 mg of phenytoin three times a day and reports to the physician that seizures are still occurring once or twice a

TABLE 1. *Impact of error in reported phenytoin concentrations*

Error (μg/ml)	Actual phenytoin concentrations (μg/ml) and impact of error on patient management					
	0	5	10	20	40	100
0.5	none	none	none	none	none	none
2.0	none	none	minor	minor	none	none
5.0	minor	minor	major	major	minor	none
30.0	major	major	major	major	minor	minor

week. In the absence of an actual phenytoin concentration, a laboratory report of 0.5 μg/ml does not mislead the physician because the patient is either not complying or not absorbing the medication. A report of 2 μg/ml would still not mislead the physician because he must first make sure that the patient is taking the prescribed dose. If the reported value is 5 μg/ml, the physician might be misled and increase the dosage if he thinks the patient is poorly absorbing or rapidly metabolizing the drug. If the previously noncomplying patient now begins taking the prescribed three capsules a day plus a fourth capsule, there is a minor possibility of intoxication because of the dose dependency of phenytoin. If the reported value is 30 μg/ml, the physician might conclude that phenytoin is of no value in this patient and change to another drug at a time when phenytoin would actually have been effective. He might also conclude that it is very strange that the patient has no nystagmus, slurred speech, or ataxia at 30 μg/ml.

When the patient with an actual phenytoin concentration of 5 μg/ml reports to the physician that he is still having one or two generalized tonic-clonic seizures a week, reported concentrations of 4.5, 5.5. 3, or 7 μg/ml would not be misleading. However, with an error of 5 μg/ml, resulting in a reported value of either 0 or 10 μg/ml, the physician might conclude that the patient is not taking the medication or that the drug is ineffective. Increasing the medication in the former case might lead to toxic side effects, whereas in the latter case adding a second drug on the assumption that phenytoin is ineffective would be unnecessary when only an increase in dosage would be important. A reported value of 35 μg/ml might lead to a lowering of dosage with increased seizure frequency, when actually the dosage should be increased.

For the patient with phenytoin concentration of 10 μg/ml who continues to have two seizures a week, reported values of 9.5 and 10.5 μg/ml would not be deceptive. A finding of 12 μg/ml would cause no trouble, but there would be minor difficulty if the concentration were reported as 8 μg/ml. This would result in an increase in the dosage, which could produce intoxication. With a reported level of 5 μg/ml, the dosage would be increased, resulting in toxic side effects, whereas a value of 15 μg/ml would cause the physician to be overcautious about increasing the medication to an adequate level for seizure control. With a reported concentration of either 0 or 40 μg/ml, the patient will suffer intoxication from an increased dosage or an increase in seizures from a reduction in medication.

A reported value of 19.5 or 20.5 μg/ml would be of no consequence in a patient with an actual phenytoin concentration of 20 μg/ml who still has one or two generalized tonic-clonic seizures a week. A reported concentration of 18 or 15 μg/ml would probably lead to an increase in medication and could result in toxic side effects, whereas a value of 22 or 25 μg/ml might make the physician reluctant to increase the medication even if the patient denied any toxic side effects. A report of the absence of a serum phenytoin concentration would certainly lead to an increase in medication with resultant intoxication, whereas a reported value of 50 μg/ml would cause the physician to be very reluctant to increase the phenytoin and he would probably turn toward a second drug.

When the patient with an actual phenytoin concentration of 40 μg/ml reports to the physician that he has slurred speech and staggering, a reported value of 39.5 or 38 μg/ml, as well as 40.5 or 42 μg/ml, would be of no consequence in the patient's management. A reported concentration of 35 μg/ml might lead the physician to reduce the medication more slowly and prolong the toxic side effects, whereas a value of 45 μg/ml might lead the physician to reduce the medication too fast and precipitate seizures, as the therapeutic drug level is not maintained. With a reported value of 10 μg/ml, the physician would be puzzled at the toxic side effects and might search for another drug or CNS dysfunction as a cause for the slurred speech and staggering. With a reported value of 70 μg/ml, the phenytoin dosage would be reduced excessively and could result in the reappearance of seizures.

Values of 99.5, 100.5, 98, 102, 95, or 105 μg/ml would have little impact on the management of a patient with an actual phenytoin concentration of 100 μg/ml who is admitted to the hospital with severe depression, ataxia, slurred speech, and nystagmus. However, with a reported concentration of 70 μg/ml, the physician might restart the discontinued drug too soon, and with a reported value of 130 μg/ml, it might be reinstituted too late.

The examples given above are only a few of the many that could be listed. It is important to remember that the impact of errors in reported antiepileptic drug concentrations will be reduced when those values are used in the context of all other information known about the patient. The physician should consider the reliability of the patient's history, the description of the reported seizures, the account of toxic side effects, an examination for evidence of toxicity or other neurological abnormalities, and the time the blood was drawn in relation to administration of the drug. The values shown in Table 1 and in the examples given above for phenytoin represent results from samples obtained at the lowest diurnal level, that is, from fasting patients in the morning. Many factors contribute to the inter- and intrapatient variability of serum drug concentrations in relation to the prescribed dosage, and often these cannot be controlled or identified. It is therefore extremely important that reported serum concentrations of antiepileptic drugs be as error-free as possible.

In summary, errors in reports of serum antiepileptic drug concentrations can lead to a delay in controlling epileptic seizures or can cause a relapse in patients whose seizures are controlled. The result may be unnecessary morbidity and human suffering through the occurrence of brain damage from recurrent seizures, which in turn leads to inability to work, attend school, or participate in recreation for a normal social life. Furthermore, such errors may cause unnecessary intoxication of the patient, with similar consequences. Access to reliable determination of antiepileptic drug concentrations will enable the skillful physician to bring many more patients' seizures under control and to reduce or eliminate impairing toxic side effects.

REFERENCES

1. Kutt, H., and Penry, J. K. (1974): Usefulness of blood levels of antiepileptic drugs. *Arch. Neurol.,* 31:283–288.
2. Lund, L. (1974): Anticonvulsant effect of diphenylhydantoin relative to plasma levels. A prospective three-year study in ambulant patients with generalized epileptic seizures. *Arch. Neurol.,* 31:289–294.
3. Pippenger, C. E., Penry, J. K., White, B. G., Daly, D. D., and Buddington, R. (1976): Interlaboratory variability in determination of plasma antiepileptic drug concentrations. *Arch. Neurol.,* 33:351–355.

ANALYTICAL TECHNIQUES

Antiepileptic Drugs: Quantitative Analysis and Interpretation, edited by C. E. Pippenger, J. K. Penry, and H. Kutt, Raven Press, New York, © 1978.

Chapter 2
Quantitative Methods for Antiepileptic Drug Analysis: An Overview

Harvey J. Kupferberg

Phenobarbital was introduced in 1912 as the first effective, organically synthesized anticonvulsant. Nearly two decades passed before it was supplanted by phenytoin (diphenylhydantoin) as a major drug in the treatment of seizures. Recently, carbamazepine, clonazepam, and sodium valproate have been introduced as effective antiepileptic agents. Along with the development of new and more potent agents has come an understanding of the relationship between seizure control and blood levels of drugs. Buchthal and co-workers (6) demonstrated this relationship for phenytoin in 1960. Since then, the demand for measuring antiepileptic drug concentrations in biologic fluids has increased. The development of methods for determining drug levels parallels the development of new analytical techniques.

Spectrophotometry was initially used for the determination of antiepileptic agents. Chromatography soon followed, first thin-layer chromatography, then gas-liquid chromatography, and now high-pressure liquid chromatography. With these chromatographic techniques came the ability for the simultaneous analysis of several drugs in a single run. Along with the general advancement in chromatography came the development of more specific and sensitive detectors. Thermal conductivity gave way to the more sensitive flame ionization detector. Now, more sensitive and specific detectors such as electron capture and nitrogen-phosphorus detectors have been developed. Mass spectrometry has been combined with chromatography, thus adding a new dimension to sensitivity and specificity of drug analysis. Immunological techniques, for example, radioimmunoassay and homogeneous enzyme immunoassay, have recently been introduced.

Clinical laboratories have adapted all of these techniques to the analysis of antiepileptic drugs consistent with time, equipment, and personnel available. The purpose of this chapter is to present an overview of the various methods in use today, with their advantages and disadvantages. Emphasis is placed on new methods of analysis. An excellent review of earlier methodology and pharmacology can be found in a monograph by Woodbury et al. (46).

SPECTROPHOTOMETRY-FLUOROMETRY

Most clinical laboratories are asked to determine one or more of the major drugs used in the treatment of epileptic seizures, that is, phenobarbital, primidone, ethosuximide, phenytoin, and carbamazepine. Phenytoin and phenobarbital were initially quantitated by spectrophotometry. The methods of Plaa and Hine (40) and Svensmark and Kristensen (44) developed ultraviolet spectrophotometric techniques for the analysis of phenytoin. Because phenobarbital can interfere with the analysis, differential extraction procedures were devised to remove the phenobarbital, but the possibility of other interfering substances still exists. Dill and associates (13) developed a colorimetric method for the analysis of phenytoin. This is probably the most commonly used spectrophotometric method for phenytoin and has been expanded to measure parahydroxy diphenylhydantoin (HPPH), the drug's major metabolite (10). Berlin and co-workers (4) compared the Dill colorimetric method with a more specific gas-liquid chromatographic method. They found similar results in patients who were taking phenytoin alone. Many drugs can interfere with this method, for example, acetylsalicylic acid, methyl phenobarbital, primidone, and phenylbutazone.

A more specific spectrophotometric method for phenytoin is its oxidation to benzophenone. Wallace (45) first used a permanganate oxidation of phenytoin followed by the extraction of the benzophenone into *n*-heptane. Dill and associates (11), Morselli (34), and Bock and Sherwin (5) have modified this basic method to use smaller sample sizes with an increase in sensitivity. Unfortunately, several other drugs, such as methadone and diphenyhydramine, are also oxidized to benzophenone and can possibly interfere with the analysis. The basic oxidation of phenytoin to benzophenone has been adapted to fluorometry (12). Recently, Dill and co-workers (14) have simplified the fluorometric benzophenone procedure for phenytoin by eliminating the need for the preliminary extraction of phenytoin from plasma with an organic solvent. Assays are done directly on 0.2 ml of plasma. The assay is sensitive enough to detect 1 μg/ml.

CHROMATOGRAPHY

Thin-Layer Chromatography

Thin-layer chromatography (TLC) was the first technique adapted to multiple anticonvulsant analysis. The various drugs were separated on the chromatographic plate rather than by solvent partition extraction. Gardner-Thorpe and colleagues (21) and Pippenger et al. (39) separated and measured semiquantitatively a number of antiepileptic drugs in blood. Olesen (35) described the quantitation of phenytoin following separation by TLC and detection by reaction with piperidine-$CuSO_4$ to form a yellow complex. Spraying with 4-pyridyl-pyridinium chloride increased the sensitivity 10-fold (36). Simon and co-workers (41) separated phenytoin on TLC plates. The phenytoin was scraped off the chromatogram and quantitated by the colorimetric procedure. Huisman (26) was the first to quantitate primidone, phenobarbital, phenytoin, mephenytoin, and mephobarbital by TLC. Plasma extracts were nitrated prior to TLC separation. The nitro compounds were placed under an ultraviolet lamp, scraped off, and estimated by a modification of the Dill technique. Carbamazepine does not form a stable nitro derivative and therefore cannot be estimated by this method. Hundt and Clark (27) have adapted TLC for the analysis of carbamazepine and its metabolites.

Gas-Liquid Chromatography

Gas-liquid chromatography (GLC) soon followed TLC as the primary method for the analysis of antiepileptic drugs in biologic fluids. The combination of temperature programming, a variety of liquid phases, and specialized detectors allows for sensitive, specific multiple drug analysis. The main qualifications of GLC are (a) that the compound can be volatilized and (b) that it is thermally stable.

Early GLC methods of analysis were carried out by extraction of drugs from plasma into an organic solvent, usually chloroform or ethylene dichloride, evaporation of the solvent, and injection into the GLC. When proper internal standards were incorporated into this type of method, quantitation of a series of antiepileptic drugs could be accomplished in a relatively short period of time. During the early development of GLC, when the art of producing highly efficient columns was not available, interaction occurred between the more polar antiepileptic drugs and the support or the liquid phase. This led to adsorption of the drug to the column and produced "tailing" peaks. Derivatives of antiepileptic drugs were made to produce peaks with little or no tailing, as well as to increase the volatility of the compounds.

Methylation is the most commonly used procedure and can be accomplished by a variety of methods. Methylation reaction with diazomethane (3) or dimethylsulfate (23) is carried out prior to analysis on the GLC. On-column or flash-heater methylation is the most widely used means of derivatizing antiepileptic agents. MacGee (32) described a method for analysis of phenytoin using tetramethylammonium hydroxide (TMAH) as a methyl donor. This procedure is based on a Hoffman degradation reaction and can be used for the production of methyl esters of carboxylic acid. Solow and Green (43) extended this method for the analysis of seven antiepileptic agents. Kupferberg (28) used trimethylphenylammonium hydroxide (TMPAH) as the methyl donor for the analysis of phenytoin, phenobarbital, and primidone. Both TMAH and TMPAH produce identical results. The injection port temperature for TMAH, however, must be higher than that for TMPAH. The extent of methylation with TMAH appears to be related to the rapidity of the injection (33). A major disadvantage to the use of these methylating agents is the remethylation of those drugs that are biologically demethylated, for example, mephobarbital, mephenytoin, and methsuximide. Recently, Friel and Troupin (20) reported the use of triethylphenylammonium hydroxide as the alkylating agent for flash-heater use. This may overcome this disadvantage.

The instability of the barbiturates and primidone in strong alkaline solutions poses a major problem in the quantitation of antiepileptic drugs. In the GLC flash-heater methylation of phenobarbital using either TMPAH or TMAH, two decomposition products are formed, N-methyl-α-phenyl butyramide and N,N-dimethyl-α-phenyl butyramide along with the expected N,N-dimethylphenobarbital (37). The amounts of these decomposition products of phenobarbital are related directly to the concentration of the base and the length of time phenobarbital is in contact with the base prior to injection into the gas chromatograph. In order to overcome this potential problem, the use of 5-ethyl-5-(*p*-methylphenyl) barbituric acid has been shown to be an excellent internal standard for phenobarbital. This compound is similar in structure to phenobarbital and therefore undergoes similar decomposition.

Extractive alkylation has been used in the analysis of phenobarbital (16), nitrazepam (17), and clonazepam (9). In this process, the acids are extracted as ion pairs with quaternary ammonium salts from alkaline aqueous phase to an organic solvent containing the alkylating reagent. The rate of alkylation increases with increasing lipophilic character and concentration of the counter ion. The organic solvent influences the alkylation rate by affecting both the degree of extraction and the reactivity of the anion. Ehrsson (16) determined phenobarbital using tetrahexylammonium hydrogen sulfate as the counter ion at pH 10. Quantitative derivatization occurred within 5 min.

Greeley (22) alkylated barbiturates using a variety of alkyl halides in a highly polar solvent system such as methanolic N,N-dimethylacetamide. The method requires that the acidic compound be converted to a soluble salt with an organic base. Tetramethylammonium hydroxide or trimethylphenylammonium hydroxide was used. Methyl, ethyl, and butyl derivatives were made quantitatively within 10 min. The *n*-butyl derivative of phenobarbital gave the best detector response of the various alkyl derivatives tried.

Silylation is another derivative formation used in antiepileptic drug analysis. Chang and Glazko (7) described a method of analysis of phenytoin and its major metabolite HPPH through the formation of trimethylsilyl derivatives. Kupferberg and colleagues have developed methods of analysis of mephenytoin (30), ethotoin (47), and carbamazepine (29), using the same derivatives. Several trimethylsilyl donors are available. The most commonly used are bis-(trimethylsilyl) acetamide (BSA) and bis-(trimethylsilyl) fluoroacetamide (BTSFA). Of the two reagents, BTSFA has advantages in its favor. It is more volatile than BSA and also more polar, which allows it to be used without a solvent in many cases. The disadvantage of these reagents is their instability in the presence of trace amounts of water or reactive solvents such as methanol. Unfortunately, the barbiturates do not form stable derivatives, whereas most hydantoins do. A practical disadvantage is that the flame ionization detector collects silicone residues and requires frequent cleaning.

High-Pressure Liquid Chromatography

High-pressure liquid chromatography (HPLC) has gained popularity in recent years as a technique for analysis of anticonvulsant drugs. The prerequisite conditions of GLC analysis, volatility and thermal stability, are not requirements for this type of chromatography. Column packing and detector technology have advanced in recent years to give resolution and sensitivity equivalent to gas chromatography. The initial reports of Evans (19) and Atwell and co-workers (2) demonstrated the use of HPLC in the analysis of phenytoin and phenobarbital. These workers used porous silica gel columns and a single wavelength detector set at 254 nm. The development of variable wavelength detectors has increased the sensitivity and allows for the detection of primidone and ethosuximide. The use of reverse phase columns allows for an aqueous mobile phase that gives elution patterns similar to GLC. Adams and Vandemark (1) and Soldin and Hill (42) extended the analysis to include primidone, ethosuximide, and carbamazepine. By varying flow rate, polarity of mobile phase, and oven temperature, a variety of separations can be achieved. Of particular significance is the analysis of the epoxide metabolite of carbamazepine by HPLC, which is extremely difficult by GLC because of its thermal instability (18).

Gas Chromatography-Mass Spectrometry

The most sensitive and accurate means of determining drug levels in biologic fluids is by gas chromatography-mass spectrometry with computer capabilities (GC-MS-COM). The mass spectrometer is used as a detector, just like the electron capture or flame ionization detectors, but in this case for charged ions of a specific molecular weight. This technique is known as mass fragmentography or selected ion monitoring. Molecular species specific to the compounds being analyzed are detected.

Both magnetic field and quadrapole mass spectrometry with either electron impact or chemical ionization can be used for the quantitation of drugs in biologic fluids. The sensitivity or lower limits of detection for most compounds by mass fragmentography is about 50 pg or 1 ng/ml. Horning and co-workers (25) have used GC-MS-COM techniques for monitoring a variety of anticonvulsants in plasma, urine, and breast milk. Stable isotope homologues of several drugs were used as internal standards, which eliminates the need to produce a standard curve. Lehrer and Karmen (31) and Hoppel et al. (24) estimated phenytoin by electron impact mass fragmentography with the lower limit of quantitation being about 20 to 50 ng/ml.

The use of such instrumentation is limited to the research laboratory because of its cost and the operating expertise required. For practical purposes, the sensitivity of the nitrogen-phosphorus and electron capture detectors is sufficient to quantitate all known antiepileptic drugs used today.

IMMUNOASSAYS

Immunoassays are now being introduced for the rapid determination of a variety of both natural and synthetic substances. At present, several antiepileptic drugs can be determined by both radioimmunoassay (RIA) and enzyme multiplied immunochemical technique (EMIT). Phenytoin (8), primidone (8), phenobarbital (8), diazepam (38), and clonazepam (15) can be determined by RIA. This type of assay is extremely sensitive and highly selective, and sample preparation is usually very simple. The sensitivity of the method depends on (a) the specific activity of the radioligand and (b) the affinity of the drug to the antibody. The specificity of the method is based on proper synthetic design of the drug-protein complex. The disadvantages of the RIA technique are (a) the need for a liquid scintillation counter and (b) the availability and stability of the antisera.

The homogeneous enzyme immunoassay (EMIT) is similar to RIA in some respects but differs in many other respects. In both cases, an antibody to the drug is necessary and the specificity is determined by the antibody. The major difference between EMIT and RIA is that a drug-enzyme complex competes with the free drug for antibody in the former method and a radiolabeled drug competes in the latter method. The catalytic activity of the drug-enzyme complex is lost when it is bound to the antibody. Unbound drug-enzyme complex is then able to convert NAD to NADH+, which can be measured spectrophotometrically and is related directly to concentration.

SUMMARY

Many different methods using a variety of analytical instrumental techniques are presently available for the analysis of antiepileptic drugs in body fluids. None of these methods is capable of determining simultaneously all drugs and their metabolites. Each method varies as to time of analysis, equipment, and expertise needed. Therefore, it is necessary for each laboratory to assess the methods and then modify them to give accurate and reproducible results.

REFERENCES

1. Adams, R. F., and Vandemark, F. L. (1976): Simultaneous high-pressure liquid-chromatographic determination of some anticonvulsants in serum. *Clin. Chem.*, 22:25–31.

2. Atwell, S. H., Green, V. A., and Haney, W. G. (1975): Development and evaluation of method for simultaneous determination of phenobarbital and diphenylhydantoin in plasma by high-pressure liquid chromatography. *J. Pharm. Sci.*, 64:806–809.
3. Baylis, E. M., Fry, D. E., and Marks, V. (1970): Micro-determination of serum phenobarbitone and diphenylhydantoin by gas-liquid chromatography. *Clin. Chim. Acta*, 30:93–103.
4. Berlin, A., Agurell, S., Borgå, O., Lund, L., and Sjöqvist, F. (1972): Micro-method for the determination of diphenylhydantoin in plasma and cerebrospinal fluid—a comparison between a gas chromatographic and a spectrophotometric method. *Scand. J. Clin. Lab. Invest.*, 29:281–287.
5. Bock, G. W., and Sherwin, A. L. (1971): The rapid quantitative determination of diphenylhydantoin in plasma, serum, and whole blood of patients with epilepsy. *Clin. Chim. Acta*, 34:97–103.
6. Buchthal, F., Svensmark, O., and Schiller, P. J. (1960): Clinical and electroencephalographic correlation with serum levels of diphenylhydantoin. *Arch. Neurol.*, 2:624–630.
7. Chang, T., and Glazko, A. J. (1970); Quantitative assay of 5,5-diphenylhydantoin (Dilantin®) and 5-(*p*-hydroxyphenyl)-5-phenylhydantoin by gas-liquid chromatography. *J. Lab. Clin. Med.*, 75:145–155.
8. Cook, C. E., Christensen, H. D., Amerson, E. W., Kepler, J. A., Tallent, C. R., and Taylor, G. F. (1976): Radioimmunoassay of anticonvulsant drugs: phenytoin, phenobarbital, and primidone. In *Quantitative Analytic Studies in Epilepsy*, edited by P. Kellaway and I. S. Petersén. Raven Press, New York.
9. de Silva, J. A. F., and Bekersky, I. (1974): Determination of clonazepam and flunitrazepam in blood by electron-capture gas-liquid chromatography. *J. Chromatogr.*, 99:447–460.
10. Dill, W. A., Baukema, J., Chang, T., and Glazko, A. J. (1971): Colorimetric assay of 5,5-diphenylhydantoin (Dilantin) and 5-(*p*-hydroxyphenyl)-5-phenylhydantoin. *Proc. Soc. Exp. Biol. Med.*, 137:674–679.
11. Dill, W. A., Chucot, L., Chang, T., and Glazko, A. J. (1971): Simplified benzophenone procedure for determination of diphenylhydantoin in plasma. *Clin. Chem.*, 17:1200–1201.
12. Dill, W. A., and Glazko, A. J. (1972): Fluorometric assay of diphenylhydantoin in plasma and whole blood. *Clin. Chem.*, 18:675–676.
13. Dill, W. A., Kazenko, A., Wolf, L. M., and Glazko, A. J. (1956): Studies on 5,5′-diphenylhydantoin (Dilantin) in animals and man. *J. Pharmacol. Exp. Ther.*, 118:270–279.
14. Dill, W. A., Leung, A., Kinkel, A. W., and Glazko, A. J. (1976): A simplified fluorometric assay for diphenylhydantoin in plasma. *Clin. Chem.*, 22:908–911.
15. Dixon, W. R., Young, R. L., Ning, R., and Liebman, A. (1975): Radioimmunoassay of the anticonvulsant agent clonazepam. *Pharmacologist*, 17:251.
16. Ehrsson, H. (1974): Gas chromatographic determination of barbiturates after extractive methylation in carbon disulfide. *Anal. Chem.*, 46:922–924.
17. Ehrsson, H., and Tilly, A. (1973): Electron capture gas chromatography of nitrazepam in human plasma as methyl derivative. *Anal. Lett.*, 6:197–210.
18. Eichelbaum, M., and Bertilsson, L. (1975): Determination of carbamazepine and its epoxide metabolite in plasma by high-speed liquid chromatography. *J. Chromatogr.*, 103:135–140.
19. Evans, J. E. (1973): Simultaneous measurement of diphenylhydantoin and phenobarbital in serum by high performance liquid chromatography. *Anal. Chem.*, 45:2428–2429.
20. Friel, P., and Troupin, A. S. (1975): Flash-heater ethylation of some antiepileptic drugs. *Clin. Chem.*, 21:751–754.
21. Gardner-Thorpe, C., Parsonage, M. J., Smethurst, P. F., and Toothill, C. (1971): A comprehensive gas chromatographic scheme for the estimation of antiepileptic drugs. *Clin. Chim. Acta*, 36:223–230.
22. Greeley, R. H. (1974): New approach to derivatization and gas-chromatographic analysis of barbiturates. *Clin. Chem.*, 20:192–194.

23. Grimmer, G., Jacob, J., and Schäfer, H. (1969): Die gaschromatographische Bestimmung von 5,5-Diphenylhydantoin und 5-(*p*-Hydroxyphenyl)-5-phenylhydantoin im Blut. *Arzneim. Forsch.,* 19:1287–1290.
24. Hoppel, C., Garle, M., and Elander, M. (1976): Mass fragmentographic determination of diphenylhydantoin and its main metabolite 5-(4-hydroxyphenyl)-5-phenylhydantoin in human plasma. *J. Chromatogr.,* 116:53–61.
25. Horning, M. G., Lertratanangkoon, K., Nowlin, J., Stillwell, W. G., Stillwell, R. N., Zion, T. E., Kellaway, P., and Hill, R. M. (1974): Anticonvulsant drug monitoring by GC-MS-COM techniques. *J. Chromatogr. Sci.,* 12:630–631.
26. Huisman, J. W. (1966): The estimation of some important anticonvulsant drugs in serum. *Clin. Chim. Acta,* 13:323–328.
27. Hundt, H. K., and Clark, E. C. (1975): Thin-layer chromatographic method for determining carbamazepine and two of its metabolites in serum. *J. Chromatogr.,* 107:149–154.
28. Kupferberg, H. J. (1970): Quantitative estimation of diphenylhydantoin, primidone and phenobarbital in plasma by gas-liquid chromatography. *Clin. Chim. Acta,* 29:283–288.
29. Kupferberg, H. J. (1972): GLC determination of carbamazepine in plasma. *J. Pharm. Sci.,* 61:284–286.
30. Kupferberg, H. J., and Yonekawa, W. (1975): The metabolism of 3-methyl-5-ethyl-5-phenylhydantoin (mephenytoin) to 5-ethyl-5-phenylhydantoin (Nirvanol) in mice in relation to anticonvulsant activity. *Drug. Metab. Dispos.,* 3:26–29.
31. Lehrer, M., and Karmen, A. (1975): Quantitative analysis of diphenylhydantoin in serum by gas chromatography mass spectrometry. *Biochem. Med.,* 14:230–237.
32. MacGee, J. (1970): Rapid determination of diphenylhydantoin in blood plasma by gas-liquid chromatography. *Anal. Chem.,* 42:421–442.
33. MacGee, J. (1971): Rapid identification and quantitative determination of barbiturates and glutethimide in blood by gas-liquid chromatography. *Clin. Chem.,* 17:587–591.
34. Morselli, P. L. (1970): An improved technique for routine determinations of diphenylhydantoin in plasma and tissues. *Clin. Chim. Acta,* 28:37–40.
35. Olesen, O. V. (1965): Determination by thin-layer chromatography of phenytoin in serum in the presence of barbiturates and other antiepileptic and various drugs. *Acta Pharmacol.* (Kbh.), 23:41–48.
36. Olesen, O. V. (1967): A simplified method for extracting phenytoin from serum, and a more sensitive staining reaction for quantitative determination by thin-layer chromatography. *Acta Pharmacol.* (Kbh.), 25:123–126.
37. Osiewicz, R., Aggarwal, V., Young, R. M., and Sunshine, I. (1974): The quantitative analysis of phenobarbital with trimethylanilinium hydroxide. *J. Chromatogr.,* 88:157–164.
38. Peskar, B., and Spector, S. (1973): Quantitative determination of diazepam in blood by radioimmunoassay. *J. Pharmacol. Exp. Ther.,* 186:167–172.
39. Pippenger, C. E., Scott, J. E., and Gillen, H. W. (1969): Thin-layer chromatography of anticonvulsant drugs. *Clin. Chem.,* 15:255–260.
40. Plaa, G. L., and Hine, C. H. (1956): A method for the simultaneous determination of phenobarbital and diphenylhydantoin in blood. *J. Lab. Clin. Med.,* 47:649–657.
41. Simon, G. E., Jatlow, P. I., Seligson, H. T., and Seligson, D. (1971): Measurement of 5,5-diphenylhydantoin in blood using thin-layer chromatography. *Am. J. Clin. Pathol.,* 55:145–151.
42. Soldin, S. J., and Hill, J. G. (1976): Rapid micromethod for measuring anticonvulsant drugs in serum by high-performance liquid chromatography. *Clin. Chem.,* 22:856–859.
43. Solow, E. B., and Green, J. B. (1972): The simultaneous determination of multiple anticonvulsant drug levels by gas-liquid chromatography. *Neurology* (Minneap.), 22:540–550.
44. Svensmark, O., and Kristensen, P. (1963): Determination of diphenylhydantoin and phenobarbital in small amounts of serum. *J. Lab. Clin. Med.,* 61:501–507.

45. Wallace, J. E. (1966): Spectrophotometric determination of diphenylhydantoin. *J. Forensic Sci.*, 11:552–559.
46. Woodbury, D. M., Penry, J. K., and Schmidt, R. P., editors (1972): *Antiepileptic Drugs*. Raven Press, New York.
47. Yonekawa, W., Kupferberg, H. J., and Cantor, F. (1975): A gas chromatographic method for the determination of ethotoin (3-ethyl-5-phenylhydantoin) in human plasma. In *Clinical Pharmacology of Anti-Epileptic Drugs,* edited by H. Schneider, D. Janz, C. Gardner-Thorpe, H. Meinardi, and A. L. Sherwin, Springer-Verlag, Berlin.

Antiepileptic Drugs: Quantitative Analysis and Interpretation, edited by C. E. Pippenger, J. K. Penry, and H. Kutt, Raven Press, New York, © 1978.

Chapter 3
Internal Standards in Gas-Liquid Chromatographic Determination of Antiepileptic Drugs

Kenneth H. Dudley

Gas chromatographs frequently used in drug determinations are equipped with some sort of detector that measures the change in composition of the effluent gas. Such a detector is classed as a *differential detector,* examples including the flame ionization, electron capture, nitrogen-phosphorous, and the thermal conductivity cell detector (17,21,43). The fundamental analytical parameter in gas-liquid chromatography (GLC), as observed on appropriate recording equipment measuring a response at this type of detector, is either the peak area or the peak height (43). The absolute peak area of a sample component is more independent of the operating conditions of a gas chromatograph than is the absolute peak height (2).

In quantitative GLC, it is imperative that all operating conditions of the instrument are maintained precisely during an experiment and are reproduced from experiment to experiment. The design of the basic components of the gas chromatograph, proper selection of column, precision control over operating conditions, and, not the least, the skill and technique of the operator, are factors that contribute to the reproducibility and accuracy of the analytical result (2,15,33,49).

MEASUREMENT OF ABSOLUTE PARAMETERS IN QUANTITATIVE GLC DETERMINATIONS

The phraseology "absolute parameter method" is used here to describe that situation in quantitative GLC analysis in which an absolute parameter, either absolute peak area or absolute peak height, is utilized to calculate the unknown amount or concentration of a component in a sample. In the absolute parameter method, only the response observed for the component is used for quantification (7,12,49). A reference material (internal standard) is not employed in this method.

A conversion factor, that is, a response factor, is predetermined experimentally and this factor is used to convert the absolute parameter measured for the component in an unknown sample to a dimension of either quantity or concentration (7,12,49). The response factor, *RF,* is therefore a number by which the absolute parameter, *P,* is multiplied, so that an amount (or concentration), *X,* of a component in a sample may be evaluated.

In the simplest case, in which the response, *P,* is equal to zero when *X* is zero, the equation for this relationship is

$$X = (RF)(P) \tag{1}$$

In practice, samples of different known values of *X* are injected into the gas chromatograph and the magnitude of the response at the detector, the absolute parameter *P,* is measured at each value of *X*. The analyst must make the choice as to which absolute parameter, peak area or peak height, is best suited for the analysis (2,7,47). If the experimental data obey Eq. 1, *RF* may be evaluated by determining the slope in a plot of *X* against *P*. Such a plot constitutes a calibration curve and permits establishment of the range of linearity. The response factor, *RF,* is a constant only within the range the absolute parameter, *P,* is linear with respect to *X*. Linearity and its range should be established experimentally, and assumptions regarding these criteria should be avoided at all cost.

Any GLC method that utilizes the measurement of an absolute parameter as the criterion for quantitative determinations is subject to the inherent and inadvertant error sources common to instrumentation and methodology. The absolute parameter method requires precise management over all instrumental conditions, most careful calibration, and a refined technical expertise of the operator. Slight fluctuations in gas flow and column temperature can alter peak characteristics (shape). Instrumental fluctuations can alter significantly absolute peak height measurements but have little effect on absolute area measurements. Accurate measurements of absolute peak areas or heights depend on the accuracies of weighing and transferring of sample and on the precision of reproducibility of the injection technique. Any loss of sample during syringe injection, whether in delivery or by "blowback" through a faulty septum, introduces error in the analytical result (20). The laborious and virtuous feat required for an accurate determination of a *single* sample by the absolute parameter method can be fully appreciated by Emery's remarks (12). He states: "This was accomplished, however, by the simple brute force of many numbers. There are very few samples upon which one can afford to spend this amount of time and effort."

USEFULNESS OF THE INTERNAL STANDARD METHOD IN QUANTITATIVE GLC DETERMINATIONS

The use of an appropriate internal standard in a quantitative GLC determination eliminates error sources common to the absolute parameter method (7,16,29,50). The internal standard method permits a laboratory to perform routinely a large number of determinations of the same kind.

In the internal standard method, a known amount of a standard is added

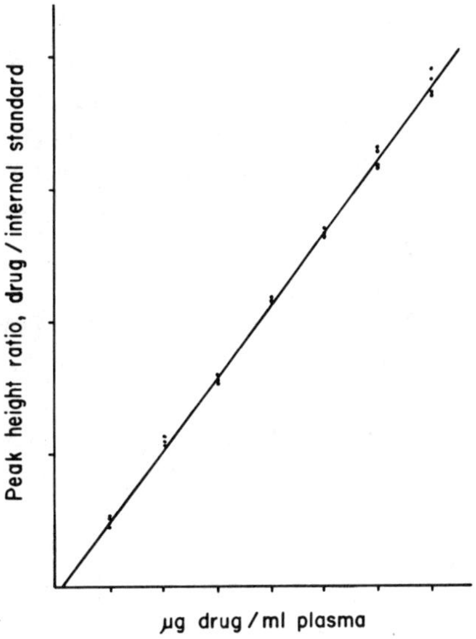

FIG. 1. Typical calibration curve for the internal standard method, in which a plot of peak height ratio (or peak area ratio) against the known concentration of the component is made.

to the component sample and a ratio is calculated from the gas chromatographic responses (peak area or peak height). Quantitation of the amount of component is based on knowledge of the relationship (calibration curve) that expresses known ratios from a series of blended samples, the amount of internal standard being held constant, as a function of different known amounts of the component (Fig. 1). The same amount of internal standard is used in the determination of the unknown amount of the component as in the experiment in which the calibration curve is established, and the determination of the unknown is performed by the same procedure as is calibration.

An expression for the internal standard method, which may be developed from Eq. 1, is

$$X_c = (X_{is}) \frac{(RF_c)}{(RF_{is})} \left(\frac{P_c}{P_{is}} \right) \tag{2}$$

If a relative response factor is defined as

$$RRF = \frac{RF_c}{RF_{is}} \tag{3}$$

then Eq. 2 may be written as

$$X_c = (X_{is})(RRF) \cdot \frac{P_c}{P_{is}} \tag{4}$$

The terms in these equations are as follows: X (weight, or concentration), RF (response factor), and P (peak area, or peak height). The subscripts, c

and *is*, refer to the component and internal standard, respectively. In quantitative GLC determinations, it is common practice to prepare a series of blended samples, as described above, and to test linearity of the method by making a plot of X_c against the ratio P_c/P_{is}. The experimental design is such that at some point in the procedure volume is held constant, so that the concentration of internal standard is constant throughout the series of samples and that the ratio (X_c/X_{is}) is known. In essence, this is an art of calibration that eliminates the need to predetermine response factors.

The premise for the use of the internal standard method is that slight variations in instrumental conditions and/or technique may affect the magnitudes of the absolute parameters, but not their ratios. An example is shown in Fig. 2, in which consecutive injections were made with different volumes of the same mixture of a component and internal standard. It may be seen that the absolute peak heights of both substances are altered by the amount injected, but that the ratio of their peak heights remains constant. This simulated example illustrates how a markedly erroneous analytical value

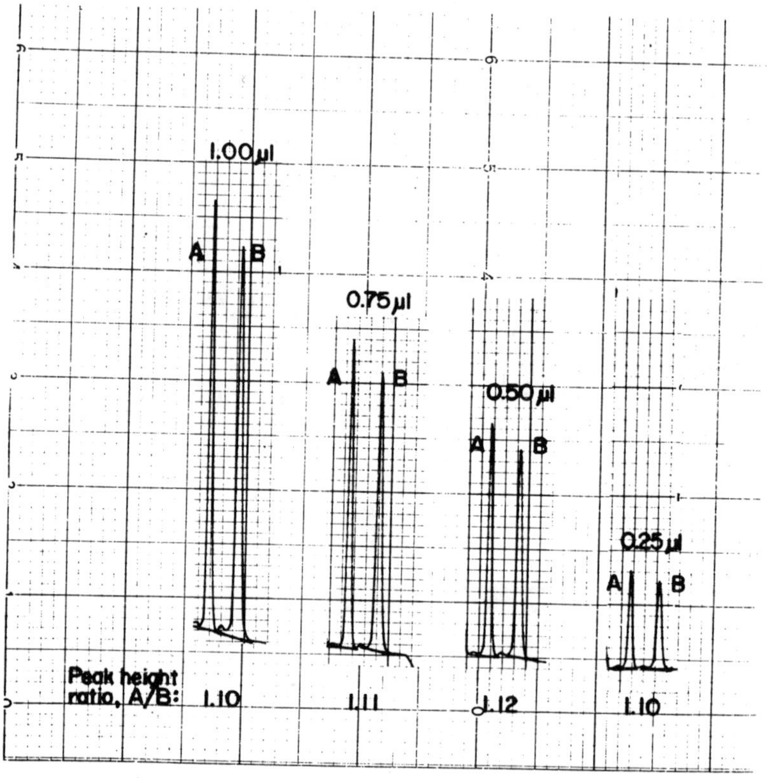

FIG. 2. The effect of sample volume on the absolute peak height of a component A and an internal standard B.

could result from faulty injection if only an absolute parameter were meaured and how such an error source can be eliminated by the use of an internal standard. The internal standard method is an excellent compensating tool, protecting the analyst from such error sources arising from "blowback" and faulty septums, fluctuations in flow rates and column conditions, and instability of detector conditions (7,16,29,50).

There are basically two places in an analytical GLC procedure at which an internal standard may be added. The different points of addition are summarized in Fig. 3. In procedure A, the internal standard is added after workup of the sample and immediately before GLC analysis; in procedure B, the standard is added prior to sample workup. With both of these procedures, a calibration curve of the type shown in Fig. 3 is required, and it is necessary that calibration be performed by carrying out the same sequence of steps as is used in the determination of the unknown quantity of the component in a sample. It should be recognized that a calibration curve con-

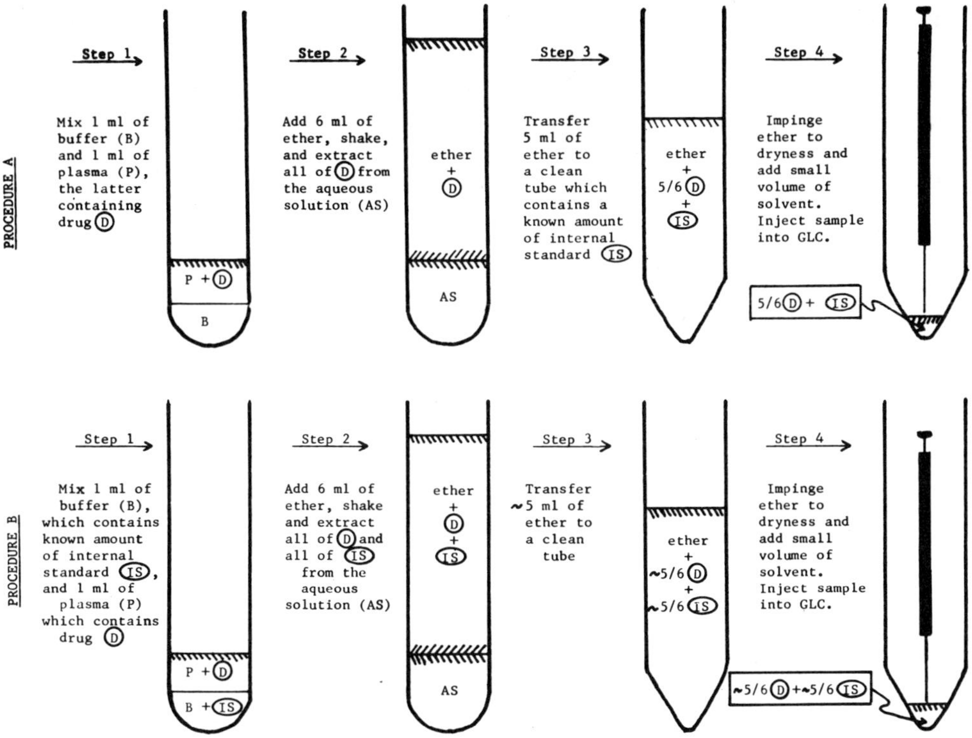

FIG. 3. Two common points in a gas chromatographic analytical method at which an internal standard might be added. In procedure A, the internal standard is added just prior to GLC analysis, necessitating accurate analytical additions and transfers in previous steps of the procedure. In procedure B, the internal standard is fixed initially and subsequent steps in the procedure do not require strict quantitative measures, provided that the solvent partitioning properties of the drug and internal standard are essentially the same.

structed by use of procedure A is of little quantitative value in the determination of an unknown quantity of a component by procedure B, and vice versa.

In routine, rapid determinations by GLC, procedure B has distinct advantages over procedure A. Both procedures require the abilities to weigh, to pipette, and to calibrate accurately. In procedure A, step 2 and step 3 require accurate addition and transfer, respectively, of organic solvent, including an accurate addition of internal standard (part of step 3). In procedure B, in which internal standard is incorporated in the buffer, the ratio of the amount of the internal standard to the amount of component is "fixed" initially. Subsequent steps, 2 and 3, do not require strict quantitative measures since the ratio of internal standard to component remains fixed at each step, provided the ether/buffer partition ratios of both the drug and internal standard (step 2) are very high or nearly equal.

Multistep extraction schemes are sometimes employed in analytical determinations in order to eliminate interfering materials. In such procedures it is desirable that the internal standard and component have similar pK_a and solvent partitioning properties, particularly if the ratio of internal standard to component is "fixed" initially (procedure B) and if the internal standard and component are to be "shuttled" together back and forth between different buffers and organic solvents. At a given step in the procedure, the *total* amount of each substance transferred from one phase to another is dependent on volumes of the phases employed, but the *ratio* of the amounts of the two substances transferred is independent of volumes.

SOME GROUND RULES FOR THE SELECTION OF AN INTERNAL STANDARD AND ITS APPLICATION TO DRUG DETERMINATIONS

The selection of an internal standard for a quantitative GLC method requires careful planning and experimental justification (16,50). The internal standard peak must be completely resolved from sample component peaks. For application of an internal standard method to quantitative determinations of drugs in biologic fluids, normal and pathologic drug-free specimens from a population of individuals should be studied for the occurrence of endogenous substances that interfere with the peak of the candidate internal standard.

An internal standard should have a retention volume, peak shape, and physical properties resembling the characteristics and properties of the component. It is these attributes of the internal standard that eliminate completely or minimize greatly error sources in quantitative GLC, for in most instances ordinary instrumental fluctuations and variations in technique affect the internal standard and the component in essentially the same manner. A satisfactory internal standard may sometimes be obtained without extensive investigation, when homologues and/or analogues of the component can be obtained commercially or synthesized conveniently. In drug determinations, however, this approach requires an awareness of the common biotransformation pathways in man and preferably, if available, the knowledge of the biotransformation pathways of the drug itself. It is an obvious error to select a drug derivative as an internal standard if there is suspicion or evidence that the derivative itself is formed by *in vivo* metabolism of the drug.

In performing routine drug-level determinations in humans, the analyst is continuously faced with the question as to what extent "other drugs," apart from those being measured, interfere with the peaks of the internal standard and component. Even though the knowledge of the physical properties of the measured drugs, internal standard, and "other drugs" can provide some clues to the specificity of the analytical method, the analyst can never rest assured until the "other drugs" are tested in the analytical procedure. The only practical approach to this problem, at least for most of us, is to have access to patients' complete drug regimens and to remain vigilant for abnormalities in the gas chromatogram.

The quantity of internal standard required for the gas chromatographic determination of a single sample is exceedingly small, and the handling of microliter volumes of an internal standard solution requires *most* strict attention (7). In a laboratory, in which an internal standard is used routinely on a daily basis for a large number of determinations, it is convenient to prepare, store, and transfer an internal standard solution on a "macro" scale (50). If an analyst wishes to incorporate the internal standard into a buffer, the internal standard can be prepared as a stable solution by dissolution in an inert and relatively nonvolatile organic solvent that is miscible with an aqueous medium (*cf.* procedure B, Fig. 3).

USE OF GLC FOR DETERMINATIONS OF ANTIEPILEPTIC DRUGS

Within the past 10 years, the usefulness of monitoring blood levels of the antiepileptic drugs in the treatment of the epilepsies has become widely recognized (10,27). The major drugs used in the clinical management of epileptic seizure disorders include phenytoin, phenobarbital, primidone, ethosuximide, and carbamazepine. The structures and pK_a values of these drugs are summarized in Fig. 4.

The development of GLC methods for measuring antiepileptic drugs in biologic fluids has received considerable attention. GLC is relatively inexpensive and, with properly designed methodology, permits rapid, simultaneous determination of multiple antiepileptic drugs in a biologic specimen. In those laboratories specializing in GLC determinations of antiepileptic drugs, the drugs are usually measured either as their native (underivatized) substances or as "permethylated" derivatives, this latter method of measurement utilizing the technique known commonly as "on-column methylation" or "flash methylation." Both methods of determination have their proponents and

MAJOR ANTIEPILEPTIC DRUGS			INTERNAL STANDARDS	
Generic Name	Structure	pK_a	Name	Structure
Phenytoin	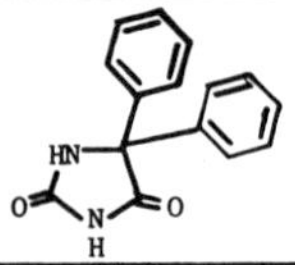	8.3	5-(p-Methylphenyl)-5-phenylhydantoin "MPPH"	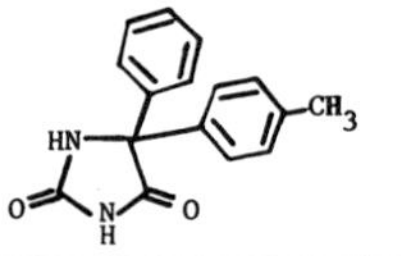
Phenobarbital	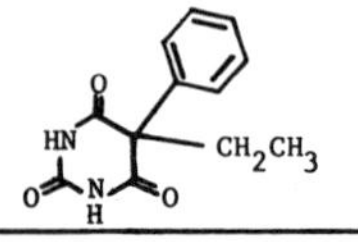	7.2 11.8	5-Ethyl-5-(p-methylphenyl)barbituric acid "MPB"	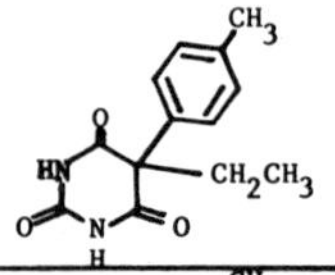
Primidone	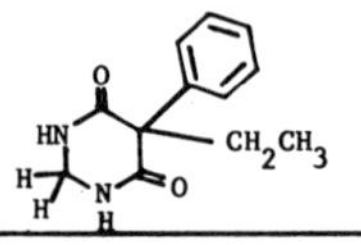	>13	5-Ethyl-5-(p-methylphenyl)hexahydropyrimidine-4,6-dione "MPD"	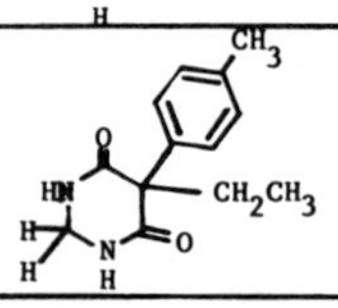
Ethosuximide	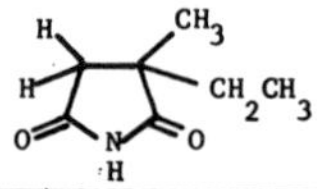	~9	α,α,β-Trimethylsuccinimide "TMS"	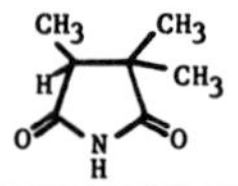

FIG. 4. A summary of the structures and pK_a's of the major antiepileptic drugs and internal standards used in their determinations by gas-liquid chromatography.

their critics. Meijer (32) has reviewed the earlier literature up to 1972, tabulating internal standards, column and instrumental conditions, and extraction conditions for 19 GLC methodologies. Other reviews and sources of GLC methodologies for major and minor antiepileptic drugs are available (26,39,48).

On-column methylation, a technique that in recent years has attracted wide interest and gained general acceptance for antiepileptic drug determinations, lends itself particularly as an example of the usefulness of the internal standard method and of the advantages in making selections of appropriate internal standards.

OVERVIEW OF THE ON-COLUMN METHYLATION TECHNIQUE AND ITS APPLICATIONS TO GLC DETERMINATIONS OF ANTIEPILEPTIC DRUGS IN BIOLOGICAL FLUIDS

The methodology of on-column methylation provides a means for rapid and facile isolation of many of the antiepileptic drugs from biologic fluids, good sensitivity, and speedy GLC measurements. The technique utilizes the principle of the Hoffmann degradation reaction, the basis for which evolved from Hoffmann's original work in 1851. The history of this chemical finding and the development and early applications of on-column methylation techniques in gas chromatography have been reviewed by MacGee (31).

MacGee (30), Kupferberg (23), and Solow and Green (41) are credited with demonstrating the usefulness of the on-column methylation technique for the rapid determination of antiepileptic drugs. MacGee's method (30) for phenytoin is described below because it demonstrates the use of an *appropriate* internal standard, 5-(*p*-methylphenyl)-5-phenylhydantoin (MPPH). The method is summarized in Fig. 5. Plasma, buffer, and toluene, of which the latter contains the set amount of MPPH, are mixed and shaken vigorously. Both phenytoin and MPPH will be largely in the organic phase, because of their partition ratios. The mixture is centrifuged and the toluene layer is transferred to a second clean tube where it is treated and extracted with 50 μl of a 24% solution of tetramethylammonium hydroxide in methanol (24% TMAH). Phenytoin and MPPH are weak acids and both are efficiently extracted from toluene by 24% TMAH. After centrifugation, the volume of the 24% TMAH is very small but sufficient to permit multiple injections of about 5 μl. The on-column methylation reaction, which is accomplished by injection of the 24% TMAH solution into a vaporizer (inlet system) maintained at 340 to 360°C, results in formation of the N_1,N_3-dimethyl derivatives of phenytoin and MPPH. Quantitation is achieved from a calibration curve in which the peak height ratios of the drug derivative to the internal standard derivative are plotted against the concentration of drug (*cf.* Fig. 1).

Without question, the on-column methylation technique involves the use

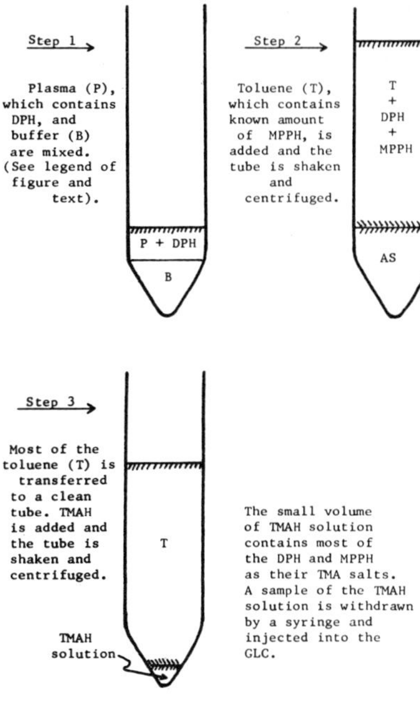

FIG. 5. A summary of MacGee's (30) on-column flash methylation method for the determination of phenytoin (DPH).

of one of the most brutal sets of thermal and environmental conditions ever imposed upon organic molecules. MPPH may be viewed as an appropriate internal standard for the determination of phenytoin, for both compounds contain the same heterocyclic nucleus and show the same tendencies for reactivity and degradation toward the methylating agent at elevated temperatures. In this application of the on-column methylation technique, the choice of MPPH as an internal standard protects the analyst not only against error sources originating from instrumental and human inconsistencies but also against error sources arising from incompleteness of the methylation reactions and degradation of the methylated derivatives during their lifetime in the inlet system.

Since the introduction of the on-column methylation technique for the determination of phenytoin (30), other investigators have elaborated the technique, modifying experimental conditions and adopting MPPH as *the* internal standard in procedures designed for the simultaneous GLC determination of multiple antiepileptic drugs. In the last few years, some investigators have begun to question such applications, the cause for concern stemming from evidence of the different chemical reactivities of the antiepileptic drugs (6,14,42,44,45).

EVIDENCES FOR DIFFERENT CHEMICAL DISPOSITIONS OF THE ANTIEPILEPTIC DRUGS IN ON-COLUMN METHYLATION REACTIONS

Ethosuximide, phenobarbital, and phenytoin are cyclic imides with pK_a's of weak acids (7.2 to ~ 9.5), but these compounds differ considerably in their behaviors, particularly in alkaline solution. Phenytoin, a 5,5-disubstituted hydantoin, is exceptionally stable in hot 5 N sodium hydroxide (5). Barbiturates and succinimides are hydrolyzed to ring-opened products by hot alkaline solution (3,11,46). It is little wonder that some analysts experience difficulties in the use of MPPH as an internal standard in the on-column methylation technique for phenobarbital and ethosuximide.

The case of phenobarbital may be cited as an example where individual laboratories have reported the presence of one, two, or three peaks appearing in the chromatogram after injection of methanolic TMAH or TMPAH (trimethylphenylammonium hydroxide) solutions of phenobarbital. Investigators have differed markedly in their opinions of the significance of the relationship of the multiple peaks to the analytical result (19,34–36,45). As evidenced by gas chromatography-mass spectrometry (34), flash methylation of a solution of phenobarbital in concentrated (1.8 M) TMPAH results in the formation of three substances. These are the "normal" derivative, N_1,N_3-dimethylphenobarbital, and two degradation products, N-methyl-α-phenylbutyramide and N,N-dimethyl-α-phenylbutyramide (34). This reaction is summarized in Fig. 6. The three peaks observed by Perchalski et al. (35)

and used by them in calculation of a phenobarbital concentration are presumably due to these substances. Van Meter and Gillen (45) and Osiewicz et al. (34) have concluded that the extent of phenobarbital degradation and, hence, the number of peaks thus formed are dependent on TMPAH concentration and, also, on the time lag between sample preparation and injection.

Carbamazepine is another example where analytical problems associated with drug degradation have been recognized in GLC. The parent drug itself, in the absence of an on-column methylating agent, is thermally unstable, decomposing in part to iminostilbene (14,24,40). Roger et al. (37), who had the benefit of an automatic sampling unit, reported that carbamazepine is quantitatively degraded in their on-column methylation technique and that quantification of the parent drug was possible by measurement of peak area ratios of iminostilbene to MPPH. At least four laboratories, all of which have used manual injection, have been unable to obtain quantitative or reproducible formation of iminostilbene in applications of an on-column methylation technique to the determination of carbamazepine (9,13,22,28). Roger et al. (37) observed that even the trimethylsilyl derivative of carbamazepine is thermally unstable.

α-Methyl-α-phenylsuccinimide and phenylethylmalondiamide, therapeutically active metabolites of methsuximide and primidone, respectively, and mephobarbital have been observed to give multiple peaks in the on-column methylation technique (38).

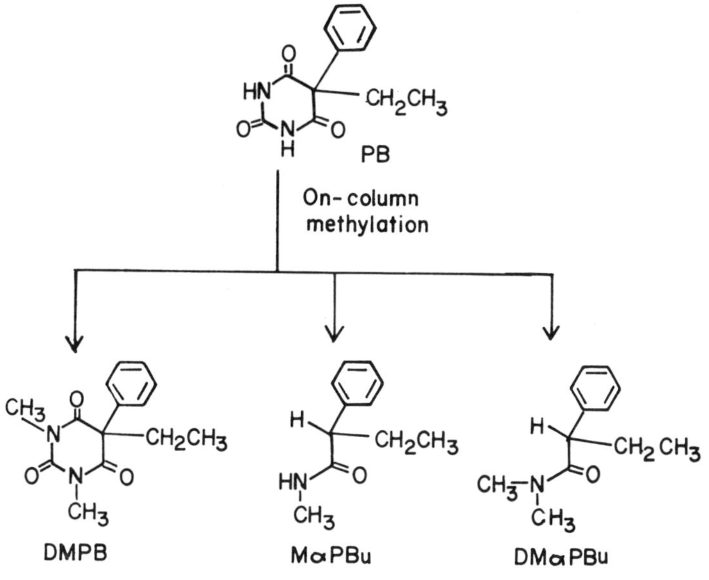

FIG. 6. A summary of the on-column methylation and degradation reactions of phenobarbital, as evidenced by the gas chromatography-mass spectrometry studies of Osiewicz et al. (34). PB: phenobarbital; DMPB: N_1,N_3-dimethylphenobarbital; MαPBu: N-methyl-α-phenylbutyramide; DMαPBu: N,N-dimethyl-α-phenylbutyramide.

USE OF MULTIPLE INTERNAL STANDARDS IN THE ON-COLUMN METHYLATION TECHNIQUE FOR THE SIMULTANEOUS DETERMINATIONS OF ANTIEPILEPTIC DRUGS

Fifteen years ago, analytical chemists argued the merits of the usefulness of the internal standard in GLC. Today, especially among specialists devoted to GLC determinations of antiepileptic drugs by an on-column methylation technique, some major arguments now rest with the questions of "What compound suffices as an *appropriate* internal standard for a given drug?" and "Are multiple internal standards useful in the simultaneous determination of multiple antiepileptic drugs in a given biologic specimen?".

Some investigators have reported the use of a single internal standard in procedures designed to permit the simultaneous determination of antiepileptic drugs (1,8,13,18,23,35,37). Early on, Solow and Green (41), in their adaptation of MacGee's on-column methylation technique (30) to the simultaneous determination of antiepileptic drugs, utilized two internal standards: α,α,β-Trimethylsuccinimide (TMS) was used for the determination of ethosuximide and MPPH for the determinations of four additional antiepileptic drugs. Gibbs is credited (42) with demonstrating the application of 5-ethyl-5-(*para*-methylphenyl)barbituric acid (MPB) as an internal standard for determination of phenobarbital by the on-column methylation technique. Solow *et al.* (42) have included MPB as an internal standard, together with TMS and MPPH, in a revised on-column methylation technique for antiepileptic drugs. It may be seen in Fig. 4 how closely the structure of each internal standard resembles that of the drug for which it is used. The structure of 5-ethyl-5-(*p*-methylphenyl)hexahydropyrimidine-4,6-dione ("*p*-methylprimidone," MPD), one of four primidone analogues synthesized and studied by Schäfer (38), is also included in Fig. 4. Schäfer (38) concluded that none of his synthetic primidone analogues offered any advantage over MPPH as an internal standard in his method for the simultaneous GLC determination of nonderivatized antiepileptic drugs. However, it has been proposed in a recent study by Dudley et al. (Chapter 4) that "*para*-methylprimidone" is an excellent internal standard for determination of primidone by an on-column methylation technique. In their on-column methylation technique, four internal standards were employed: TMS was used for the determination of ethosuximide; MPB for phenobarbital; MPD for primidone, and MPPH for phenytoin (cf. Fig. 4). It was shown also that MPPH was an adequate internal standard for the determination of 5-ethyl-5-phenylhydantoin, the active metabolite of mephenytoin (4,25).

CONCLUSIONS

As judged from the literature, the trend today in gas chromatographic analyses of antiepileptic drugs leans heavily to the use of the internal standard method. Investigators have devoted considerable effort to the design and development of GLC procedures that permit the simultaneous determinations of multiple antiepileptic drugs in a plasma sample. The use of a single internal standard for quantitation of multiple antiepileptic drugs has been the rule rather than the exception. The choice of an internal standard for a GLC method has been forced by the measure of availability rather than be permitted by rational design, particularly in the clinical setting. Only recently have reliable commercial samples of MPPH, TMS, and MPB become available. Schäfer's (38) primidone analogues, which hold much promise, are not yet commercially available. Many investigators would welcome the availability of an appropriate internal standard for carbamazepine, one that shows essentially the same tendency for thermal and/or on-column decomposition as carbamazepine itself.

No one would argue that antiepileptic drugs cannot be determined simultaneously by the use of a single internal standard. Evidence is beginning to accumulate, however, to indicate that the use of multiple, appropriate internal standards may offer a better protection against the different chemical dispositions of the antiepileptic drugs during GLC determinations and against the common error sources in gas chromatography. The use of multiple, appropriate internal standards, as judged from our own experience, can reduce the not-so-infrequent and untimely problems that disrupt the daily routine of a laboratory devoted to antiepileptic drug GLC determinations. This is not to imply that the employment of multiple, appropriate internal standards will prove the panacea for this state of the art. Above all, it is a rigorous *intra*laboratory quality control program that justifies the use and preserves the integrity of any method. An *inter*laboratory quality control program, such as that sponsored by the Epilepsy Foundation of America, is a very meaningful instrument to establish and to "watchdog" the states of arts in antiepileptic drug determinations, but it should not be construed as the ultimate test for justification of a method. An *inter*laboratory quality control program should, at most, serve as an adjunct to rigorous *intra*laboratory control.

ACKNOWLEDGMENT

The program of the Epilepsy and Anticonvulsant Drug Research Laboratory (University of North Carolina at Chapel Hill) is supported by the Developmental Disabilities, Facilities, and Construction Service Act, Grant No. P.L. 91–517, awarded by the North Carolina Council on Developmental Disabilities.

REFERENCES

1. Abraham C. V., and Joslin, H. D. (1976): Simultaneous gas-chromatographic analysis for phenobarbital, diphenylhydantoin, carbamazepine, and primidone in serum. *Clin. Chem.*, 22:769–771.

2. Ball, D. L., Harris, W. E., and Habgood, H. W. (1968): Experimental evaluation of indeterminate error in height-width and height only measurements of chromatographic peaks. *Anal. Chem.*, 40:129–134.
3. Bush, M. T., and Sanders-Bush, E. (1972): Phenobarbital, mephobarbital, and metharbital, and their metabolites: Chemistry and methods for determination. In *Antiepileptic Drugs*, edited by D. M. Woodbury, J. K. Penry, and R. P. Schmidt, pp. 293–302. Raven Press, New York.
4. Butler, T. C. (1953): Quantitative studies of the physiological disposition of 3-methyl-5-ethyl-5-phenylhydantoin (Mesantoin) and 5-ethyl-5-phenylhydantoin (Nirvanol). *J. Pharmacol. Exp. Ther.*, 109:340–345.
5. Butler, T. C. (1957): The metabolic conversion of 5,5-diphenylhydantoin to 5-(*p*-hydroxyphenyl)-5-phenylhydantoin. *J. Pharmacol. Exp. Ther.*, 119:1–11.
6. Callery, P. S., and Leslie, J. (1975): Decomposition of 1,3-dimethylphenobarbital in trimethylanilinium hydroxide. *Clin. Chem.*, 22:926–927.
7. Deans, D. R. (1968): Accurate quantitative gas chromatographic analysis, Part 1: Methods of calculating results. *Chromatographia,* 1:187–194.
8. Dorrity, F., and Linnolia, M. (1976): Rapid gas-chromatographic measurement of anticonvulsant drugs in serum. *Clin. Chem.*, 22:860–862.
9. Dudley, K. H., and Bius, D. L.: Unpublished results.
10. Eadie, M. J. (1976): Plasma level monitoring of anticonvulsants. *Clin. Pharmacokinetics,* 1:52–66.
11. Edward, J. T., and Terry, K. A. (1957): The hydrolysis of amides and related compounds. IV. Diacetylamine and succinimide in aqueous alkali. *J. Chem. Soc.*, 3527–3530.
12. Emery, E. M. (1967): The role of quantitation in gas chromatography. *J. Gas Chromatogr.*, 5:596–600.
13. Friel, P., and Green, J. R. (1973): Quantitative assay for carbamazepine serum levels by gas-liquid chromatography. *Clin. Chim. Acta,* 43:69–72.
14. Frigerio, A., Baker, K. M., and Belvedere, G. (1973): Gas chromatographic degradation of several drugs and their metabolites. *Anal. Chem.*, 45:1846–1851.
15. Goedert, M., and Guiochon, G. (1969): A study of the sources of error in quantitative gas chromatography: Reproducibility of the response of a catharometer. *J. Chromatogr. Sci.*, 7:323–339.
16. Hammarstrand, K. (1976): Internal standard in gas chromatography. *Varian Instrument Applications,* 10:10–11.
17. Hill, D. W. (1969): Detectors for gas chromatography. In *Gas Chromatography in Biology and Medicine,* A Ciba Foundation Symposium, edited by R. Porter, pp. 37–58. Churchill, London.
18. Joern, W. A. (1975): Gas-chromatography of anticonvulsant drugs, with no solvent evaporation. *Clin. Chem.*, 21:1548–1549.
19. Kananen, G., Osiewicz, R., and Sunshine, I. (1972): Barbiturate analysis—a current assessment. *J. Chromatogr. Sci.*, 10:283–287.
20. Karasek, F. W. (September 1973): Sampling techniques in chromatography. *Research/Development,* pp. 54–57.
21. Komers, R. (1966): Gas chromatography. In *Laboratory Handbook of Chromatographic Methods,* edited by O. Mikeš. Van Nostrand Co., London.
22. Kupferberg, H. J.: Personal communication.
23. Kupferberg, H. J. (1970): Quantitative estimation of diphenylhydantoin, primidone and phenobarbital in plasma by gas-liquid chromatography. *Clin. Chim. Acta,* 29:283–288.
24. Kupferberg, H. J. (1972): GLC determination of carbamazepine in plasma. *J. Pharm. Sci.*, 61:284–286.
25. Kupferberg, H. G., and Yonekawa, W. (1975): The metabolism of 3-methyl-5-ethyl-5-phenylhydantoin (mephenytoin) to 5-ethyl-5-phenylhydantoin (Nirvanol) in mice in relation to anticonvulsant activity. *Drug Metab. Dispos.*, 3:26–29.
26. Kutt, H. (1975): Carbamazepine: Chemistry and methods of determination. In *Complex Partial Seizures and Their Treatment,* Advances in Neurology, Vol. 11, edited by J. K. Penry and D. D. Daly, pp. 249–261. Raven Press, New York.

27. Kutt, H., and Penry, J. K. (1974): Usefulness of blood levels of antiepileptic drugs. *Arch. Neurol.,* 31:283–288.
28. Least, C. J., Johnson, G. F., and Solomon, H. M. (1975): Therapeutic monitoring of anticonvulsant drugs: Gas-chromatographic simultaneous determination of primidone, phenylethylmalonamide, carbamazepine, and diphenylhydantoin. *Clin. Chem.,* 21:1658–1662.
29. Lee, E. H., and Oliver, G. D. (1959): Use of two or more internal standards in gas chromatography. *Anal. Chem.,* 31:1925.
30. MacGee, J. (1970): The rapid determination of diphenylhydantoin in blood plasma by gas-liquid chromatography. *Anal. Chem.,* 42:421–422.
31. MacGee, J. (1973): The chemistry and technique of flash alkylation in gas chromatography. In *Methods of Analysis of Anti-Epileptic Drugs,* edited by J. W. A. Meijer, H. Meinardi, C. Gardner-Thorpe, and E. Van Der Kleijn, pp. 111–125. American Elsevier, New York.
32. Meijer, J. W. A. (1973): Review of methods. In *Methods of Analysis of Anti-Epileptic Drugs,* edited by J. W. A. Meijer, H. Meinardi, C. Gardner-Thorpe, and E. Van Der Kleijn, pp. 227–242. American Elsevier, New York.
33. Mikkelsen, L. (1967): Error sources in the gas chromatographic system. *J. Gas Chromatogr.,* 5:601–604.
34. Osiewicz, R., Aggarwal, V., Young, R. M., and Sunshine, I. (1974): The quantitative analysis of phenobarbital with trimethylanilinium hydroxide. *J. Chromatogr.,* 88:157–164.
35. Perchalski, R. J., Scott, K. N., Wilder, B. J., and Hammer, R. H. (1973): Rapid, simultaneous GLC determination of phenobarbital, primidone, and diphenylhydantoin. *J. Pharm. Sci.* 62:1735–1736.
36. Perchalski, R. J., and Wilder, B. J. (1973): GC assay of phenobarbital. *Clin. Chem.,* 19:788–789.
37. Roger, J.-C., Rodgers, G., and Soo, A. (1973): Simultaneous determination of carbamazepine ("Tegretol") and other anticonvulsants in human plasma by gas-liquid chromatography. *Clin. Chem.,* 19:590–592.
38. Schäfer, H. R. (1975): Some problems concerning the quantitative assay of primidone and its metabolites. In *Clinical Pharmacology of Antiepileptic Drugs,* edited by H. Schneider, D. Janz, C. Gardner-Thorpe, H. Meinardi, and A. L. Sherwin, pp. 124–130. Springer-Verlag, Berlin.
39. Schneider, H., Janz, D., Gardner-Thorpe, C., Meinardi, H., and Sherwin, A. L., editors (1975): *Clinical Pharmacology of Anti-Epileptic Drugs.* Springer-Verlag, Berlin.
40. Sheehan, M., and Beam, R. E. (1975): GLC determination of underivatized carbamazepine in whole blood. *J. Pharm. Sci.,* 64:2004–2006.
41. Solow, E. B., and Green, J. B. (1972): The simultaneous determination of multiple anticonvulsant drug levels by gas-liquid chromatography. *Neurology* (Minneap.), 22:540–550.
42. Solow, E. B., Metaxas, J. M., and Summers, T. R. (1974): Antiepileptic drugs: A current assessment of simultaneous determination of multiple drug therapy by gas-liquid chromatography on-column methylation. *J. Chromatogr. Sci.,* 12:256–260.
43. Szepesy, L. (1970): *Gas Chromatography,* edited by E. D. Morgan. Iliffe Books Ltd., London.
44. Van Meter, J. C. (1973): Problems of practical importance in the gas chromatographic assay of anti-epileptic drugs. In *Methods of Analysis of Anti-Epileptic Drugs,* edited by J. W. A. Meijer, H. Meinardi, C. Gardner-Thorpe, and E. Van Der Kleijn, pp. 99–102. American Elsevier, New York.
45. Van Meter, J. C., and Gillen, H. W. (1973): A source of variation in the gas-chromatographic assay of phenobarbital treated with trimethylanilinium hydroxide. *Clin. Chem.,* 19:359–360.
46. Walton, H. F., and Schilt, A. A. (1952): The ionization constant and rate of hydrolysis of succinimide. *J. Am. Chem. Soc.,* 74:4995–4996.
47. Williams, A. F., and Murray, W. J. (1963): The accuracy of gas chromatography. *Talanta,* 10:937–959.

48. Woodbury, D. M., Penry, J. K., and Schmidt, R. P., editors (1972): *Antiepileptic Drugs*. Raven Press, New York.
49. Young, I. G. (June 1975): Postrun calculation techniques in gas chromatography, Part II. *American Laboratory,* pp. 37–44.
50. Young, I. G. (August 1975): Postrun calculation techniques in gas chromatography, Part III. *American Laboratory,* pp. 11–21.

Antiepileptic Drugs: Quantitative Analysis and Interpretation, edited by C. E. Pippenger, J. K. Penry, and H. Kutt, Raven Press, New York, © 1978.

Chapter 4
Multiple Internal Standards in Determination of Antiepileptic Drugs by a Gas-Chromatographic On-Column Methylation Technique

Kenneth H. Dudley, Daniel L. Bius, Betsy L. Kraus, and Larry W. Boyles

An on-column methylation technique that utilizes multiple, appropriate internal standards has been developed. This on-column methylation technique is employed for the simultaneous determination of blood levels of ethosuximide (ES), phenobarbital (PB), primidone (PD), phenytoin (DPH), and 5-ethyl-5-phenylhydantoin (EPH). EPH is the therapeutically important, N-demethylated metabolite of mephenytoin (Mesantoin) (1,3). Four internal standards are used in the on-column methylation technique. These are α,α,β-trimethylsuccinimide, TMS (for ES) 5-ethyl-5-(*p*-methylphenyl)barbituric acid, MPB (for PB), 5-ethyl-5-(*p*-methylphenyl)hexahydropyrimidine-4,6-dione, MPD (for PD), and 5-(*p*-methylphenyl)-5-phenylhydantoin, MPPH (for DPH and EPH). These internal standards were obtained commercially (Aldrich Chemical Co., Milwaukee, Wisc.). The sample of MPD used in the present study was kindly furnished by Dr. H. R. Schäfer (2).

EXTRACTION METHOD

The method is shown in Fig. 1. Plasma (1 ml) and 0.25 M phosphate buffer of pH 7.6 (1 ml), with the aid of MLA pipettes, are mixed. The buffer contains all of the internal standards. Ether (8.0 ml), which has been previously equilibrated with buffer, is added to the buffered plasma, and this mixture is shaken. The tube is centrifuged briefly and the organic layer is transferred to a Concentratube®. Trimethylphenylammonium hydroxide (TMPAH 0.3 M, 100 μl), is added to the Concentratube®, and the mixture is shaken vigorously and again centrifuged, this latter step being carried out at 10°C. If the five drugs mentioned above are present originally in the plasma sample, the final TMPAH solution contains ES, PB, PD, DPH, EPH, and the four internal standards used in their determinations. The overall recovery of PD is adequate, about 34%. If carbamazepine (CBZ) is present together

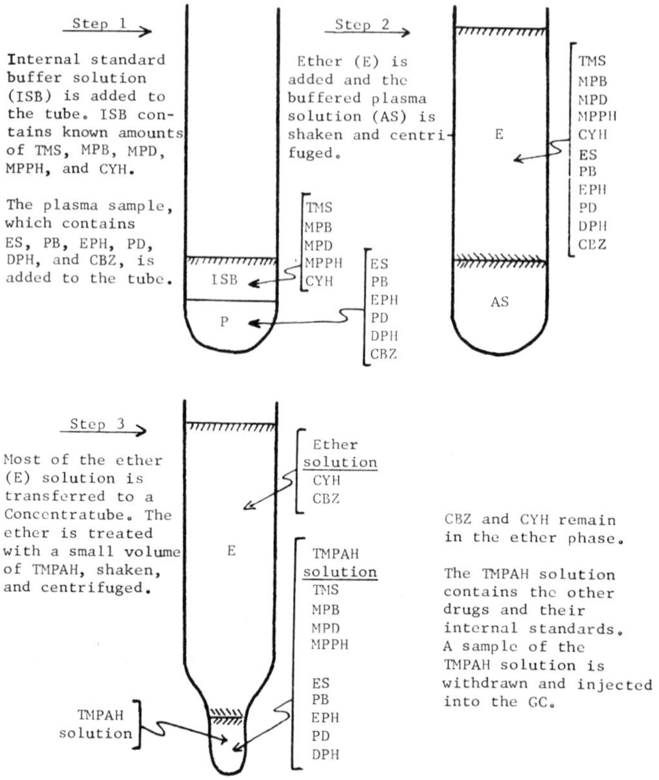

FIG. 1. Extraction procedure for on-column methylation technique in which a buffered solution of multiple internal standards is added initially to a plasma sample.

with the other drugs in the original plasma sample, as shown in Fig. 1, and if its internal standard, cyheptamide (CYH) is included in the buffer solution, these two substances remain in the ether layer at the final step of the extraction procedure. After on-column methylation is carried out, the ether layer may be removed and worked up for the determination of CBZ by a procedure of choice.

GAS CHROMATOGRAPHY

Typical chromatograms obtained with the on-column methylation technique are shown in Fig. 2. The 0.3 M TMPAH extract, obtained as shown in Fig. 1, was injected (0.5 to 1.0 μl) directly into the inlet port.

The conditions for gas chromatography were as follows. A Hewlett-Packard Model 5711 gas chromatograph was used, being equipped as described below for the accumulation of data used in Figs. 3 through 6. Each 6-ft silanized glass column (6 mm o.d., 2 mm i.d.) was packed with 3%

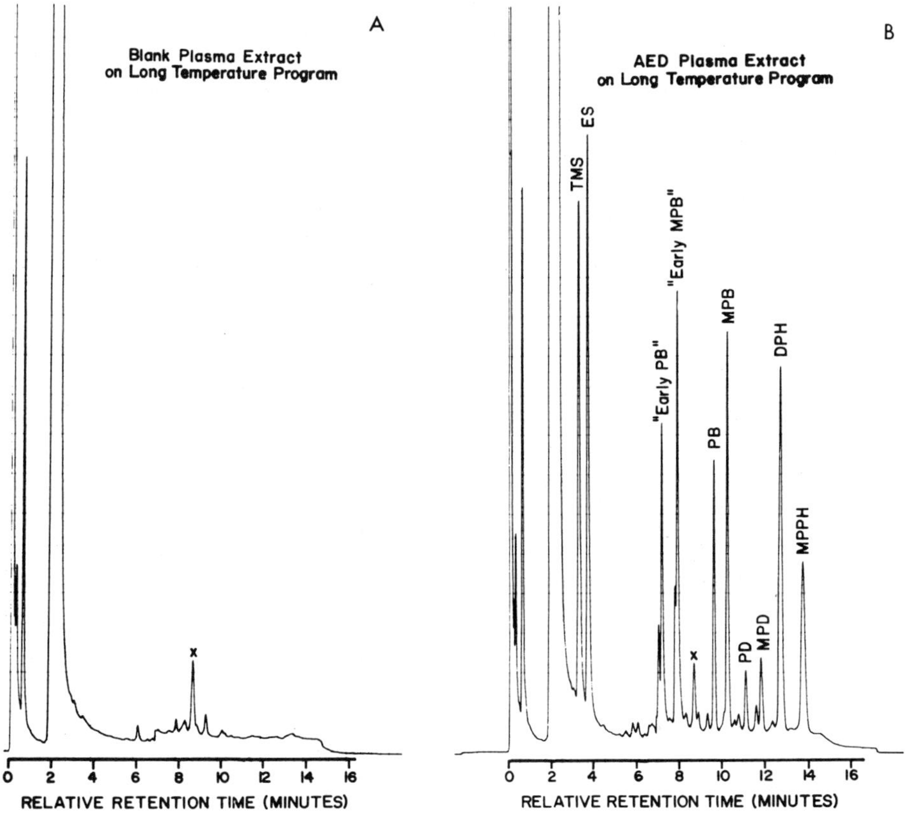

FIG. 2. A. Gas chromatogram of blank plasma. B. Gas chromatogram of plasma containing antiepileptic drugs and their internal standards (cf. text for explanations of abbreviations).

OV-17 on 100/120 mesh Gas Chrom Q (Applied Science Labs., State College, Pa.). Gas flows were as follows: nitrogen, 40 cm^3/min; hydrogen, 40 cm^3/min; and air, 250 cm^3/min. Columns were conditioned at a temperature of 100°C, which was maintained for 1 hr, and then the temperature was raised to 250°C at a rate of 1°/min and maintained at 250°C for 48 hr.

The temperature program for all determinations was as follows: Initial temperature, 100°C with a 2-min hold time; the rate of temperature rise was 16°C/min; and the final temperature was 240°C with a 4-min hold time.

In Fig. 2, the peak designated as "x" in each chromatogram is attributable to a plasma constituent or to methylating agent. It is assumed that the labeled peaks are the "*per*methylated" derivatives of the parent drugs. The peak for EPH is not shown in this record, but it elutes just shortly before the PB peak and it may be quantitated by use of MPPH as the internal standard. The presence of EPH does not interfere with the determination of PB; nor does PB interfere with the determination of EPH. "Early PB" and "early MPB"

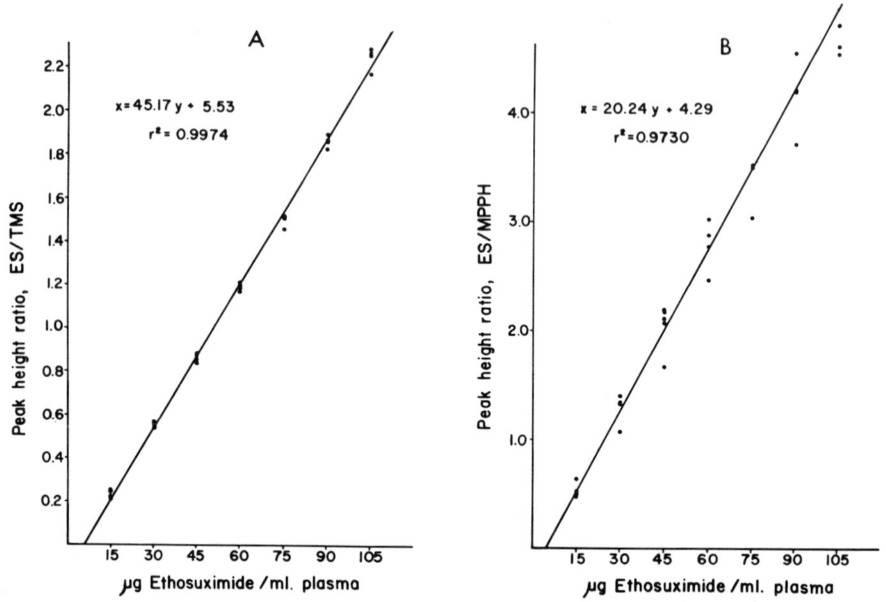

FIG. 3. Comparison of the calibration data for the determination of ethosuximide (ES), as obtained by the use of A, *α,α,β*-trimethylsuccinimide (TMS); and B, 5-(p-methylphenyl)-5-phenylhydantoin (MPPH) as internal standards.

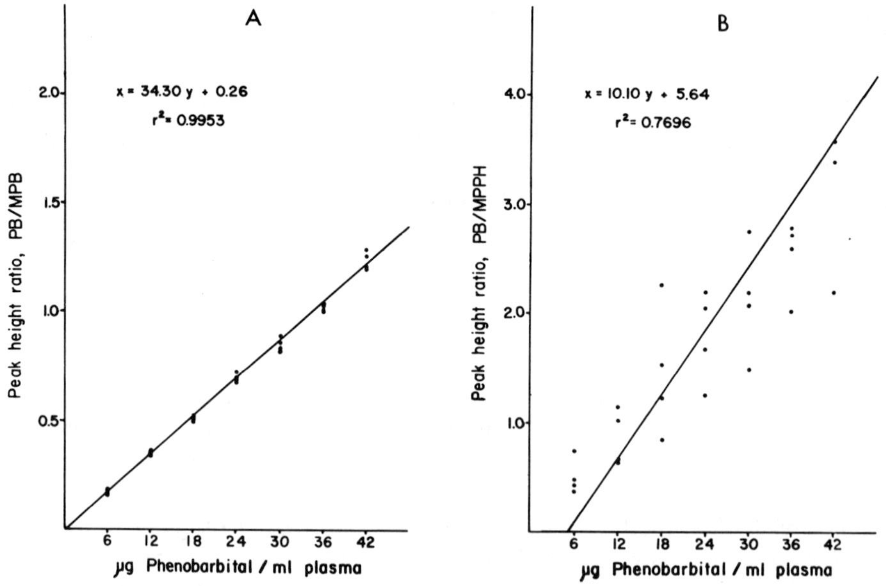

FIG. 4. Comparison of the calibration data for the determination of phenobarbital (PB), as obtained by the use of A, 5-ethyl-5-(*p*-methylphenyl)barbituric acid (MPB); and B, 5-(*p*-methylphenyl)-5-phenylhydantoin (MPPH) as internal standards.

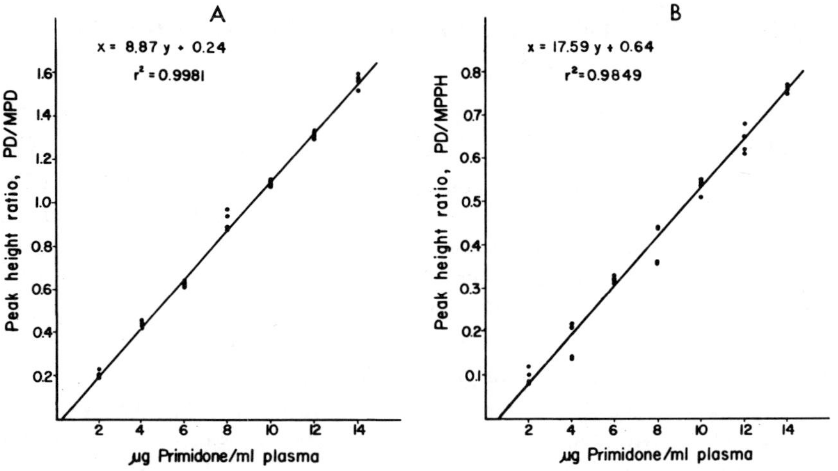

FIG. 5. Comparison of the calibration data for the determination of primidone (PD), as obtained by the use of A, 5-ethyl-5-(p-methylphenyl)hexahydropyrimidine-4,6-dione (MPD); and B, 5-(p-methylphenyl)-5-phenylhydantoin (MPPH) as internal standards.

are degradation products of PB and MPB, respectively. Experiments have shown that a plot of the peak height ratio, "early PB"/"early MPB", against PB concentration is linear. This calibration may be used to certify a PB result, if such is desired when PB is present together with EPH in a plasma sample, and it may be used also to quantitate PB, if PB is present together with glutethimide in a plasma sample. The peak for glutethimide interferes with the "normal PB peak" in this on-column methylation technique.

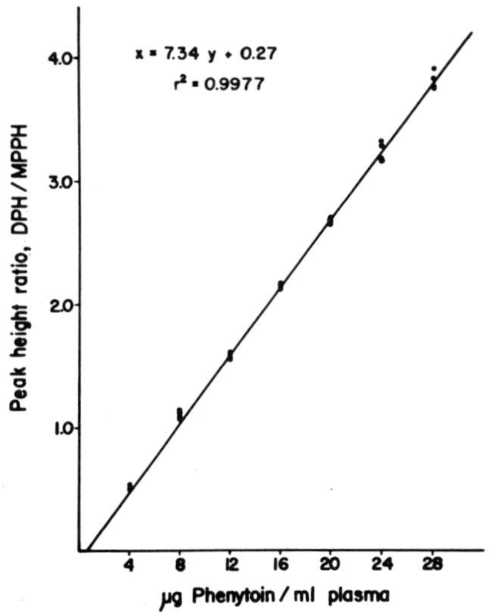

FIG. 6. Calibration data for the determination of phenytoin (DPH), as obtained by the use of 5-(p-methylphenyl)-5-phenylhydantoin (MPPH) as the internal standard.

RELEVANCE OF THE USE OF MULTIPLE, APPROPRIATE INTERNAL STANDARDS

Data shown in Figs. 3 through 6 point to some of the advantages in employing multiple, appropriate internal standards in an on-column methylation technique. The data were derived from chromatograms, such as that shown in Fig. 2B, at a time when two instruments (four columns) were being routinely calibrated. To obtain these data, two Hewlett-Packard 5711 instruments were used, each instrument being equipped with dual columns, dual flame ionization detectors, dual input-output electrometers, and dual pen recorders. Two technicians participated in these experiments, each person working on one instrument and preparing her own series of "blended plasma-calibration samples" from the same stock mixtures. The columns were packed by different individuals. Each series of blended plasma-calibration samples contained a different known amount of each of four drugs, ES, PB, PD, and DPH. Each blended sample in a series also contained a set known amount of each of the four internal standards, TMS (for ES), MPB (for PB), MPD (for PD), and MPPH (for DPH). All injections were performed manually.

In Figs. 3A through 5A and 6, in which peak height ratios of a given drug to its *appropriate* internal standard are plotted against the concentration of the drug, it is evident that there is very little, if any, variation in the data obtained on four different columns (two dual-column instruments) under the same conditions. The figures show that the same calibration curve may be used to quantitate a given drug regardless of which column is used for the determination.

The data summarized in Figs. 3B through 5B show the "intercolumn variation" of four columns (two dual-column instruments) when MPPH was used as the internal standard for ES, PB, and PD. In each figure are plotted the peak height ratios of a given drug to MPPH against the known concentration of the drug. The same peak heights of the drugs were used in the calculation of peak height ratios (drug/MPPH) for these figures, as were used in Figs. 3A through 5A. In some of the examples on individual columns (e.g., Fig. 4B) the correlations between peak height ratio and known drug concentration amount to "unacceptable calibration curves."

The excellent correlation of the calibration data in Fig. 4A may be attributed to the similarity of the chemical structures of MPB and PB and to the likelihood that MPB and PB have the same dispositions toward the alkaline methylating reagent (see Chapter 3). Comparison of data in Fig. 4A against those in Fig. 4B supports the conclusion that, although the absolute value of the proportion of the degradation reaction of PB may vary from injection to injection, the proportions (fractional amounts) of PB and MPB degraded are the same and, hence, the ratio of their concentrations, as obtained in terms of a peak height ratio, is a constant.

One might argue the case that if only one column were used, MPPH is an acceptable internal standard for the determinations of ES and PD. In our experience, this has not been the case. In determinations of ES and PD with MPPH as the internal standard, the "real-world problem" has been the reproducibility of their calibration curves on a day-to-day basis. Even with a single column, we find that their calibration curves either "fall apart" at the higher drug concentrations or that the slopes of the curves change significantly. The use of multiple appropriate internal standards reduces the incidence of untimely problems that disrupt the normal routine of the laboratory.

ACKNOWLEDGMENT

The program of the Epilepsy and Anticonvulsant Drug Research Laboratory (University of North Carolina at Chapel Hill) is supported by the Developmental Disabilities, Facilities, and Construction Service Act, Grant No. P.L. 91–517, awarded by the North Carolina Council on Developmental Disabilities.

REFERENCES

1. Butler, T. C. (1953): Quantitative studies of the physiological disposition of 3-methyl-5-ethyl-5-phenylhydantoin (Mesantoin) and 5-ethyl-5-phenylhydantoin (Nirvanol). *J. Pharmacol. Exp. Ther.,* 109:340–345.
2. Kupferberg, H. J., and Yonekawa, W. (1975): The metabolism of 3-methyl-5-ethyl-5-phenylhydantoin (mephenytoin) to 5-ethyl-5-phenylhydantoin (Nirvanol) in mice in relation to anticonvulsant activity. *Drug Metab. Dispos.,* 3:26–29.
3. Schäfer, H. R. (1975): Some problems concerning the quantitative assay of primidone and its metabolites. In *Clinical Pharmacology of Antiepileptic Drugs,* edited by H. Schneider, D. Janz, C. Gardner-Thorpe, H. Meinardi, and A. L. Sherwin, pp. 124–130. Springer-Verlag, New York.

Antiepileptic Drugs: Quantitative Analysis and Interpretation, edited by C. E. Pippenger, J. K. Penry, and H. Kutt, Raven Press, New York, © 1978.

Chapter 5

Use of the Partition Ratio in Studies of Antiepileptic Drugs

Kenneth H. Dudley

The partition coefficient, K, is a constant that defines the distribution of a solute between two immiscible phases in equilibrium with one another. Although the thermodynamics of partitioning systems, linear free-energy relationships, and the energy requirements for phase transfer are theoretical elements of interest to the state of this art (18,23), these topics are beyond the scope of most practical applications of the partition coefficient in the development of routine analytical methodologies.

THE DISTRIBUTION LAW

Henry's law, expressed by Eq. 1, defines the equilibrium at constant temperature between a gas and its solution in a solvent:

$$\frac{m}{p} = K \qquad (1)$$

In this expression, m is the mass of gas dissolved per unit volume of solvent and p is the pressure of the gas phase at constant temperature. K is a distribution constant, usually referred to as the partition coefficient. Because the number of gas molecules (or mass of gas) per unit of volume (gas phase) is proportional to pressure, p can be expressed as a concentration term, C_g (mass of gas per unit volume of gas phase). Likewise, m may be replaced by a similar term, C_s (mass of gas per unit volume of solvent phase). Equation 1 may be rewritten as

$$\frac{C_s}{C_g} = K \qquad (2)$$

Equation 2, a simple restatement of Henry's law, governs the distribution of an ideal solute between two immiscible solvents at equilibrium. In contemporary usage, the partition coefficient, K, is defined as

$$\frac{C_1}{C_2} = K \qquad (3)$$

where C_1 and C_2 are the *concentrations* of the solute in the lighter and heavier phase, respectively.

The concept of the distribution law, as stated by Nernst in 1891 (24), is that a solute will distribute itself between two immiscible phases so that at equilibrium the ratio of the concentrations in the two phases is a constant at a given temperature.

ASSOCIATION, DISSOCIATION, AND IONIZATION OF SOLUTES IN TWO-PHASE SOLVENT SYSTEMS

Any system more complex than rare gases in either water or pure hydrocarbon solvents becomes impossible to define precisely at the molecular level (23). The distribution law (Eq. 3) is obeyed and can be treated by

TABLE 1. *A summary of the laws defining the distribution between two immiscible phases of solutes subject to association, ionization, and dissociation*[a]

Case	Condition	Distribution law[b]
1	Phase I: No molecular change occurring Phase II: No molecular change occurring	$\frac{C_1}{C_2} = K$
2	Phase I: Dissociation occurring[c] Phase II: No molecular change occurring	$\frac{C_1(1-\alpha)}{C_2} = K$
3	Phase I: No molecular change occurring Phase II: Association occurring	$\frac{C_1}{C_2\alpha'} = K$
4	Phase I: Dissociation occurring[c] Phase II: Association occurring	$\frac{C_1(1-\alpha)}{C_2\alpha'} = K$

[a] Craig and Craig (18) have included Hill's summary (22) in their review of these laws, but they inadvertently misquoted Hill's definition, which reads "α and α' as the degree of dissociation," to read as "α and α' as the degree of association."

[b] α and α' represent fractions of dissociation, but the assignments of α and α' to the processes of cases 3 and 4 are different from those of Hill (22).

The laws summarized for cases 3 and 4 are rearranged expressions also. If the reader refers elsewhere (18,22), it can be noted that other reviewers use K in cases 1 and 2 to represent a ratio of concentrations and then employ the same symbol K in cases 3 and 4 to represent a ratio of concentrations multiplied by the square root of a dissociation constant. For example, if K is defined as the ratio of concentrations for case 3, and if the symbols and definitions adopted in the text are employed, the following equation may be derived:

$$\frac{C_1}{\sqrt{C_2(1-\alpha')K_D}} = K$$

It follows that

$$\frac{C_1}{\sqrt{C_2(1-\alpha')}} = \sqrt{K_D}\cdot K = K''$$

Other reviewers (18,22) employ K in place of K'' in their laws for cases 3 and 4. Such usage of K is incorrect by definition and inconsistent with the correct usage of K in cases 1 and 2.

[c] If dissociation is defined as a process such as $HA \rightleftharpoons A^- + H^+$, an equivocal process also governed by this law would be ionization, such as $B + H^+ \rightleftharpoons BH^+$, where B is the simple molecule that is distributed between the two phases.

classical thermodynamics only if the same single molecular species of the solute exists in each of the two immiscible phases. Solutes of interest to the analytical chemist seldom obey the distribution law in the strictest sense, because of their propensities to associate (e.g., self-association of molecules of solute to form dimer, trimer, etc.), dissociate (e.g., loss of a proton from a molecule of solute), and ionize (e.g., gain of a proton by a molecule of solute) in either one or both of the two phases. Another source of deviation of a solute from ideal behavior can result from hydration of a solute, for example, the propensity of a solute in an aqueous phase to form complex hydrated species with water molecules and to carry one or more bound water molecules into the nonaqueous phase. With any solute whose behavior deviates from ideality, it is impractical, if not virtually impossible, to determine the exact molecular species distributed between two immiscible phases.

Nernst (24) has derived generalizations to define the distributions of some nonideal solutes between two immiscible phases, the laws being useful in simple cases of association and dissociation of solute. The laws, which have been summarized by Hill (22), are tabulated in Table 1 (see footnotes to table for explanation of the modifications of these laws). Theoretically, the laws governing dissociation of a solute (Table 1, case 2 and case 4), should be applicable to define the distribution of a solute that ionizes by gain of a proton.

In Table 1, C_1 and C_2 are the concentrations of the solute in the lighter phase I and the heavier phase II, respectively, as determined by an analytical method that accounts for total solute in a phase. α represents the fractional dissociation of a solute of C_1 (phase I) by a mechanism involving a loss of a proton. α' represents the fractional dissociation of a solute of C_2, which exists in some proportion as a dimer (association). The values of α and α' are determined by methods specific for the processes. In the derivation of these laws (Table 1), it is assumed that the distributed species is the simple molecule and that the degree of dissociation obeys the mass law.

DISTINCTION BETWEEN THE USAGE OF PARTITION COEFFICIENT AND PARTITION RATIO

K is a symbol used to denote the partition coefficient of a single species, after the experimental data have been corrected for dissociation, ionization, association, and other solution phenomena. The symbol P is also used widely in place of K, in order to avoid confusions with other equilibrium constants often encountered in treatment of data. Leo et al. (23) have suggested that distinction be made between the usage of "partition coefficient" and "partition ratio," the former term being reserved for corrected data that define the distribution of a presumed single species between two phases, the latter to define uncorrected distribution of solute in a two-phase system. The symbol K' will be used below to define the partition ratio, as shown by Eq. 4.

$$\frac{C'_1}{C'_2} = K' \qquad (4)$$

The symbols C'_1 and C'_2 refer to the total concentration of solute in the lighter and heavier phase, respectively, and are inclusive of all species of solute present, for example, solute present as simple species, dissociable dimer, conjugate acid and/or base, and hydrated complexes.

The partition ratio of a solute, rather than the refined partition coefficient, can be an important tool for the analyst whose mission is the separation and quantification of a solute. Because the analyst is concerned primarily with the percentage of the total solute recovered in one of the phases of an extraction process, there is often little to be gained in the accumulation of data to define the distribution of a solute more precisely than that offered by the value of K' itself.

SOME FACTORS AFFECTING THE DISTRIBUTIONS OF SOLUTES

As pointed out earlier, solutes other than rare gases seldom show ideal behavior in solution. Most solvents used in liquid-liquid extraction of a solute are not totally immiscible. The concentration of water miscible with common organic solvents at saturation can vary considerably, from 2.5×10^{-3} M for cyclohexane to 9.4 M for butan-1-ol (23). A nonideal solute, except at very low concentrations, can markedly alter solvent character, viz., the proportion of water miscible with an organic phase. With a solute very soluble in the aqueous phase, K (or K') may become variable, differing significantly at low and near-saturation concentrations of solute.

Association of a solute in one of the phases is thought to be the principal cause of deviation from a linear partition isotherm (i.e., deviation of the partition ratio as the concentration of solute is varied). Craig and Craig (18) have reviewed several cases in which the choice of organic solvent, the compounding of solvents, and the addition of amounts of small polar molecules, such as ethanol or acetic acid, have resulted in marked reduction of deviations from ideality, even in observation of apparent ideal behaviors of some strongly associated solutes.

The partition ratio of a solute that dissociates (e.g., by loss of a proton) or ionizes (e.g., by gain of a proton) in an aqueous medium will be dependent on pH. Table 2 summarizes the apparent partition ratios of phenobarbital between ether and some 0.2 M glycine buffers of different pH. The values of K' in Table 2 were calculated from data reported by Butler (5). The partition ratio of phenobarbital, a weak dibasic acid with $pK'_1 = 7.2$ (10) and $pK'_2 = 11.8$ (15), decreases with increasing pH. Bush (2) has studied the distribution of several barbiturates between organic solvents and buffers of different pH.

The "carrier effect" is a phenomenon by which a highly water-soluble

TABLE 2. *The effect of pH on the partition ratio (K′) of phenobarbital (PB) between ether and some 0.2 M glycine buffers*

pH of 0.2 M glycine buffer	$K'^{a,b}$
8.8	1.3
9.2	0.7
9.6	0.3
10.0	0.1

[a] $K' = [PB]_{ether}/[PB]_{buffer}$, where $[PB]_{ether}$ is the concentration of undissociated PB in ether and $[PB]_{buffer}$ is the total concentration of dissociated and undissociated PB in the buffer.

[b] The initial concentration of PB in the ether phase, prior to shaking with buffer, was 6 μg/ml.

organic acid or base, buffered as its conjugate ion, may be rendered extractable by the presence of an organic cation or anion, respectively. Craig and Craig (18) and Titus (27) have summarized several examples in the literature in which the formation of certain salts of acids and bases ("ion-pair extraction") results in more favorable partition ratios.

Another phenomenon affecting the distribution of a solute is the "salting in effect" (18). By this phenomenon, a slightly water-soluble substance is rendered readily soluble in an aqueous solution by an agent such as sodium benzoate.

DETERMINATION OF PARTITION RATIOS

In the development of a methodology for quantification of a solute, the principal concerns are the percentage of recovery of the desired solute and the avoidance of solutes that interfere with the analytical method. In a quantitative determination, it is advantageous to know the true value of the partition ratio under the experimental conditions of the determination, with care being taken to avoid any condition that may cause the value of the constant to vary. The chief points to be considered are the composition of the phases, the temperature of equilibration, and the final concentrations of the solute being partitioned (18). In the design of an extraction procedure for quantification of a solute by an analytical method, a certain amount of deviation from constant partition ratios can be tolerated because standardization of the analytical method compensates for small losses and gains in the recoveries of a solute at different initial concentrations.

Solutes differ in their time requirements to attain equilibrium in distribution experiments. Craig and Craig (18) suggest that 50 simple inversions during a period of about 1.5 min are sufficient to bring about equilibrium of a solute between two phases. Leo et al. (23) recommend that about 100 inversions during a span of 5 min produces consistent results. Vigorous shaking, which may cause some degree of emulsification, is to be avoided. Before measurements are made on either of the phases, centrifugation is performed to ensure complete separation of the two phases.

A partition ratio accurate to 10% is sufficient to permit a rational design of an extraction method for recovery of a solute. However, when the partition ratio is to be used as a means for identification of a solute, a constant with accuracy within 1% is desirable (2,18). The partition ratio, like the micromelting point, has been used extensively in past years for identification purposes, but this application has waned with the advent of recent sophisticated instrumental techniques.

The simplest method for the measurement of a partition ratio is to determine the concentration of the solute in each of the two phases. With solutes that possess characteristic ultraviolet and/or visible light absorption properties, the distribution experiment can be readily designed for spectrophotometry with very small quantities of solute. Gas chromatography is also useful when only small quantities of a solute are available. Preferably, the concentration of solute in both phases should be determined, although it is common practice among investigators to determine the concentration of solute in one phase and to obtain that of the other phase by difference. The practice of single-phase analysis can be hazardous if adsorption of solute to glass occurs (21).

A common procedure for estimating a partition ratio, requiring only an analytical balance, is to equilibrate a solute between a two-phase system and to transfer a portion of the organic solvent to a tared tube. After evaporation of the solvent, drying of the residue, and equilibration of the tube at ambient temperature, the residue is weighed and the concentration of the solute in the organic phase is calculated. If an aqueous buffer is employed as the second phase, the concentration of solute is determined by difference. Detergents and organic amine buffers that tend to distribute between both phases preclude the application of this technique.

In order to obtain a reliable partition ratio, due consideration must be given jointly to the amount being measured in a phase and to the accuracy of the measurement (18,23). Assume, as shown in Table 3, that a total of 3.00 mg of a solute with a true partition ratio of 74 is equilibrated between equal 60-ml volumes of ether and an aqueous buffer and that all of the ether can be removed for the determination of the weight of solute in the organic phase. Theoretically, 2.96 mg of solute should be present in the ether phase and 0.04 mg in the aqueous phase. If the sensitivity of the analytical balance is 0.01 mg, the experimental value of K' can vary from 59 to 99. In Table 3, it may be seen that the experimental range of K' for this example may be

TABLE 3. *Approximation of the experimental range of the partition ratio (K′) of a solute with a true partition ratio of 74 between ether and an aqueous buffer*[a]

Total initial quantity of solute, x_t (mg)	Volume of ether phase, V_1 (ml)	Volume of buffer phase, V_2 (ml)	Quantity of solute in ether phase, x_1 (mg)	Quantity of solute in buffer phase, x_2 (mg)	Approximate range of K'[b]
3.00	60	60	2.96	0.04	59–99
3.00	30	60	2.92	0.08	65–83
3.00	10	60	2.78	0.22	72–80
18.00	60	60	17.76	0.24	71–77

[a] If the definitions in the text and Table 3 are employed, the relationships,

$$x_t = x_1 + x_2$$

and

$$K' = \frac{C'_1}{C'_2} = \frac{x_1/V_1}{x_2/V_2}$$

can be used to derive the following equation, which is useful in estimating x_1 when the true value of K' is known. This equation may then be used to estimate the experimental value of K' when x_1 is altered by the limits of the analytical measurement, e.g., the sensitivity of the analytical balance or the accuracy of the method:

$$K' = \left(\frac{V_2}{V_1}\right)\left(\frac{x_1}{x_t - x_1}\right)$$

[b] The approximate range of K' was calculated on the assumption that the weighing of the amount of the solute (x_1) in the total ether phase was performed on an analytical balance with an accuracy of ± 0.01 mg.

reduced within acceptable limits of error (10% of true K') by simply decreasing the volume of ether to 10 ml or by increasing the initial quantity of solute to 18.00 mg.

Partition ratios may be calculated from counter current distribution data, an advantage being that several values of the partition ratios can be obtained from a single experiment. When the experimental range of the values is small, an accurate estimate of the true partition ratio is obtained. If the values of the partition ratio differ significantly, either a single solute is present that does not obey its distribution law over the studied concentration range, or two or more solutes with significantly different partition ratios are being extracted simultaneously (18).

PRACTICAL SIGNIFICANCES AND USES OF PARTITION RATIOS

The distribution of phenobarbital between benzene and 0.1 M sodium dihydrogenphosphate solution and between ether and 0.1 M sodium dihydrogenphosphate solution is summarized in Fig. 1. In a dihydrogenphosphate solution of pH 4.2, phenobarbital exists essentially as its undissociated species (99.90%). The experimentally determined K' of phenobarbital in the ben-

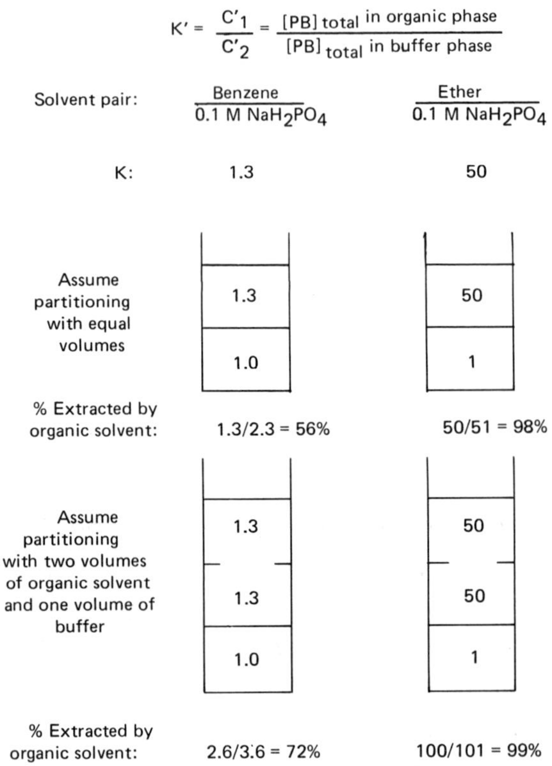

FIG. 1. Distribution of phenobarbital (PB) between 0.1 M sodium dihydrogenphosphate solution (pH 4.2) and different organic solvents.

zene system is 1.3, and in the ether system, 50. Figure 1 shows that an equal volume of benzene removes about 56% of the amount of phenobarbital present originally in the aqueous dihydrogenphosphate solution. If the volume of benzene is doubled, 72% of the drug may be recovered. Extraction of the aqueous dihydrogenphosphate solution with an equal volume of ether results in a 98% recovery of phenobarbital. If the volume of ether is doubled, there is no significant increase in the recovery of phenobarbital.

It is seldom appreciated that a weakly acidic or basic drug can be extracted by an appropriate solvent from an aqueous medium in which the drug is present largely in an ionic form. In a buffer of pH 8.80, phenobarbital (pK'_1 7.2) exists as its monobasic anion to the extent of 97.5%. Yet, as shown in Table 2, the partition ratio of phenobarbital between ether and a glycine buffer of pH 8.80 is 1.3. With an equal volume of ether, 56% of the initial amount of phenobarbital in the buffer may be recovered; with a twofold volume of ether, 72%; and with a threefold volume of ether, 80%. The underlying factor that determines the ability of an organic solvent to extract phenobarbital, or any weakly acidic or basic drug, from a medium in which the drug is largely ionized, is the magnitude of K' of the *undissociated* form of the drug between the solvent and aqueous buffer. As shown in Fig. 1, the K' of undissociated phenobarbital between ether and an aqueous medium is 50/1. In a buffer phase of pH 8.80, it may be estimated by use of the Henderson-Hasselbalch equation that the ratio of the monobasic anionic form to the undissociated form of phenobarbital is 40/1. With these numerical values, it may be further calculated that the ratio of undissociated phenobarbital in the ether phase to total phenobarbital in the pH 8.80 buffer phase is 50/41, or 1.2. This calculated K' of 1.2 compares favorably with the experimental value of 1.3 in Table 2.

APPLICATIONS OF PARTITION RATIOS IN STUDIES OF THE DISPOSITION AND METABOLISM OF ANTIEPILEPTIC DRUGS

In 1953, Butler (6) devised a method by which the pK' and the partition coefficient of the undissociated form of a weak acid could be determined simultaneously. The method can be used as a test of the specificity of an extraction scheme applied to biological fluids, as well as a tool for identification purposes. His method is based on Eq. 5, which was derived by assuming that the ionic form of the compound is confined entirely to the aqueous phase and that the undissociated form is distributed between the organic and aqueous phases with a constant partition coefficient.

$$\log (C_a/C_o - 1) = \mathrm{pH} - \mathrm{p}K' \tag{5}$$

In Eq. 5, C_a is the partition coefficient of the undissociated form between organic and aqueous phases and C_o is the observed partition ratio for the distribution of total solute. Measurement of C_o at two values of pH permits calculation of C_a and pK'.

Many classical studies of the antiepileptic drugs have been based on a spectrophotometric method designed with the knowledge of a partition ratio. These include: Drug accumulation in patients on chronic antiepileptic drug therapy (4,5,7,9,14,16,17); the metabolic conversion of short-lived, parent antiepileptic drugs to more persistent therapeutically active metabolites (4,5,9,13,16); the isolation and identification of inactive metabolites (3,8,10–12); and the concept of phenobarbital tolerance (14).

Svensmark and Kristensen (26) studied the distribution of phenytoin [pK' 8.3 (1)] and phenobarbital [pK' 7.2 (5)] between equal volumes of chloroform and borate buffers of different pH. At pH 8.80, about 88% of the phenobarbital was present in the aqueous buffer phase and 88% of the phenytoin was present in the chloroform phase. When two such partitions were performed successively, 77% of each drug was recovered and the contamination by the other drug amounted to only 1.4%. Based on this knowledge, the authors designed a separation scheme for the determination of the drugs when both were present in the same plasma sample.

Ethotoin (3-ethyl-5-phenylhydantoin, **1**) is one of the less widely prescribed antiepileptic drugs. The metabolic fate of ethotoin in the dog has been studied (19). The primary metabolite, formed by metabolic deethylation, was 5-phenylhydantoin **(2)**. The greater proportion of the metabolically formed 5-phenylhydantoin **(2)** was further converted by a stereospecific ring-opening reaction to (*R*)(—)-2-phenylhydantoic acid **(3)**. With the knowledge of the physical constants summarized in Table 4, a scheme for the stepwise isolation of **2** and **3** was devised. Urine from dogs receiving either ethotoin or 5-phenylhydantoin was adjusted to pH 6.0 and was extracted continuously (liquid-liquid extractor) with ether for 48 hr. This step selectively removed **2** from the urine. After the removal of **2** was complete, the pH of the urine sample was lowered to 4.0 and the urine was extracted continuously with a fresh portion of ether for 450 to 500 hr. During this lengthy period, (*R*)-2-phenylhydantoic acid was slowly removed from the urine, crystallizing directly as it accumulated in the ether reservoir flask.

The partition ratios summarized in Table 4 were the basis for the design of the stepwise gas-liquid chromatographic determinations of 5-phenylhydantoin **(2)** and 2-phenylhydantoic acid **(3)** in quantitative studies of the enzymatic ring-opening reaction (20). In incubations of **2** with the 100,000 × *g* supernatant of a rat liver homogenate at pH 7, the unmetabolized proportion of **2** was removed by ether extraction and was quantitated by gas-liquid chromatography (GLC). The 2-phenylhydantoic acid **(3)**, formed by the enzymatic reaction, remains in the buffered aqueous phase at pH 7. The hydantoic acid **3** was then reconverted to the hydantoin **2** by acid-catalyzed cyclodehydration, a reaction that was made essentially quantitative by adding mineral acid directly to the aqueous incubation phase and by heating the mixture. The reconstituted hydantoin **2** was extracted with ether and was quantitated in terms of **3** by GLC. The same principles in these isolation and analytical techniques have been applied to studies of the metabolic fate and disposition of ethotoin in epileptic patients (28).

TABLE 4. *Ionization exponents (pK′) and partition ratios (K′) of 5-phenylhydantoin and 2-phenylhydantoic acid (19)*

Compound	pK'_a	K′ Ether/pH 6 buffer[a]	K′ Ether/pH 4 buffer[a]
(*RS*)-5-Phenylhydantoin	8.5[b]	2.10	2.00
(*RS*)-2-Phenylhydantoic acid	3.4[c]	0.00	0.03
(*R*)-2-Phenylhydantoic acid	3.4[c]	0.00	0.04

[a] 1.0 M potassium phosphate solution.
[b] In 5% acetone.
[c] In water.

Schäfer (25), in designing a GLC method for the simultaneous determination of underivatized antiepileptic drugs, made a systematic study of the partitioning properties of six antiepileptic drugs relative to that of his internal standard, 5-(*p*-methylphenyl)-5-phenylhydantoin (MPPH). His multiple-step extraction scheme resulted in excellent recoveries of the drugs, the lowest recovery being about 75%.

The use of partition ratios, like that described in Schäfer's study (25), is rarely employed today in the design of GLC determinations of antiepileptic drugs. GLC, because of its greater sensitivity, is less demanding than spectrophotometry on the need for recovery of a solute. Investigators frequently express the efficiency of their overall extraction scheme for GLC determinations as "percentage recovery." Percentage recovery of a drug is, in essence, a summation of the partitioning properties of a drug, defining the fractional amount of the drug recovered at the final step of the procedure. However, one can find in the literature, as pointed out by Schäfer (25), misleading and conflicting statements about the percentage recovery of a particular drug by essentially the same extraction scheme. The paucity of information devoted to explanation of a recovery experiment and the ambiguous usage of "percentage recovery" by investigators contributes to this present state of confusion. Both the student and expert of GLC antiepileptic drug determinations could gain a better understanding of extraction schemes if investigators were to concur on the definition and usage of "percentage recovery" and were to provide adequate explanation of their recovery experiments in scientific publications.

ACKNOWLEDGMENT

The program of the Epilepsy and Anticonvulsant Drug Research Laboratory (University of North Carolina at Chapel Hill) is supported by the Developmental Disabilities, Facilities, and Construction Service Act, grant no. P.L. 91–517, awarded by the North Carolina Council on Developmental Disabilities.

REFERENCES

1. Agarwal, S. P., and Blake, M. I. (1968): Determination of the pK_a' value for 5,5-diphenylhydantoin. *J. Pharm. Sci.,* 57:1434–1435.
2. Bush, M. T. (1961): Extraction and identification of barbiturates. *Microchem. J.,* 5:73–90.
3. Bush, M. T., Butler, T. C., and Dickinson, H. L. (1953): The metabolic fate of 5-(1-cyclohexen-1-yl)-1,5-dimethyl barbituric acid (hexobarbital, Evipal) and of 5-(1-cyclohexen-1-yl)-5-methyl barbituric acid ("Nor-evipal"). *J. Pharmacol. Exp. Ther.,* 108:104–111.
4. Butler, T. C. (1952): Metabolic demethylation of 3-methyl-5-ethyl-5-phenyl hydantoin (Mesantoin). *J. Pharmacol. Exp. Ther.,* 104:299–308.
5. Butler, T. C. (1952): Quantitative studies of the metabolic fate of mephobarbital (N-methyl phenobarbital). *J. Pharmacol. Exp. Ther.,* 106:235–245.
6. Butler, T. C. (1953): Quantitative studies of the demethylation of trimethadione (Tridione). *J. Pharmacol. Exp. Ther.,* 108:11–17.

7. Butler, T. C. (1953): Quantitative studies of the physiological disposition of 3-methyl-5-ethyl-5-phenyl hydantoin (Mesantoin) and 5-ethyl-5-phenyl hydantoin (Nirvanol). *J. Pharmacol. Exp. Ther.*, 109:340–345.
8. Butler, T. C. (1954): Metabolic oxidation of phenobarbital to *p*-hydroxyphenobarbital. *Science,* 120:494.
9. Butler, T. C. (1955): Metabolic demethylation of 3,5-dimethyl-5-ethyl oxazolidinedione (paramethadione, Paradione). *J. Pharmacol. Exp. Ther.*, 113:178–185.
10. Butler, T. C. (1956): The metabolic hydroxylation of phenobarbital. *J. Pharmacol. Exp. Ther.*, 116:326–336.
11. Butler, T. C. (1956): The metabolic conversion of 3-methyl-5-ethyl-5-phenyl hydantoin (Mesantoin) and of 5-ethyl-5-phenyl hydantoin (Nirvanol) to 5-ethyl-5-(*p*-hydroxyphenyl) hydantoin. *J. Pharmacol. Exp. Ther.*, 117:160–165.
12. Butler, T. C. (1957): The metabolic conversion of 5,5-diphenyl hydantoin to 5-(*p*-hydroxyphenyl)-5-phenyl hydantoin. *J. Pharmacol. Exp. Ther.*, 119:1–11.
13. Butler, T. C., Mahaffee, D., and Mahaffee, C. (1952): The role of the liver in the metabolic disposition of mephobarbital. *J. Pharmacol. Exp. Ther.*, 106:364–369.
14. Butler, T. C., Mahaffee, C., and Waddell, W. J. (1954): Phenobarbital: Studies of elimination, accumulation, tolerance, and dosage schedule. *J. Pharmacol. Exp. Ther.*, 111:425–435.
15. Butler, T. C., Ruth, J. M., and Tucker, Jr., G. F. (1955): The second ionization of 5,5-disubstituted derivatives of barbituric acid. *J. Am. Chem. Soc.*, 77:1486–1488.
16. Butler, T. C., and Waddell, W. J. (1956): Metabolic conversion of primidone (Mysoline) to phenobarbital. *Proc. Soc. Exp. Biol. Med.*, 93:544–546.
17. Butler, T. C., and Waddell, W. J. (1958): N-methylated derivatives of barbituric acid, hydantoin, and oxazolidinedione used in the treatment of epilepsy. *Neurology* (Minneap.), 8:106–112.
18. Craig, L. C., and Craig, D. (1956): In *Technique of Organic Chemistry,* 2nd ed., edited by A. Weissberger, Vol. III, Part 1, pp. 149–393. Interscience Publishers, New York.
19. Dudley, K. H., Bius, D. L., and Butler, T. C. (1970): Metabolic fates of 3-ethyl-5-phenylhydantoin (ethotoin, Peganone), 3-methyl-5-phenylhydantoin and 5-phenylhydantoin. *J. Pharmacol. Exp. Ther.*, 175:27–37.
20. Dudley, K. H., Butler, T. C., and Bius, D. L. (1974): The role of dihydropyrimidinase in the metabolism of some hydantoin and succinimide drugs. *Drug Metab. Dispos.*, 2:103–112.
21. Fogh, J., Rasmussen, O. H., and Skadhauge, K. (1954): Colorimetric method for quantitative microdetermination of quaternary ammonium compounds. *Anal. Chem.*, 26:392–395.
22. Hill, A. E. (1930): In *Treatise on Physical Chemistry,* 2nd ed., edited by H. S. Taylor, Vol. I, pp. 467–589. Van Nostrand Co., New York.
23. Leo, A., Hansch, C., and Elkins, D. (1971): Partition coefficients and their uses. *Chem. Rev.*, 71:525–616.
24. Nernst, W. (1891): Verteilung eines Stoffes zwischen zwei Lösungsmitteln und zwischen Lösungsmittel und Dampfraum. *Z. Phys. Chem.*, 8:110–139.
25. Schäfer, H. R. (1975): Some problems concerning the quantitative assay of primidone and its metabolites. In *Clinical Pharmacology of Antiepileptic Drugs,* edited by H. Schneider, D. Janz, C. Gardner-Thorpe, H. Meinardi, and A. L. Sherwin, pp. 124–130. Springer-Verlag, New York.
26. Svensmark, O., and Kristensen, P. (1963): Determination of diphenylhydantoin and phenobarbital in small amounts of serum. *J. Lab. Clin. Med.*, 61:501–507.
27. Titus, E. O. (1971): Isolation procedures—Liquid extraction and isolation techniques. In *Fundamentals of Drug Metabolism and Drug Disposition,* edited by B. N. LaDu, H. G. Mandel, and E. L. Way, pp. 419–436. Williams & Wilkins, Baltimore.
28. Yonekawa, W., Kupferberg, H. J., Cantor, F., and Dudley, K. H. (1975): Ethotoin distribution and metabolism in epileptic patients. *Pharmacologist* 17:193 (abstr.).

Antiepileptic Drugs: Quantitative Analysis and Interpretation, edited by C. E. Pippenger, J. K. Penry, and H. Kutt, Raven Press, New York, © 1978.

Chapter 6

Instrumentation for Gas-Liquid Chromatographic Analysis of Antiepileptic Drugs: Quality Control

Erich L. Gibbs and Trudy J. Gibbs

The antiepileptic drug level came of age about 8 years ago with the development of gas-liquid chromatographic (GLC) methods for the convenient, accurate analysis of the more common antiepileptic drugs. Now, essentially all of the hydantoins, barbiturates (including primidone), succinimides, diones, carbamazepine, and their active metabolites can be determined selectively and accurately with little or no interference from other drugs or the plasma matrix (Fig. 1). Because all of these drugs can be determined with a single basic methodology, the quantitative analysis of three or four drugs in a single sample costs only slightly more than a complete blood count (5,7,9,15). The effectiveness of these drugs and their active metabolites at concentrations well above 1 μg/ml of plasma allows them to be measured with stable, wide-range GLC equipment, using flame ionization detectors (FID). The fact that a single methodology is applicable to all of these drugs has made it convenient to refer to them as "Type 1" antiepileptic drugs. The development of stable nitrogen-phosphorous flame ionization detectors (N-P FID) may soon make it possible to use GLC for the routine determination of the benzodiazepines, which have therapeutic ranges nearly an order of magnitude lower than the Type 1 drugs (2,4,14).

The accuracy of an antiepileptic drug-level determination is more a function of the competence and dedication of the staff than of the specific hardware or methodologies employed, but there are important differences nonetheless. Thin-layer chromatographic (TLC) or spectrophotometric procedures are, by their nature, not as quantitative or specific as other approaches. GLC, used in conjunction with a variety of detection devices, is currently the primary method used in most laboratories that are researching the pharmacology or clinical effectiveness of the antiepileptic drugs. The wide variety of drugs that can be analyzed specifically is a major reason for this choice, because it is important that the benefits of the antiepileptic drug-level determination not be restricted to only a few of the effective medications. Confidence in the specificity of GLC is another key reason for selecting it. GLC is basically a scanning methodology, and interferences are far more likely to be detected than in the targeted methodologies such as radioimmunoassays (RIA), enzymatically coupled antibody assays (EMIT) (Syva,

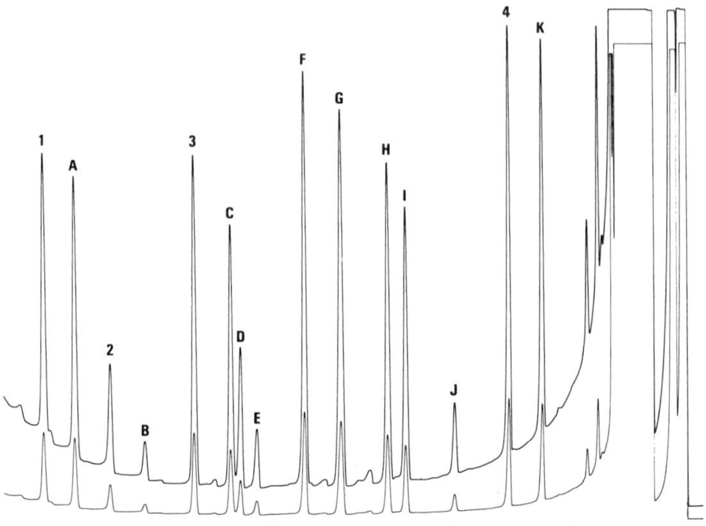

FIG. 1. A GLC temperature-programmed scan of a number of antiepileptic drugs in a plasma matrix. The peaks are as follows: (1) 5,5-(p-tolyl)phenylhydantoin; (A) 5,5-diphenylhydantoin; (2) 5,5-ethyl(p-tolyl)-2,4-hexahydropyrimidinedione; (B) 5,5-ethylphenyl-2,4-hexahydropyrimidinedione; (3) 5,5-ethyl(p-tolyl) barbituric acid; (C) 5,5-ethylphenylbarbituric acid; (D) 5,5-ethylphenylhydantoin; (E) 5,5-methylphenylhydantoin; (F) 3,3-methylphenylsuccinimide; (G) 5,5-allyl(l-methylbutyl)barbituric acid; (H) 5,5-ethyl(sec-butyl) barbituric acid; (I) 5,5-allyl(isopropyl)barbituric acid; (J) 5,5-diethylbarbituric acid; (4) 3,3-methylpropylsuccinimide; (K) 3,3-ethylmethylsuccinimide. Column OV-17.

Palo Alto, Calif.), or spectrophotometric assays (see Chapter 18). High-pressure liquid chromatography (HPLC) also offers the advantages of scanning and great flexibility, and in time it may parallel GLC, but it has yet to be thoroughly seasoned with routine use (1,12). The immunoassays have important adjunctive applications, especially when the 0.5-ml serum sample required for a GLC assay may be difficult to obtain or the number of samples is so great that automated equipment can be used in a cost-effective manner (3). Unfortunately, many laboratories have developed the mistaken impression, nurtured by advertising, that the immunoassays are less expensive and more accurate than GLC and, above all, practically foolproof by comparison. The fact that "EMIT laboratories," participating in the Epilepsy Foundation of America Quality Control Program (EFA-QCP) have, on the average, scored somewhat better than "GLC laboratories" (10) will doubtless be used as evidence for the superiority of EMIT even though the EFA-QCP has not yet examined quality control during the intervals between sample mailings. This laboratory has the distinct impression that a headlong rush to use the "simple" immunoassays will result in better quality control data and lower routine quality. All of the antiepileptic drug-level methodologies are sensitive and complex in a fundamental sense, and shifting responsibility to a commercial source by using fully automatic, self-adjusting instruments or prepared reagents does not make a method foolproof and can increase the extent of any errors that may occur. Furthermore, if less experienced or less dedicated technicians are given the responsibility for performing an assay that is considered foolproof, the results can be unbelievably poor. These points are stressed so that the following frank discussion of errors associated with GLC hardware does not become a carelessly thrown boomerang that contributes to the destruction of the key methodology it is intended to improve.

LABORATORY COMMITMENT

A 20% change in a patient's plasma drug concentration can make the difference between ideal control and seizures or side effects; it stands to reason, therefore, that the error associated with antiepileptic drug-level measurements should be kept to 5% or less within the therapeutic range, if the values are to be clinically useful (5,6,10,11). It is not enough to maintain precision alone; results must be accurate with respect to absolute standards or it will be necessary to establish correction factors for every laboratory in order to make use of suggested optimal therapeutic levels. Such accuracy requires a major commitment in instrumentation and personnel and is not likely to be achieved in laboratories lacking specialized technologists or in laboratories that use their GLC instruments for a variety of assays requiring significant changes in the operating conditions. Assuming that a laboratory could start with a thoroughly tested GLC method and instruments that have worked for other operational laboratories, it is likely to take at least 300 hr of shakedown and training of key personnel before the 5% error level can be met on a regular basis. Unfortunately, so few methods have been exhaustively tested and accepted for publication in sufficient detail that a laboratory could be reasonably certain of encountering pitfalls unless at least key personnel are trained at an experienced laboratory. Establishing tolerance limits for the elements of an assay and gaining practical knowledge of interfering drugs or matrix effects can take years, but many laboratories, encountering difficulty with a method, have made modifications without revalidation and without making the effort to discuss the modifications with the original investigators.

Once in operation, a laboratory with a single GLC system should expect to spend 20% of its effort repairing, tuning, and standardizing the instruments, testing reagents, and challenging the method. Specializing and increasing the sample load can greatly improve efficiency; duplication of instrumentation reduces downtime and simplifies service by permitting substitution checks. Duplicate instruments can also be standardized and tuned in groups.

THE GLC COLUMN

The column is the heart of the GLC instrument (8). The choice of support and liquid phase can greatly affect the quality of the end results. Chemical or adsorptive interaction between sample and support must be negligible, but the support must also provide an enormous surface area, on the order of meters per gram, with good uniformity of particle and pore sizes. As though in contradiction to these requirements, however, it must not be so friable that it breaks up with handling and use, producing fines that would contaminate a GLC detector or plug the column to the free flow of the gas phase. Currently, the most widely used and effective support is acid-washed, silane-treated, flux-calcinated diatomite material screened to 100/120 mesh. This material gives high plating efficiencies with a minimum of polar interaction and is sold under a number of trade names such as Chromsorb W HP (Johns-Manville, Denver, Col.), Gas-Chrom Z (Applied Sciences Laboratories, Inc., State College, Pa.), and Anakrom Q (Analabs, North Haven, Conn.). All must meet published general quality control specifications, but such specifications do not necessarily guarantee uniformity for a specific application. It is important to remember that diatomite materials are mined natural products.

Relatively few liquid phases have been studied or compared in the antiepileptic drug-level field. This is not because of any herd instinct on the part of antiepileptic drug-level laboratories; rather it is a reflection of the fact that of some 250 liquid phases that can be found in most catalogues, only a few meet the high-temperature, low-viscosity, and stability requirements of the antiepileptic drug-level field. With the exception of several largely unknown possibilities, only the phenyl/methyl silicones will operate well at temperatures of up to 300°C, are neutral, and offer the right range of polarity for good separation. OV-17 (Ohio Valley Specialty Co., Marietta, Ohio) has been one of the most widely used and effective liquid phases, but other, potentially equivalent phases, may offer some advantages or pose problems and should eventually be compared under controlled conditions. Regardless of the phase selected, it is important to request detailed information on the date of manufacture and the lot number. Some lots may be inferior or superior, and it is good practice to stay in close contact with the original manufacturer.

The use of phenyl/methyl silicone liquid phases, and even the best supports, requires the derivatization of the antiepileptic drugs in order to mask reactive groups that would result in unacceptable tailing of GLC peaks. The possibility of determining the underivatized drugs on an acidic column is currently being studied (13), but the potential for fouling these columns with basic material should be weighed carefully against the relative simplicity of derivatization steps that may simultaneously serve as necessary stages of concentration and cleanup of the sample.

Coating the solid support with the liquid phase can be a major source of error, and many laboratories would be well advised to purchase precoated column packing from quality-conscious suppliers. The liquid phase must be dissolved in a volatile solvent and added to the solid support in a manner that minimizes trapped air in the voids of the support. Then the solvent must be evaporated under conditions that leave a thin film of the liquid phase covering a maximum surface area without filling the voids of the support with the liquid phase. The amount of liquid phase added will depend primarily on the type of support and liquid phase selected. If too much liquid phase is added, the voids will fill and the rate of equilibration between the gas and liquid phases will decrease. This will result in a loss of resolution. A variety of coating methods have been recommended, but all involve a good deal of technique and even experienced individuals will suffer occasional failures. The best advice is to quality control batches of coated support well before they will be needed. There is a feeling among some that the phenyl/methyl silicone phases may not all be stable over long periods of time when applied to diatomite supports. However, there appears to be no reason for concern in a time span of a year or so. Chromsorb W HP coated with OV-17 has not shown any sign of deterioration over a 2-year period and, in any case, deterioration is not likely to be abrupt (7). Most of the reported column failures are more likely to be due to improper coating, loading, or conditioning than to defective support or liquid phases.

The design of the GLC column should minimize sharp bends that can result in an uneven path length and tailing. Because well-designed FIDs can accurately detect 0.1 μg of drug, fine bore (1 to 2 mm) columns can be used and a column 1 to 2 m long will usually give excellent resolution. A GLC assay should be considered as a system of interacting stages and each stage must be matched at the interface. Thus, the sensitivity and linearity of the detector determine how much drug should be placed on the column and this in turn dictates the diameter of the column, which cannot be so great that the drug is "lost" in the column packing. The wall thickness of glass columns must be thin if the column is to be temperature programmed, or the interior of the column may not track the changes in oven temperature faithfully.

When the column is loaded with packing, great care must be taken to obtain a solid pack, so that the column will not compress and leave a large gas space in the injector end of the column. However, this must be accomplished without producing fines that can work their way into a tight spot in the packing to produce a block and prevent the even flow of the gas phase. Ideally, the best resolution will be obtained when the pressure drop of the gas phase across the column is minimized, but in practice excellent resolution can be attained with pressure drops as high as 2 kg/cm^2. The volume of gas space in the injector end of the column should be kept to a minimum from the standpoint of peak symmetry, but injection directly onto the column packing is not recommended for on-column derivatization. In fact, the geometry of the injector end of the column can be a major variable when on-column derivatization is employed, and plugging the injector end of the column with silanized glass wool to prevent the packing material from blowing out of the column, when the pressure is suddenly released from the injector, is not recommended either. It is better practice to turn off the carrier gas and wait for the pressure to drop in the column before opening the injector.

Chemically resistant glass appears to be the best construction material for the column itself. Stainless steel tends to break down the antiepileptic drugs, especially the barbiturates, and, if the analytical procedure involves on-column derivatization, stainless steel is completely unsatisfactory. The on-column methylation of phenobarbital with tetramethylammonium hydroxide (TMAH) produces such extensive breakdown when a metal column is used that the breakdown peaks are larger than the drug peaks. Glass also has the advantage of being transparent, thereby permitting visual inspection of the column packing. An uneven column bore can cause "log jams" and interruptions in the packing. Simple interruptions of the liquid phase have surprisingly little practical effect, but, if fines become jammed in a constriction, they may create an uneven pressure gradient in the gas phase and spoil column performance. Subjecting the column to sudden wide temperature swings greatly increases the rate at which column packing compresses and crumbles into fine material. Vibration, perhaps from an oven fan, can also hasten the break up of column packing, and when breaks do occur in a column, care must be taken to use a minimum of tapping. Increased column back-pressure, resulting from column compression and trapped fines, probably explains at least as many column failures as deterioration of the liquid phase.

COLUMN INSTALLATION

The packed column must be installed and conditioned before it is ready for use. Installation may sound trivial, but the seals that hold the column in place are critical. If they leak, the leak is likely to be temperature dependent, and when the GLC assay involves temperature programming, there will be a relatively greater loss of the more volatile drugs. Assuming the use of a glass column, metal compression ferrules must be ruled out because they do not provide the necessary elasticity to make up for the differential expansion between glass and metal. Teflon ferrules compress and must be tightened and replaced frequently. Graphite ferrules can be messy and they too compress, and silicone rubber is not recommended at oven temperatures above 200°C. Vespel (Alltech Associates, Arlington Heights, Ill.) ferrules represent an excellent solution provided that they are properly installed. Vespel will seize on the glass column and compression nut simultaneously, so that rotation of the nut twists the column. To avoid this problem, a thin Teflon washer can be placed between the Vespel ferrule and the compression nut, a little item without which there can be no success. It is important to learn to recognize the signs of a leaking injector-column seal from the shape of the "front" on the output chart, because even Vespel will loosen with repeated temperature cycling and it is not a good idea to tighten column nuts on a routine preventive maintenance basis. Excessive torquing of the nuts will distort the threads of all but specially hardened, high-temperature stainless steel fittings. The injector and detector ends of a glass column should be placed as far as possible into the injector and detector to prevent the drugs from contacting more metal than is absolutely necessary.

COLUMN CONDITIONING

A loaded GLC column must be conditioned in order to remove volatile fractions in the liquid phase and to obtain maximum resolution and stability. Conditioning a column, employing a phenyl/methyl silicone liquid phase, involves heating it to about 10°C above the maximum temperature of the assay for 8 to 10 hr, with the carrier gas flowing at the assay rate. Other types of liquid phases may have different requirements, but heating a silicone liquid phase above 250°C in the presence of oxygen will degrade the phase, and conditioning an OV-17 liquid phase on Chromsorb W HP, without a flow of oxygen-free, dry carrier gas will probably spoil the column irreversibly. For this reason, and to prevent excessive temperature cycling, it may be wise never to shut off the flow of carrier gas, except for septum changes, and to maintain an intermediate oven temperature when the column is not in use. Under these conditions, a column may meet rigid specifications even after months of use. The detector should not be connected, or at least not completely assembled, during conditioning, because the initial bleed from the column would coat the detector elements and make it necessary to clean them anyway.

Further conditioning may be necessary for on-column derivatization. The TMAH on-column methylation of the antiepileptic drugs will proceed as expected the first few times a new column is used, but then the barbiturates may suffer astonishingly selective degradation, which will persist for 5 to 10 more injections before subsiding. This effect can go unnoticed if specific barbiturate internal standards are not employed. Some laboratories have completed standardizing a new column during this phase and, without barbiturate internal standards, had no way of detecting an error that subsequently affected many results. Class-specific loss or degradation of the antiepileptic drugs can result from a number of GLC assay variables, so no laboratory should work without at least one internal standard for each class of drugs. A further, striking example of such an effect occurs when impure toluene is used in the drug extraction procedures. Pesticide-grade or reagent-grade toluene from a number of suppliers contains far more impurities than one would expect. It is not uncommon to filter 20 liters and find literally spoonfuls of varnish and plastic residues that probably came from storage and handling equipment. Some lots of such toluene have specifically suppressed barbiturate peaks in

TMAH on-column methylation methods by as much as 70%. It is best to purchase high-quality, glass-distilled solvents from specialty suppliers that rigorously control quality.

GAS FLOW CONTROLS

A GLC column cannot operate without a substantial amount of support instrumentation, everything from low flow gas controls and linear temperature controls to linear chart recorders or other outputs. It is necessary that the 20 or so instrument-support systems, many of them interdependent, be optimized for sensitivity, resolution, and stability; and, naturally, the controls themselves must be stable and dependable. In many cases, it may be necessary to modify equipment extensively in order to obtain the desired level of stability or control. For instance, many GLC instruments are equipped with pressure-regulating constant-flow controls, which do not work in practice. If the flow controls are not well insulated from the heat of the GLC oven, gas flows may drift extensively as the oven temperature is programmed. Such drifting will go undetected if gas flows are only spot checked with a bubble meter. Rotameters are a relatively inexpensive means of monitoring flows continuously, but low-flow rotameters have very light floats that tend to stick to the wall of the meter tube as static charges build up in the dry gas. Heat-transfer (mass) flow meters represent a better solution. Failure to maintain reproducible and stable gas flows will seriously affect the stability of the detector and efficiency of the column.

INJECTOR PORT

The design of the injector port, temperature-stabilizing heater block, and heater controls can be especially important when on-column derivatization is employed. Manufacturers frequently suggest that the injector temperature be set somewhat higher than the maximum column temperature employed. In the antiepileptic drug-level field, the maximum temperatures of a programmed run may be as high as 290°C. But injector temperatures above 260°C will result in extensive breakdown of many of the antiepileptic medications during on-column derivatization. On the other hand, injector temperatures below 250°C will result in inadequate vaporization of the less volatile compounds, such as 5,5-(*p*-tolyl)-phenylhydantoin, a hydantoin internal standard. Moreover, a 5°C shift of the injector temperature can significantly affect standardization when on-column methylation procedures are employed. Having to operate the injector within a narrow, stable temperature range was not contemplated by many manufacturers. Often injector blocks are too small or the heater controls too insensitive, perhaps lacking feedback, to provide adequate temperature stability for on-column derivatization. Another injector design problem is reflected in the fact that many authors have reported using injection port temperatures on the order of 300°C for on-column derivatization with much more success than would be expected at such temperatures. Some instruments do not provide for preheating the carrier gas stream or permit the injection septum to remain much cooler than the rest of the injection chamber. In other cases, the injector geometry has not been arranged so that the carrier gas sweeps through the injector in a path that minimizes dead volume. The net result is very uneven temperatures or gas flows, or both, within the injector, despite what the monitors may indicate.

SEPTUMS

When samples are derivatized prior to injection onto the GLC column, the tolerance limits for temperature control of the injector are much less critical. However, injector temperatures should still be minimized or injector port septum life will be greatly reduced. The selection of septum materials is also important; the wrong type of septum can be a source of error and an efficiency-robbing nuisance. Many septum materials "bleed" continuously or they are so tough as to be nearly impenetrable, damaging syringes. Bleeding will produce a sequence of peaks in the background when the GLC oven temperature is programmed, and the height of the peaks will be variable, depending on such factors as the sharpness of the syringe needle or how long the oven was kept at its lower temperature before beginning the program. Teflon-faced silicone septums are soft and relatively durable, provided that they are operated at temperatures below 270°C. However, most of these septums will bleed, despite claims to the contrary, unless they are conditioned in a vacuum at about 250°C for 8 to 10 hr.

OVEN TEMPERATURE CONTROLS

It is obvious that the temperature of the GLC column oven must be uniform and must track the rate of temperature programming accurately. Step temperature differences of as little as 1°C can alter the height of a peak and defeat the most ideal internal standards. Perhaps it is for this reason that many laboratories believe peak height measurement to be unreliable and prefer to use averaging equipment to determine the area under the curve. Unfortunately, measuring the area under the curve can also result in errors if an interfering peak distorts the shoulder of the drug peak. As a general rule, electronic outputs that reduce the reliance on competent visual inspection of a primary chart output or claim to filter out or correct for uncontrolled variables may do an astonishingly good job, but they are no substitute for first-order stability and freedom from interference.

No GLC instrument would be produced without specifications indicating linear oven temperature control and accurate initial temperature control, but specifications are no guarantee that an instrument will actually perform as hoped, even when it is brand new. An inexpensive chart recorder, monitoring the flow of electric current to the oven heaters, is a sensitive means of detecting step deviations in the normal profile. Such a monitor is of practical importance, because the conventional motor-driven slide-wire controls will develop rough spots on the slide wire with time. Designing the automatic temperature limit controls to trip prematurely if the slide wiper loses contact with the wire altogether is commendable, but not adequate because complete loss of contact is rarely the first sign of trouble. When slide wires do go bad, they can be easily and inexpensively replaced in the field. The newer "all solid state" temperature-programming controls are more elegant, but they are also far more complex and difficult to service in the field.

DETECTORS

Detector systems based on mass spectrograph equipment or electron capture equipment are temperamental, even in the most experienced hands, and a discussion of the potential sources of error would be too lengthy and esoteric for the purposes of the present discussion. However, even the simple FID and related amplification systems can fail in ways that are likely to baffle the inexperienced and result in expensive downtime or reporting errors. A crack in the glass insulator, separating the burner tip from the detector base, can result in oven temperature-dependent changes of sensitivity. Such a crack can be so small as to be almost invisible to the naked eye and can be easily caused by sudden temperature changes such as might be produced by an ignition coil positioned too close to the seal. Again, the best defense against errors is the visual inspection of a primary chart output by an experienced technologist. The cracked seal will give itself away by causing negative changes in relative baseline early in a temperature program run. A dirty insulator can also cause unstable detector sensitivity. With care, the burner, anode, and cathode elements can be cleaned with diluted hydrogen fluoride without unduly shortening the useful life of the parts.

Fuel and oxidant flows should be optimized, insofar as possible, within plateau ranges in order to minimize the need for critical flow control. Temperature control of an FID is not critical as long as the internal surfaces of the detector exceed the maximum oven temperature of the oven program by 10 to 20°C. Of course, excessive temperatures will shorten the life of the FID elements, especially the heater. When an FID is marginally cool, the peaks at the high-temperature end of the curve will be unstable. High-temperature peak material will condense on cold detector surfaces before being burned.

The detector fuel, often hydrogen, should never be turned on when a column is not in place. The oven space might fill with a sufficient volume of combustible material to do real damage. As a matter of general safety, it is wise to minimize connections in the lines carrying the fuel and to use the smallest diameter soft copper refrigeration tubing or stainless steel tubing commensurate with the requirements for flow rate and pressure drop. Leak checks should also be performed on a regular basis, especially on cylinder valves.

SUMMARY

Although this discussion has only hedgehopped through a small part of the field of antiepileptic drug-level technology, we hope that it has shed a little light on the importance of experience and quality control in this, as in any branch of laboratory medicine, and helped to explain the gap between promise and practice in the clinical use of the antiepileptic drug level for the treatment of the epilepsies. GLC instrumentation is complex, and its effective use requires considerable technical skill, but in competent hands it is the most powerful, accurate, and flexible means of determining the antiepileptic drugs and the many other drugs and biologically important substances currently available.

ACKNOWLEDGMENT

The authors are grateful to Cathy A. Meyer and Julia M. Simons for their excellent technical support.

REFERENCES

1. Adams, R. F., and Vandemark, F. L. (1976): Simultaneous high-pressure liquid chromatographic determination of some anticonvulsants in serum. *Clin. Chem.,* 22:25–31.
2. Burgett, C. A., Smith, D. H., Bente, B., Wirfel, J. C., and Goodhart, S. E. (1976): Chromatographic capabilities of the nitrogen-phosphorous selective detector. Hewlett Packard Applications Note ANGC 2–76. Avondale, Pa.
3. Finley, P. R., Williams, R. J., and Byers, J. M., III (1976): Assay of phenytoin: Adaptation of "EMIT" to the centrifugal analyzer. *Clin. Chem.,* 22:911–914.
4. Garattini, S., Mussini, E., and Randall, L. O. (Editors) (1973): *The Benzodiazepines.* Raven Press, New York.
5. Gibbs, E. L. (1974): Anti-epilepsy blood levels, sister field of EEG. *Clin. Electroencephalogr.,* 5:152–160.
6. Gibbs, E. L., and Gibbs, T. J. (1974): What is the meaning of antiepilepsy drug blood drug level measurements? Gibbs Laboratories, Wilmette, Ill.
7. Gibbs, E. L., and Gibbs, T. J. (1977): *AEDL (Anti-Epilepsy Drug Level),* Vol. 1: *Methodology.* Gibbs Laboratories, Wilmette, Ill. (in press).
8. McNair, H. M., and Bonelli, E. S. (1969): *Basic Gas Chromatography.* Consolidated Printers, Berkeley, Calif.
9. Penry, J. K., Smith, L. D., and White, B. G. (Editors) (1972): Blood level determinations of antiepileptic drugs: clinical value and methods. A bibliography with key-word and author indexes. DHEW Publication No. (NIH) 73–396; U.S. Government Printing Office, Washington, D.C.
10. Pippenger, C. E. (1976): Interlaboratory variability. Presented at the Symposium on the Reliable Quantification of Antiepileptic Drugs, November 29, 1976, Kansas City, Mo.

11. Pippenger, C. E., Penry, J. K., White, B. G., Daly, D. D., and Buddington, R. (1976): Interlaboratory variability in determination of plasma antiepileptic drug concentrations. *Arch. Neurol.,* 33:351–355.
12. Soldin, S. J., and Hill, J. G. (1976): Rapid micromethod for measuring anticonvulsant drugs in serum by high performance liquid chromatography. *Clin. Chem.,* 22:856–859.
13. Thoma, J. J., and Ottenstein, D. (1976): Anticonvulsant drug determination by GLC without derivatization—A new development in packed column stationary phases. Presented at the Symposium on the Reliable Quantification of Antiepileptic Drugs, November 29, 1976, Kansas City, Mo.
14. Vandemark, F. L., and Adams, R. F. (1976): Ultramicro gas-chromatographic analysis for anticonvulsants, with use of a nitrogen-selective detector. *Clin. Chem.,* 22:1062–1065.
15. Woodbury, D. M., Penry, J. K., and Schmidt, R. P. (Editors) (1972): *Antiepileptic Drugs.* Raven Press, New York.

Antiepileptic Drugs: Quantitative Analysis and Interpretation, edited by C. E. Pippenger, J. K. Penry, and H. Kutt, Raven Press, New York, © 1978.

Chapter 7

Gas-Liquid Chromatographic Quantitation of Phenytoin, Phenobarbital, Primidone, and Carbamazepine

Barbara A. Darcey, Elizabeth B. Solow, and C. E. Pippenger

This chapter provides an overview of the three most commonly used gas-liquid chromatographic (GLC) techniques for the analysis of phenytoin, phenobarbital, primidone, and carbamazepine. In establishing gas-liquid chromatographic procedures, the choice of methodology is left to the individual laboratory, based on the experience of others in the field, as well as their own developmental efforts.

ANALYSIS WITHOUT DERIVATIZATION

The determination of antiepileptic drug levels by direct injection of underivatized serum extracts most efficiently takes advantage of the ability of a gas chromatograph to separate and quantitate individual members of a mixture of molecular species. The approach is simple and a minimum of steps are required (i.e., extraction and injection). Thus, the potential for both operator and system error is minimized. If good technique is followed during the extraction, problems that arise with direct injection are almost always associated with poor column performance.

Derivatization introduces an additional step (chemical alteration of the molecule) and enhances the possibility of errors. Trimethylsilyl derivatives will not form in the presence of moisture, and the yield of some derivatives is low unless long reaction times are allowed (9). On-column methylation is not as subject to interference from moisture, but incomplete methylation and multiple peaks are a source of problems. Phenobarbital, for example, may yield two peaks when methylated (18).

Direct injection requires higher operating temperatures than derivatization, decreases sensitivity, and increases the potential for peak tailing. With thermally stable packing and properly adjusted operating conditions, linearity can be attained for all of the antiepileptic drugs over the ranges encountered in clinical materials, and these levels are easily measured by direct injection. This is true even in older models of gas chromatographs. Reproducibility for direct injection procedures is the same as that reported for derivatization procedures. Our coefficient of variation for phenobarbital, phenytoin, and ethosuximide are consistently less than 5%, and for primidone and carbamazepine it is 5 to 10%.

Because problems of direct injection can often be attributed to decreased column performance, trouble shooting is simplified. A good column can only be attained with high-quality packing material. However, the preparation of packing is an art, and not all lots of packing produces satisfactory chromatograms. Ask the supplier to replace the packing if a new lot of a previously satisfactory packing does not yield good chromatograms. Stock solutions, prepared in methanol because of the low aqueous solubility of most antiepileptic drugs, can be used to evaluate column performance. For example, a solution of phenobarbital, primidone, phenytoin, and internal standard (5 mg/ml of each in methanol) can be used to judge a new column or to make a daily check on an older column. On a good column, injection of 1 to 2 μl of this solution will produce sharp peaks, with baseline separation of the drugs and a phenytoin peak equal in height to the primidone peak. On an unsatisfactory column, the same solution will yield a distorted phenobarbital peak and a much lower, broader, and tailing phenytoin peak, which is poorly separated from the primidone peak.

If a column is used for alkaline drugs (i.e., amphetamines, benzodiazepines, phenothiazines), the sensitivity and separating ability of the column for acidic drugs may decrease. Several injections of the stock solution of acidic drugs or heating the column overnight at 280°C will usually recondition the column. Extra peaks, wider peaks, tailing, and poor separation can often be corrected by cleaning the injection end of the column. We use a pipe cleaner saturated with chloroform to scrub the glass. The glass wool and 6 to 8 cm of packing are removed and replaced with fresh materials. The column is ready for use as soon as the gas chromatograph is at operating temperature. If these measures fail to improve column performance, the column must be thoroughly cleaned and repacked.

The extraction of antiepileptic drugs from biological materials is not a problem. The recoveries are high, and following a cleanup step the extracts can be concentrated and injected. Some methods utilize a single chloroform extraction of drugs from acidified serum. Back-washing of the drugs into alkali followed by acidification and reextraction into chloroform offers several advantages for the simultaneous determination of phenobarbital, primidone, and phenytoin. Several normally occurring serum constituents present in the single extraction are removed by the double extraction technique. The injection of the cleaner extract will lengthen column life. Although these compounds do not elute with the drugs, late eluting compounds from one injection may produce peaks in the following injections, which could be misinterpreted. Carbamazepine, diazepam, and phenylethylmalonamide (PEMA), a major metabolite of primidone, remain in the first chloroform extract. Carbamazepine and diazepam may interfere with the quantitation of phenytoin or could be identified as phenytoin on some columns. PEMA elutes very close to or with phenobarbital on some columns and could cause falsely elevated phenobarbital levels.

A major difficulty in the determination of carbamazepine is the instability of the molecule at high temperatures (3,12). The choice of column packing is critical because the determination must be carried out at the lowest possible temperature. It is extremely important to maintain the flash heater and detector at the same temperature as the column to prevent decomposition at these sites. Higher temperatures at any site may produce peak splitting. The column used for carbamazepine is very sensitive to exposure to compounds such as amines, which create active sites on the packing. Greatest sensitivity, linearity, and column life will be attained with limited use of the column for other analyses.

Ethosuximide is one of the easiest of the antiepileptic drugs to quantitate, because the analysis is carried out at such a low temperature that many of the endogenous compounds that could interfere with other determinations are not eluted from the column. Drugs such as hydantoins, barbiturates, and other succinimides which may be administered in conjunction with ethosuximide also are not eluted at low column temperatures. Ethosuximide has a low boiling point and low vapor pressure, and losses can be encountered if extracts are evaporated to dryness. It is possible to extract a large volume of serum with a small volume of solvent and inject the solvent without concentration, but the extraction is not efficient and emulsions frequently occur. Greater sensitivity using a much smaller sample is attained by extracting the serum with larger volumes of solvent and concentrating the extract, being careful not to evaporate to dryness. Ethosuximide is used in the treatment of absence seizures, primarily a disorder of children. Because these children often receive other antiepileptic drugs, however, which have to be determined from a small serum specimen, the microethosuximide assays are preferable.

Some of the precautions that must be taken to obtain reliable and reproducible antiepileptic drug levels, with a minimum of variation, are the same as those needed for any laboratory procedure. The specimens must be properly collected and labeled, and clean glassware, a clean, dry air supply, and high-purity solvents and reagents are imperative. (Sodium hydroxide is a prime source of extraneous peaks in a chromatogram because it absorbs contaminants from the air.) Inaccurate standards are a major source of gross errors. Compounds must be pure, anhydrous, and stored dessicated. It is very important to use internal standards and to run standards prepared in serum before and after every group of unknowns. If more than 8 to 10 unknowns are done in one run, it is advisable to inject a standard midway through the run. With direct injection, it is possible to use the same standard extracts for several injections, because the compounds are stable in the solvent.

ANALYSIS WITH DERIVATIZATION

Tetramethylammonium Hydroxide

The degradation of quaternary ammonium compounds was first demonstrated by Hofmann (4). He subjected tetramethylammonium hydroxide (TMAH) to heat and the reaction proceeded to trimethylamine and methyl alcohol:

$$(CH_3)_4N^+OH^- \rightarrow (CH_3)_3N + CH_3OH$$

He also showed that trimethylphenylammonium hydroxide (TMPAH) decomposed to yield dimethylaniline and methyl alcohol:

$$C_6H_5N(CH_3)_3{}^+OH^- \rightarrow C_6H_5N(CH_3)_2 + CH_3OH$$

The TMPAH is the same compound that Brochmann-Hanssen and Oke (1) prepared and named trimethylanilinium hydroxide. Robb and Westbrook (11) were the first to show that solutions of quaternary ammonium compounds could yield methyl esters of various compounds when injected into the gas chromatograph.

The polarity of functional groups of anticonvulsant drugs makes the task of gas chromatography difficult because of low vapor pressures and the absorptive property these groups contribute. MacGee (7) demonstrated that the technique of flash alkylation improved the separation of phenytoin when using TMAH. Kupferberg (6) used TMPAH for the simultaneous separation of phenobarbital, primidone, and phenytoin. Later, Solow and Green (14) demonstrated that TMAH and flash alkylation could be used for ethosuximide quantitation. Solow and colleagues (15,16) described a method using TMAH for simultaneous quantitation of a broad spectrum of anticonvulsant drugs.

Kananen and co-workers (5) used TMAH to quantitate barbiturates, as well as phenytoin and primidone. MacGee (8) reported that tetraethylammonium hydroxide (TEMH) could decrease the degradation of some barbiturates and improve separation characteristics. Friel and Troupin (2) used TEMH for flash-heater alkylation of anticonvulsant drugs.

There are some differences between the methods using TMAH and TMPAH as methyl donors. The temperature of the vaporization chamber is lower with TMPAH than with TMAH. For example, the suggested inlet temperature is 280°C for TMPAH and 300 to 350°C for TMAH, depending on the design of the injection port.

Van Meter and Gillen (18) observed that TMPAH was responsible for fragmentation of phenobarbital into two major peaks and postulated the degradation to 2-ethyl-2-phenylmalondiamide (PEMA). They associated the strength of TMPAH as a critical factor in reducing fragmentation and also attributed variable decomposition to the length of time the combined extractions were exposed to TMPAH before injection.

Skinner and associates (13) reported on a study of barbiturates with a gas chromatograph-mass spectrometer and showed that the underivatized drugs decompose on-column after injection. However, they used TMPAH to produce methyl derivatives of the compounds and obtained better stability with this technique. Osiewicz et al. (10) have confirmed by GC-mass spectrometer the fragmentation patterns of phenobarbital associated with TMPAH. Wu (19) also demonstrated the degradation of phenobarbital to butyramides.

Thompson (17) in a report on permethylation of barbiturates using a GC-mass spectrometer concluded that methylating agents such as diazomethane, TMPAH, or TMAH are preferred for derivatizing this group of compounds prior to gas-liquid chromatographic or mass spectrometric analysis.

Which of the methyl donors, TMAH or TMPAH, is preferable for antiepileptic drug analysis remains a matter of individual choice.

Trimethylphenylammonium Hydroxide

Brochmann-Hanssen and Oke (1) first introduced trimethylphenylammonium hydroxide as an alkylating reagent for the quantitation of barbiturates by gas-liquid chromatography. Kupferberg (6) expanded the application of TMPAH to the antiepileptic drugs in 1970. The major advantages of TMPAH as a methylating agent include: improved GLC response to antiepileptic drugs as a consequence of increased volatility following methylation; minimal decomposition of barbiturates; and shorter analysis time. During the same year, MacGee (7) described the application of tetramethylammonium hydroxide as a methylating agent for the analysis of phenytoin. Both TMPAH and TMAH gained rapid acceptance as the reagents of choice for on-column methylation in many laboratories performing routine antiepileptic drug analysis.

On-column methylation provides an accurate and reproducible system for the quantitation of antiepileptic drugs while eliminating some of the problems associated with peak tailing and long retention times commonly encountered with underivatized assays. However, it does introduce other technical problems, including erratic decomposition of barbiturates and remethylation of desmethyl metabolites to their parent compounds.

There are certain factors related to on-column methylation that must be considered in the analysis of antiepileptic drugs with TMPAH. The decomposition of barbiturates in both TMPAH and TMAH is related to the alkalinity of the methylating solution, as well as to the high injection port temperatures needed to drive the reactions to completion. The presence of small amounts of water in a methanolic TMPAH solution will enhance the decomposition of phenobarbital. Inappropriate extraction conditions, such as excessive heat during evaporation under vacuum, can also enhance phenobarbital decomposition. The decomposition products of phenobarbital following on-column methylation have been identified (17,19).

Low concentrations of TMPAH (0.05 to 0.1 M) have been reported to decrease phenobarbital decomposition (18). Although methylation of antiepileptic drugs in aqueous solutions is complete under these conditions, extraneous materials in serum extracts use some of the available methylating reagent, so that the concentration of TMPAH may be insufficient to completely methylate all of the drugs present. With low concentrations of TMPAH, the first compound to be incompletely methylated will be primidone, followed by carbamazepine, phenobarbital, and phenytoin. Incomplete methylation is evidenced by multiple gas chromatographic peaks, which represent mixtures of the mono- and dimethylated derivatives of the respective antiepileptic drugs.

Successful elimination of the potential errors introduced by phenobarbital decomposition in TMPAH is readily achieved by use of the appropriate internal standard, *p*-tolylphenobarbital, which has the same extraction characteristics and also undergoes the same decomposition reactions as phenobarbital (see Chapter 3). *p*-Tolylphenobarbital significantly reduces extraneous errors associated with phenobarbital decomposition in both TMPAH and TMAH.

Another major problem encountered with on-column methylation is in the quantitation of carbamazepine. Roger and associates (12) reported the quantitation of carbamazepine based on its breakdown to iminostilbene in the presence of TMPAH. Carbamazepine is decomposed to iminostilbene in an alkaline medium at elevated temperatures. Decomposition of carbamazepine in the presence of TMPAH yields the two end products iminostilbene and methyliminostilbene. The ratio of iminostilbene to methyliminostilbene depends on the concentration of the TMPAH solution, the length of time the sample is in the injection port, the injection port temperature, and the geometry of the port. It has been our experience that the quantitation of carbamazepine by decomposition to iminostilbene is carried out most successfully in laboratories that have automatic injectors on their gas chromatographs. With automatic injection, each sample is injected at the same speed and depth. Manual injections of carbamazepine in TMPAH may yield unreproducible results because of the lack of consistency between injections. Thus, if decomposition to iminostilbene is used to quantitate serum carbamazepine concentrations, it is imperative that the same technician makes every injection, a standard curve is constructed daily, and the ratio of iminostilbene to methyliminostilbene is assessed in each sample.

The metabolism of several antiepileptic drugs is such that methylation procedures present additional problems for clinical interpretation. Methylation converts the demethylated metabolites of certain drugs to the parent compound (Table 1), producing both parent drug and N-demethylated metabolite. Because the N-demethylated metabolites often represent the active therapeutic principle and exhibit different pharmacokinetic properties than the parent drugs, it is most helpful for the clinician to know the level of both

TABLE 1. *Antiepileptic drugs with active metabolite derived by N-demethylation*

Parent drug	Metabolite
Trimethadione	Dimethadione
Paramethadione	N-desmethylparamethadione
Methsuximide	N-desmethylmethsuximide
Phensuximide	N-desmethylphensuximide
Mephobarbital	Phenobarbital
Mephenytoin	5-Ethyl-5-phenylhydantoin
Diazepam	N-desmethyldiazepam
Metharbital	Barbital

parent drug and metabolite. The half-life of N-demethylated metabolites is usually considerably longer than the half-life of the parent drug, and the metabolite therefore accumulates to a much higher level. Thus, a high serum level of parent drug usually indicates drug intake over the past 2 to 3 days, whereas elevated metabolite levels indicate drug intake over the past 2 to 3 weeks. Low metabolite levels in the presence of known patient compliance could suggest a metabolic problem.

Because methylation negates the possibility of analyzing demethylated antiepileptic drug metabolites, the laboratory must pay particular attention to specimens containing the drugs listed in Table 1. For example, some laboratories quantitate mephenytoin (Mesantoin) using TMPAH. However, 5-ethyl-5-phenylhydantoin (Nirvanol), the major metabolic product of mephenytoin, is converted to mephenytoin in the presence of TMPAH. Methylation of both mephobarbital and phenobarbital yields the same end product, dimethylphenobarbital. Therefore, these two compounds cannot be separated by routine methylation techniques and mephobarbital will be quantitated as phenobarbital. When patients are receiving anticonvulsant drugs that are metabolically demethylated, ethylation (2) or some other derivative reaction may be successfully employed to separate the parent compound from its metabolite.

Methylation has distinct advantages over underivatized assays. Nevertheless, laboratories engaged in the analysis of antiepileptic drugs, whether using TMPAH or TMAH, must consider the ramifications of these derivatization techniques, particularly the decomposition of phenobarbital, the conversion of active metabolites to parent compounds, and the possibility of interference from drugs with similar chemical structures.

REFERENCES

1. Brochmann-Hanssen, E., and Oke, T. O. (1969): Gas chromatography of barbiturates, phenolic alkaloids, and xanthine bases: Flash-heater methylation by means of trimethylanilinium hydroxide. *J. Pharm. Sci.*, 58:370–371.
2. Friel, P., and Troupin, A. S. (1975): Flash-heater ethylation of some antiepileptic drugs. *Clin. Chem.*, 21:751–754.

3. Frigerio, A., Baker, K. M., and Morselli, P. L. (1973): Gas chromatographic-mass spectrometric studies on carbamazepine. *Adv. Biochem. Psychopharmacol.,* 7:125–134.
4. Hofmann, A. W. (1881): Ueber die Einwirkung der Wärme auf die Ammoniumbasen. *Ber. Dtsch. Chem. Ges.,* 14:494–496.
5. Kananen, G., Osiewicz, R., and Sunshine, I. (1972): Barbiturate analysis—A current assessment. *J. Chromatogr. Sci.,* 10:283–287.
6. Kupferberg, H. J. (1970): Quantitative estimation of diphenylhydantoin, primidone, and phenobarbital in plasma by gas-liquid chromatography. *Clin. Chem. Acta,* 29:283–288.
7. MacGee, J. (1970): Rapid determination of diphenylhydantoin in blood plasma by gas liquid chromatography. *Anal. Chem.,* 42:421–422.
8 MacGee, J. (1971): Rapid identification and quantitative determination of barbiturates and glutethimide in blood by gas liquid chromatography. *Clin. Chem.,* 17: 587–591.
9. Meijer, J. W. A. (1971): Simultaneous quantitative determination of antiepileptic drugs, including carbamazepine, in body fluids. *Epilepsia,* 12:341–352.
10. Osiewicz, R., Agarwal, V., Young, R. M., and Sunshine, I. (1974): The quantitative analysis of phenobarbital with trimethylanilinium hydroxide. *J. Chromatogr.,* 88:157–164.
11. Robb, E. W., and Westbrook, J. J., III (1963): Preparation of methyl esters for gas liquid chromatography of acids by pyrolysis of tetramethylammonium salts. *Anal. Chem.,* 35:1644–1647.
12. Roger, J., Rodgers, G., Jr., and Soo, A. (1972): Simultaneous determination of carbamazepine ("Tegretol") and other anticonvulsants in human plasma by gas-liquid chromatography. *Clin. Chem.,* 19:590–592.
13. Skinner, R. F., Gallagher, E. G., and Predmore, D. B. (1973): Rapid determination of barbiturates by gas chromatography-mass spectrometry. *Anal. Chem.,* 45: 574–576.
14. Solow, E. B., and Green, J. B. (1971): The determination of ethosuximide in serum by gas chromatography. *Clin. Chim. Acta,* 33:87–90.
15. Solow, E. B., and Green, J. B. (1972): The simultaneous determination of multiple anticonvulsant drug levels by gas-liquid chromatography. Method and clinical application. *Neurology* (Minneap.), 22:540–555.
16. Solow, E. B., Metaxas, J. M., and Summers, T. R. (1974): Antiepileptic drugs: A current assessment of simultaneous determination of multiple therapy by gas-liquid chromatography-on column methylation. *J. Chromatogr. Sci.,* 12:256–260.
17. Thompson, R. M. (1976): Permethylation of barbiturates: Variation in product ratios with varying methylsulfinylmethide carbanion. *J. Pharm. Sci.,* 65:288–290.
18. Van Meter, J. C., and Gillen, H. W. (1973): A source of variation in the gas-chromatographic assay of phenobarbital treated with trimethylanilinium hydroxide. *Clin. Chem.,* 19:359–360.
19. Wu, A. (1974): Concerning on-column methylation of phenobarbital. *Clin. Chem.,* 20:630.

Antiepileptic Drugs: Quantitative Analysis and Interpretation, edited by C. E. Pippenger, J. K. Penry, and H. Kutt, Raven Press, New York, © 1978.

Chapter 8

Evaluation of On-Column Methylation in Gas-Liquid Chromatographic Quantitation of Antiepileptic Drugs

Robert J. Perchalski and B. Joe Wilder

The determination of plasma concentrations of antiepileptic drugs has become a desirable and, in some areas of this country, a routine control measure available to assist physicians in the treatment of patients with convulsive disorders (18). Kutt and Penry (8) recently summarized the information necessary for interpreting blood-level data for the primary anticonvulsant drugs. MacGee's (9) novel incorporation of a concentrated on-column methylating reagent into the extraction procedure for phenytoin contributed greatly to the simplification of the gas-liquid chromatographic assay of anticonvulsants (4,11,13–15). These rapid methods are as efficient as much longer techniques (3,6,7), and results are available in one-fourth to one-tenth the time.

The primary controversy over on-column methylation with the concentrated reagents, methanolic trimethylphenylammonium hydroxide (TMPAH) and tetramethylammonium hydroxide (TMAH), lies in the production of multiple derivatives with phenobarbital. This was reported in 1966 by Stevenson (16) and in recent years by a number of other authors (5,10–13,17). The "early phenobarbital" peaks (5) were recognized as significant in the precise quantitation of phenobarbital by Perchalski and Wilder (12), who used three peaks for quantitation, one of which had been identified as N,N-dimethylphenobarbital (1). The two unidentified peaks were recently found to be N,N-dimethyl-α-phenylbutyramide and N-methyl-α-phenylbutyramide by Wu (19) and Osiewicz et al. (10), who reported that the major peak, N-methyl-α-phenylbutyramide could be used alone for the precise quantitation of phenobarbital. The identification of these two components clears up the notion that these peaks were simple methylated derivatives of phenylethylmalonamide (PEMA) (11,12,17). This finding also explains why the mass spectral study of Solow et al. (15) revealed no intact PEMA in plasma that contained phenobarbital and was extracted and subjected to methylation with 2.0 M TMAH. However, since on-column methylation of PEMA also produces these two peaks, the exact mechanism of this degradation of phenobarbital is not yet known.

In this study we have evaluated the various extraction procedures and methods of quantitation of phenobarbital to determine the optimum combination of all factors. Only concentrated methylating reagents are considered, since very precise results can be obtained with these, and longer extractions are required for use of reagents less concentrated than 1.5 M.

EXPERIMENTAL

Apparatus

Two four-column Varian 2100 gas chromatographs equipped with flame ionization detectors were used in this study. All columns (91.5 cm × 2 mm i.d. glass U-tube) were packed with 10% OV-17 on 100/120 mesh Gas Chrom Q (Applied Science Laboratories, State College, Pa.) and were conditioned overnight at 300°C with low carrier gas flow. The flow rate of nitrogen was adjusted to about 15 ml/min to give a retention time of 4.0 ± 0.2 min for phenytoin at 240°C. The injection port was heated to 325°C. The detector temperature was 270°C.

Reagents

Tetramethylammonium hydroxide, a 2.0 M solution in methanol, was used as purchased (Southwestern Analytical Chemicals, Inc., Austin, Texas). Trimethylphenylammonium hydroxide was made as a 1 M solution in methanol by the following procedure:

After recrystallization of trimethylphenylammonium iodide (Eastman Kodak Co., Rochester, N.Y.) from absolute methanol in an amber bottle, 15.8 g is slurried in 60 ml of absolute methanol. The slurry is transferred with methanol rinses to a 125-ml gas washing bottle (#7166–10, Ace Glass, Inc., Vineland, N.J.) that contains a magnetic stirring bar and that has been wrapped with aluminum foil to exclude light. A low flow of dry nitrogen is maintained through the side arm to keep the slurry from filtering through the glass frit. The lower portion of the bottle is wrapped with heating cord or tape to keep the temperature of the solution at 40 to 45°C. The apparatus is placed on a magnetic stirrer operating at about 200 to 300 rpm. Silver oxide (Matheson, Coleman, and Bell, Raleigh, N.C.) (7.0 g) is then cut to a fine powder and, with the N_2 flow momentarily cut off, added to the bottle at the surface of the solution through a long-stemmed funnel. The N_2 flow is resumed, and the ground-glass top is placed on the bottle. The reaction is allowed to proceed for about 2 hr with addition of methanol, if necessary. The solution is then filtered into an amber bottle.

The TMPAH solution was titrated with standardized 0.1 N HCl and adjusted to the desired concentration, 1.5 M or 2.0 M, by evaporation of the excess methanol at 50°C under a stream of nitrogen. All solvents used for extraction were analytical reagent grade. Phenobarbital, primidone, and phenytoin were recrystallized from absolute ethanol plus water, methanol, and absolute ethanol, respectively. The internal standards, 5-(*p*-methylphenyl)-5-

phenylhydantoin and 5-ethyl-5-(*p*-methylphenyl) barbituric acid were used as purchased (Aldrich Chemical Co., Milwaukee, Wisc.). The hydantoin internal standard was made up in 0.1 N NaOH to a concentration of 40 μg/ml. The barbiturate standard was made by dissolving about 25 mg in 25 ml of methanol and adding this solution to 475 ml of 0.1 M ascorbic acid.

PROCEDURE

Comparison of 1.5 M and 2.0 M TMPAH. Simultaneous Analysis of Single Phenobarbital Samples on Eight Columns

Two plasma samples from patients who were taking phenobarbital, primidone, and phenytoin were chosen to cover a broad range of phenobarbital

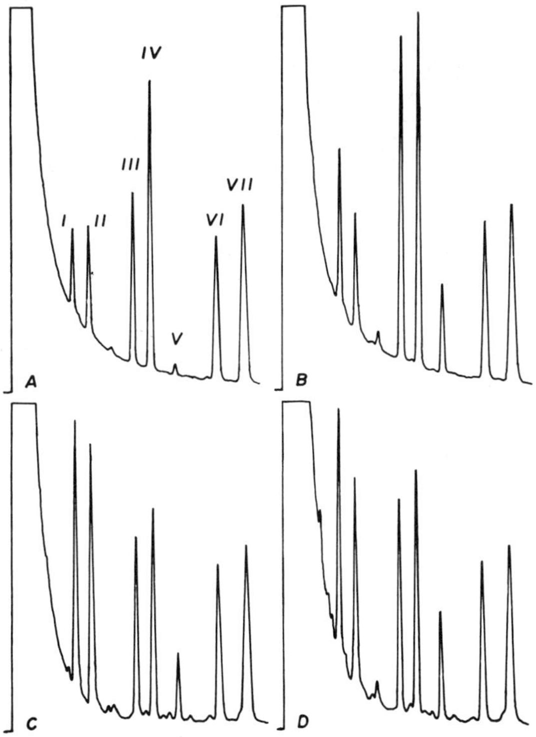

FIG. 1. Pooled plasma sample containing 25.0 μg/ml of phenobarbital, 8.33 μg/ml of primidone, and 13.0 μg/ml of phenytoin extracted by four different methods. A. Plasma extracted with toluene, toluene extracted with 2.0 M TMAH. B. Plasma extracted with ether, ether residue dissolved in toluene, toluene extracted with 2.0 M TMAH. C. Plasma extracted with ether (saturated with phosphate buffer), ether extracted with 0.3 M TMPAH. D. Plasma extracted with ether, ether residue dissolved in toluene, toluene extracted with 1.5 M TMPAH. Peaks are (I) mono- and dimethyl-α-phenylbutyramide; (II) mono- and dimethyl-α-(p-methylphenyl) butyramide; (III) N,N-dimethylphenobarbital; (IV) N,N-dimethyl-5-ethyl-5-(p-methylphenyl) barbituric acid; (V) N,N-dimethylprimidone; (VI) N,N-dimethyldiphenylhydantoin; (VII) N,N-dimethyl-5-(p-methylphenyl)-5-phenylhydantoin.

concentrations, the low level being about 20 μg/ml and the high level about 125 μg/ml. The samples were extracted in duplicate according to the procedure of Perchalski et al. (11), the final extractions being done with 1.5 M TMPAH for one sample and with 2.0 M TMPAH for the replicate. Each sample was injected simultaneously (within 10 sec) on all eight columns, and the column temperature was programmed from 150 to 240°C at 10°C/min. Peak height ratios were calculated for the two phenobarbital peaks, separately, and for the corrected sum of the two peaks, given by Eq. 1:

$$h_{Pb-T} = \frac{w_{\mathrm{I}}}{w_{\mathrm{III}}} h_{\mathrm{I}} + h_{\mathrm{III}} \tag{1}$$

in which h and w are the heights and widths at half-height of the phenobarbital peaks I and III (Fig. 1). The concentrations of phenytoin and primidone were also calculated for each sample on the eight columns.

Comparison of 1.5 M TMPAH and 2.0 M TMAH

A. Reproducibility

Eight replicate samples of a patient's plasma, containing phenobarbital, primidone, and phenytoin at concentrations of 31.4, 4.20, and 17.2 μg/ml, respectively, were extracted as above. The toluene phases of four samples were extracted with 1.5 M TMPAH and those of the other four samples were extracted with 2.0 M TMAH. All samples were chromatographed on a single column, using the temperature program described above. Peak height ratios for the single and total phenobarbital peaks and the primidone and phenytoin peaks were calculated for each sample.

B. Recovery

An extraction scheme (Table 1) was set up with five groups of four replicate samples each, which would allow evaluation of absolute recoveries of phenobarbital, primidone, and phenytoin extracted from plasma with ether or toluene, and relative recoveries of these drugs extracted from toluene with 1.5 M TMPAH or 2.0 M TMAH. A drug standard solution was made up in methanol so that 20 μl of solution added to a sample would give concentrations of 23.8, 7.76, and 14.4 μg/ml in plasma of phenobarbital, primidone, and phenytoin, respectively. An internal standard solution was also made up so that 20 μl would give 20 μg/ml of 5-(*p*-methylphenyl)-5-phenylhydantoin in plasma. The drug reference samples were made by adding 20-μl aliquots of the drug standard and internal standard solutions to each of four tubes, evaporating the methanol, and adding 25 μl of 1.5 M TMPAH. Each of the 20 samples was injected on the same column.

TABLE 1. *Comparison of 1.5 M TMPAH and 2.0 M TMAH. Recovery of phenobarbital, primidone, and phenytoin with various extractions and methylation reagents*

	Peak height ratio														
	Group A[b,d,f]			Group B[b,e,f]			Group C[b,d,g]			Group D[c,d,f]			Group E[h]		
Sample[a]	Pb-T	M	D	Pb-T	M	D	Pb-T	M	D	Pb-T	M	D	Pb-T	M	D
1	2.73	0.627	0.974	2.56	0.888	1.02	1.96	0.509	0.928	1.16	0.068	0.742	2.55	0.815	1.05
2	2.46	0.606	0.982	2.43	0.801	1.02	1.98	0.442	0.929	1.08	0.073	0.738	2.52	0.822	1.10
3	2.36	0.608	0.970	2.29	0.865	1.06	1.86	0.530	0.909	1.17	0.069	0.740	2.34	0.804	1.03
4	2.36	0.561	0.984	2.47	0.857	1.06	1.92	0.433	0.947	1.10	0.074	0.732	2.24	0.765	1.11
$\bar{x}$	2.48	0.601	0.978	2.44	0.85	1.04	1.93	0.48	0.928	1.13	0.071	0.738	2.41	0.801	1.07
σ	0.18	0.028	0.007	0.11	0.04	0.03	0.05	0.05	0.016	0.05	0.003	0.004	0.15	0.026	0.04

[a] Replicate extractions according to *b-h*.
[b] Plasma extracted with ether.
[c] Plasma extracted with toluene.
[d] Drugs added to plasma before extraction.
[e] Drugs added to organic phase after extraction and transfer.
[f] Drugs and internal standard extracted from toluene with 1.5 M TMPAH.
[g] Drugs and internal standard extracted from toluene with 2.0 M TMAH.
[h] Drug reference standards in 1.5 M TMPAH.

Peak height ratios were calculated for phenobarbital (total), primidone, and phenytoin for all samples, and the average ratios were calculated for replicate extractions. Relative recoveries were calculated, assuming equal (100%) efficiency of extraction of the internal standard by 1.5 M TMPAH and 2.0 M TMAH and quantitative methylation of all drugs by both reagents. Standard deviations for recovery were calculated, using the standard formula for error propagation.

Comparison of Methods of Phenobarbital Quantitation

A quality control sample was made up by pooling plasma from patients taking phenobarbital to give a sample containing about 40 μg/ml. This plasma was analyzed over a 44-day period by the method of Perchalski et al. (11) except that the barbiturate internal standard for phenobarbital (2,15) was also added. Peak height ratios for phenobarbital were calculated using the modified summation technique with 5-(*p*-methylphenyl)-5-phenylhydantoin as the internal standard, and by comparing peaks within each set of barbiturate derivatives, using 5-ethyl-5-(*p*-methylphenyl) barbituric acid as the internal standard.

RESULTS AND DISCUSSION

In this discussion and in the tables, the following symbols will be used: The butyramide derivatives of phenobarbital, which elute as a single peak on the 3-ft (91.5-cm) columns used here are designated as Pb-1, the N,N-dimethyl derivative of phenobarbital is designated as Pb-2, and the summation of all phenobarbital derivatives as Pb-T. Primidone and diphenylhydantoin are denoted by M and D, respectively.

Comparison of 1.5 M and 2.0 M TMPAH. Simultaneous Analysis of Single Phenobarbital Samples on Eight Columns

The results are shown in Table 2. This study has demonstrated that identical columns, whether in the same or different chromatographs, do not produce identical phenobarbital methylation patterns, even with the same sample. Also, the concentration of TMPAH, even as high as 2.0 M, does little to produce constant ratios of N-methyl-α-phenylbutyramide to N,N-dimethylphenobarbital in glass injection ports. One must bear in mind that in the quantitative study reported by Osiewicz et al. (10), stainless steel columns and, presumably, a stainless steel injection port were used. However, since it is widely accepted that drug analysis, especially with on-column methylation, should be done with at least a glass-lined injection port, an all-glass system was used for these studies. Results for both phenobarbital concentrations and both TMPAH concentrations indicate that the use of either Pb-1

TABLE 2. Comparison of 1.5 M and 2.0 M TMPAH. Simultaneous analysis of single phenobarbital samples on eight columns

	Peak height ratio											
	Sample 1[a,c]			Sample 2[a,d]			Sample 3[b,c]			Sample 4[b,d]		
Column	Pb-1	Pb-2	Pb-T	Pb-1	Pb-2	Pb-T	Pb-1	Pb-2	Pb-T	Pb-1	Pb-2	Pb-T
1	1.16	1.29	2.22	0.893	1.08	1.79	7.67	6.43	12.5	8.51	3.91	10.7
2	1.35	0.892	1.97	1.00	0.951	1.75	5.88	7.16	11.8	6.64	6.32	11.6
3	1.28	0.950	1.97	1.17	0.715	1.65	8.48	4.33	11.1	8.48	3.25	10.0
4	1.23	1.13	2.11	1.24	0.598	1.58	9.03	5.46	12.7	8.16	4.27	10.8
5	0.816	1.30	1.94	0.823	1.40	2.06	4.57	7.58	11.2	4.76	9.21	13.0
6	0.966	1.31	2.08	1.10	1.14	2.02	6.42	6.20	11.3	7.22	7.19	12.9
7	0.862	1.18	1.87	0.968	1.10	1.87	5.57	6.49	10.9	6.92	6.61	12.1
8	0.927	1.15	1.89	0.782	1.36	1.98	4.73	6.54	10.3	5.68	7.00	11.5
$\bar{x}$	1.07	1.15	2.01	0.977	1.04	1.84	6.54	6.27	11.5	7.05	5.97	11.6
RSD (%)	19	14	6	17	27	10	26	16	7	19	34	9

[a] 22.2 μg phenobarbital/ml of plasma.
[b] 124 μg phenobarbital/ml of plasma.
[c] Toluene extracted with 1.5 M TMPAH.
[d] Toluene extracted with 2.0 M TMPAH.

or Pb-2 alone for quantitation is not sufficiently precise, whereas the corrected (Eq. 1) total of the two peaks gives acceptable relative standard deviations (<10%) in all cases. In an earlier work (11), this modified summation of peaks was shown to be chromatographically and quantitatively valid, based on molar response ratios over the normal range of plasma phenobarbital concentrations, and reproducible during the 2-hr period after the drug was extracted into the methylating reagent.

Concentration values and relative standard deviations for the eight simultaneous determinations of primidone and diphenylhydantoin in each of the samples were also calculated. All relative standard deviations were within an acceptable limit of 10%, except the determination of the lower primidone concentration with 2.0 M TMPAH. This may indicate that there should be an upper limit to the concentration of TMPAH used for multiple antiepileptic drug determinations. However, this may apply only if samples are processed in large volume, necessitating the use of more than one or two columns or instruments.

Comparison of 1.5 M TMPAH and 2.0 M TMAH for Reproducibility and Recovery

Reproducibility was evaluated using eight replicate extractions of a patient's plasma that contained phenobarbital, primidone, and phenytoin at concentrations of 31.4, 4.20, and 17.2 μg/ml, respectively. The extraction of four replicates was completed with 1.5 M TMPAH and that of the other four replicates with 2.0 M TMAH. Relative standard deviations for phenobarbital, primidone, and phenytoin were 1.2%, 2.6%, and 0.5%, respectively, for the samples extracted with 1.5 M TMPAH; and 2.8%, 7%, and 1.1%, respectively, for the samples extracted with 2.0 M TMAH. Although all of the relative standard deviations are lower for replicates extracted with 1.5 M TMPAH than for those extracted with 2.0 M TMAH, the most striking difference in the comparison of the two reagents is in the relative standard deviation of the primidone concentration, which is almost three times higher for the TMAH than for TMPAH.

The values in Table 3 were calculated from the data in Table 1. This study was designed to give the relative recoveries of phenobarbital, primidone, and phenytoin when extracted with 1.5 M TMPAH and 2.0 M TMAH, and also to show the effect of eliminating the initial ether extraction. These are not absolute recovery values in all cases because for all groups except E the internal standard was carried through the final extraction from toluene into the methylating reagent. The calculations are based on the assumptions that the efficiency of extraction of the internal standard was the same for group A as for group C and that no loss of internal standard occurred through extraction from toluene with 1.5 M TMPAH. A comparison of the phenytoin ratios for groups A and C shows that the first assumption is probably valid, and a comparison of the phenobarbital and phenytoin ratios for groups B and E proves that the second assumption is valid. In any case, recovery of the internal standard cannot be greater for group B than for group E, nor can it be greater for groups A, C, and D than for group B. Therefore, the values given in Table 3 will at least set an upper limit on recoveries by the various reagents and extractions.

In Table 3 the ratios of the drugs of group A to the corresponding drugs of group B give the absolute recovery for the ether extraction, since no assumptions about the recovery of the internal standard are necessary. The

TABLE 3. *Comparison of 1.5 M TMPAH and 2.0 M TMAH. Percent recovery of phenobarbital, primidone, and phenytoin with various extractions and methylation reagents*

	Percent recovery[a]		
Group ratio	Pb-T	M	D
A:B[b]	102 ± 9	71 ± 5	94.0 ± 2.8
D:B[c]	46.3 ± 2.9	8.4 ± 0.5	71.0 ± 2.1
B:E[d]	101 ± 8	106 ± 6	97 ± 5
C:A[e]	78 ± 6	80 ± 9	94.9 ± 1.8

[a] Calculated from Table 1.
[b] Absolute efficiency of ether extraction.
[c] Absolute efficiency of toluene extraction.
[d] Relative efficiency of 1.5 M TMPAH extraction.
[e] Relative efficiency of 2.0 M TMAH extraction.

absolute efficiencies of extraction of the three drugs from plasma with toluene are given as the ratios of the drugs of group D to those of group B. The relative efficiencies of extraction of the drugs from toluene with 1.5 M TMPAH and 2.0 M TMAH are given by the ratios B:E and C:A, respectively.

By combining the various recoveries and assuming a lower limit of detection of 0.5 μg of drug/ml of plasma at 100% recovery, a lower limit can be calculated for each drug extracted with the different solvents and reagents.

The chromatograms in Fig. 1 show various extractions of the same pooled sample, which contained 25.0 μg/ml, 8.33 μg/ml, and 13.0 μg/ml of phenobarbital, primidone, and phenytoin, respectively, and illustrate the results given in Tables 1 and 3. Injection volumes and attentuation settings were varied to make the hydantoin standard peak approximately the same size in all cases. Sample A was extracted with toluene, and the toluene was extracted with 2.0 M TMAH. Sample B was extracted with ether. The ether residue was taken up in toluene, which was then extracted with 2.0 M TMAH. The attenuation setting was increased by a factor of 2 in going from A to B, so that there was actually a considerable increase in recovery of all drugs. The most striking increase was in the recovery of primidone, which went from a barely visible peak to a peak consistent with its concentration. Sample D was extracted with ether; however, the toluene was extracted with 1.5 M TMPAH. This change of methylating reagent resulted in maximum recovery of each drug, which, when calculated from the results of Table 1, is 100% for phenobarbital, 75% for primidone, and 91% for phenytoin. Sample C was extracted using a new technique introduced by Dudley (Chapter 3), in which ether previously saturated with phosphate buffer is used to extract the drugs from plasma, and then the ether is extracted directly with 0.3 M TMPAH. The primary disadvantage of this technique is the reduction of primidone recovery to about 45%, necessitating the introduction of a third internal standard, specific for primidone. However, the advantages include reduction of the solvent front, elimination of the ether evaporation step, and simplification of the synthesis of the methylating reagent.

Comparison of Methods of Phenobarbital Quantitation

A sample of pooled plasma, containing about 40 μg/ml of phenobarbital, was run 17 times over a 44-day period. Results based on the modified summation of the butyramide and N,N-dimethyl derivatives of phenobarbital with 5-(*p*-methylphenyl)-5-phenylhydantoin as the internal standard had a relative standard deviation of 7%. Those based on the ratio of the butyramide derivative of phenobarbital to that of 5-ethyl-5-(*p*-methylphenyl) barbituric acid had a relative standard deviation of 6%, whereas results based on the ratio of the N,N-dimethyl derivative of phenobarbital to that of methyl phenobarbital had a relative standard deviation of 5%.

CONCLUSIONS

As these results show, the most efficient extraction technique for the primary anticonvulsants involves ether extraction of acidified plasma; evaporation of the ether phase; dissolution of the residue in toluene; and, finally, extraction of the drugs into 1.5 M TMPAH. All attempts to shorten this procedure have resulted in reduced recovery, particularly that of primidone. This decrease in recovery is generally accompanied by a decrease in precision and accuracy.

The controversy over the formation of multiple derivatives with phenobarbital during on-column methylation has become largely academic since the introduction of 5-ethyl-5-(*p*-methylphenyl) barbituric acid by Gibbs and Gibbs (2) as an internal standard, specific for phenobarbital. This compound, which differs from phenobarbital only in the addition of a methyl group at the para position of the phenyl ring, undergoes the same reaction with the concentrated methylating reagents as evidenced by peaks II and IV in the chromatograms of Fig. 1. As with phenobarbital, the extent of formation of each of these products is inconsistent and unpredictable; however, when both compounds are together in the same sample, the ratios of one butyramide derivative to the other and one dimethyl derivative to the other are concentration-dependent, linear over the range of phenobarbital plasma levels and constant with time and reagent concentration. As the results indicate, the most precise method for quantitating phenobarbital is now by comparison of the dimethyl derivative of phenobarbital to that of its internal standard. The presence of the butyramide derivative, however, is still a good qualitative confirmation, so it should not be totally eliminated from the chromatogram.

REFERENCES

1. Brochmann-Hanssen, E., and Oke, T. O. (1969): Gas chromatography of barbiturates, phenolic acids and xanthine bases: Flash heater methylation by means of trimethylanilinium hydroxide. *J. Pharm. Sci.*, 58:370–371.
2. Gibbs, E. L., and Gibbs, T. J. (1974): Gas-liquid chromatographic determination of anti-epilepsy drugs and their active metabolites in blood. Gibbs Laboratory Reports, Evanston, Ill., February 20.
3. Hammer, R. H., Wilder, B. J., Streiff, R. R., and Mayersdorf, A. (1971): Flash methylation and GLC of diphenylhydantoin and 5-(*p*-hydroxyphenyl)-5-phenylhydantoin. *J. Pharm. Sci.*, 60:327–329.
4. Joern, W. A. (1975): Gas chromatography of anticonvulsant drugs with no solvent evaporation. *Clin. Chem.*, 21:1548–1550.
5. Kananen, G., Osiewicz, R., and Sunshine, I. (1972): Barbiturate analysis—a current assessment. *J. Chrom. Sci.*, 10:283–287.
6. Kupferberg, H. J. (1970): Quantitative estimation of diphenylhydantoin, primidone and phenobarbital in plasma by gas-liquid chromatography. *Clin. Chim. Acta*, 29:283–288.
7. Kupferberg, H. J. (1972): GLC determination of carbamazepine in plasma. *J. Pharm. Sci.*, 61:284–286.

8. Kutt, H., and Penry, J. K. (1974): Usefulness of blood levels of antiepileptic drugs. *Arch. Neurol.,* 31:283–288.
9. MacGee, J. (1970): Rapid determination of diphenylhydantoin in blood plasma by gas-liquid chromatography. *Anal. Chem.,* 42:421–422.
10. Osiewicz, R., Agarwal, V., Young, R. M., and Sunshine, I. (1974): The quantitive analysis of phenobarbital with trimethylanilinium hydroxide. *J. Chromatogr.,* 88:157–164.
11. Perchalski, R. J., Scott, K. N., Wilder, B. J., and Hammer, R. H. (1973): Rapid, simultaneous GLC determination of phenobarbital, primidone and diphenylhydantoin. *J. Pharm. Sci.,* 62:1735–1736.
12. Perchalski, R. J., and Wilder, B. J. (1973): GC assay of phenobarbital. *Clin. Chem.,* 19:788–789.
13. Perchalski, R. J., and Wilder, B. J. (1974): GLC microdetermination of plasma anticonvulsant levels. *J. Pharm. Sci.,* 63:806–807.
14. Solow, E. B., and Green, J. B. (1972): The simultaneous determination of multiple anticonvulsant drug levels by gas-liquid chromatography: Method and clinical application. *Neurology,* 22:540–550.
15. Solow, E. B., Metaxas, J. M., and Summers, T. R. (1974): Antiepileptic drugs: A current assessment of simultaneous determination of multiple drug therapy by gas-liquid chromatography-on column methylation. *J. Chromatogr. Sci.,* 12:256–260.
16. Stevenson, G. W. (1966): On column methylation of barbituric acids. *Anal. Chem.,* 38:1948–1949.
17. Van Meter, J. C., and Gillen, H. W. (1973): A source of variation in the gas chromatographic assay of phenobarbital treated with trimethylanilinium hydroxide. *Clin. Chem.,* 19:359–360.
18. Wilder, B. J., and Perchalski, R. J. (1974): How assay methods can guide drug therapy for epileptic patients. *Mod. Med.,* 43:68–71.
19. Wu, A. (1974): Concerning on column methylation of phenobarbital. *Clin. Chem.,* 20:630.

Antiepileptic Drugs: Quantitative Analysis and Interpretation, edited by C. E. Pippenger, J. K. Penry, and H. Kutt, Raven Press, New York, © 1978.

Chapter 9

Gas-Liquid Chromatographic Quantitation of Ethosuximide

Christine D. Harvey and Allan L. Sherwin

The rapid development in the past decade of practical techniques to determine the levels of various antiepileptic drugs in blood has resulted in renewed interest, among neurologists, in the therapy of the epilepsies. A recent prospective study in our Institute (9) showed that regular monitoring of plasma ethosuximide levels in a large group of patients with absence seizures led to striking improvement in seizure control. The number of patients with seizures was reduced by one-half as a result of the recognition of noncompliance and the individualization of drug requirements. Improved control of absence seizures was also demonstrated by Browne et al. (1) with plasma ethosuximide levels ranging from 40 to 100 μg/ml being observed in controlled patients.

It is essential to realize that the *"therapeutic window"* (i.e., the range of plasma drug levels usually found to be effective) of this particular drug is significantly *larger* than that of other antiepileptic drugs. Unfortunately, as with many other such agents, it is not possible to predict accurately a given patient's plasma concentration from the ethosuximide dose (1). Some idea of the regularity of drug intake or a hint of the presence of an absorptive or metabolic defect can be obtained by the use of dose-plasma level regression curves (9, Chapter 25). Nevertheless, careful titration of plasma levels is frequently required to obtain seizure control, as a number of patients can only be controlled near, or sometimes, somewhat above the usual upper plasma level limit. As absence (petit mal) seizures almost always begin in childhood, the physician frequently has to make appropriate dosage increases in order to account for the weight gain of maturing children. The "fine tuning" required to maximize the control of absence seizures by means of ethosuximide is thus as equally dependent on reliable plasma levels as other antiepileptic drugs.

HISTORICAL REVIEW

In 1958, ethosuximide was reported by Zimmerman and Burgemeister (14) to be particularly effective in the treatment of absence seizures with a low incidence of harmful side effects. Ethosuximide (Zarontin®) is known chemically as 2-ethyl-2-methylsuccinimide. It has a molecular weight of 141.17, is highly soluble in water, and exhibits at pH 7 a partition coefficient of 9.0 between an aqueous layer and chloroform (8). The first assay for ethosuximide was a spectrophotometric procedure, reported by Hansen in 1963 (5). It was based on the ultraviolet absorbance of extracted ethosuximide at 218 nm. Because of interference from barbiturates, a second reading at 240 nm was required to permit appropriate corrections. The method, unfortunately, lacked sensitivity and specificity.

A highly specific gas-liquid chromatographic method (GLC) was described in 1965 by Dill et al. (3). The extraction procedure required the addition of an internal standard, α,α-dimethyl-β-methylsuccinimide. This made precise measurements of the solvents unnecessary. Unfortunately, the addition of a small amount of an equimolar mixture of K_2HPO_4/KH_2PO_4 required time in the weighing and the addition of these salts. In addition, 2-ml samples were required for this extraction procedure, which was not always feasible in the case of children and infants, from whom only a small amount of blood could be taken. The assay was performed by means of a 6-ft glass column (¼ in.) packed with 5% XE-60 on Gas Chrom Z using a GLC equipped with flame ionization detector. In 1967, Wechselberg and Hubel (13) reported a thin-layer chromatographic method for the detection of ethosuximide; however, it lacked sensitivity. A semiquantitative thin-layer chromatographic method was also developed by Vedso et al. (12). In 1969, Buchanan et al. (2) described a GLC procedure for routine estimation of ethosuximide in plasma. The extraction method required only 1 ml of sample and has proved to be very reliable. Glazko and Dill (4) later devised a micro method for pediatric work, allowing fingertip blood specimens of 0.2 ml to be extracted, and good peaks were observed with as little as 0.1 μg of ethosuximide.

Solow and Green (10) in 1971 reported a gas-liquid chromatographic procedure using flash-heater methylation for the determination of ethosuximide in serum. They employed α,α-dimethyl-β-methylsuccinimide as an internal standard and tetramethylammonium hydroxide as the methylating reagent and did not concentrate their samples. Flash methylation was performed on a 6-ft glass column packed with 5% OV-17 on Gas Chrom Q, 100/120 mesh. Another gas-liquid chromatographic method was published by Meijer in 1971 (7). The internal standard chosen, however, was phthamide, a compound that does not resemble ethosuximide as closely as α,α-dimethyl-β-methylsuccinimide. The procedure required 2 ml of plasma, which was then acidified and extracted with ethyl acetate. The chromatographic analysis was performed with a column packed with 10% QF-1/XE-60.

Van der Kleijn et al. (11) reported a simple, rapid method utilizing columns packed with 3% OV-17 on Supelcoport 80–100 mesh and maintained at 125°C. The internal standard employed was naphthalene, which had a longer retention time than ethosuximide. Plasma samples of 1 ml, to which

1 ml of saturated KH_2PO_4 solution was added, were extracted with only 100 μl of chloroform containing 5 μg of naphthalene.

ASSAY FOR THE DETERMINATION OF ETHOSUXIMIDE IN PLASMA OR SERUM

Ethosuximide is assayed in our laboratory by a modification of the revised gas-liquid chromatographic technique described by Buchanan et al. (2). To a round-bottomed glass-stoppered test tube (14 × 100 mm) is added the following in exact order: 0.1 ml of the internal standard, α,α-dimethyl-β-methylsuccinimide (200 μg/ml in distilled water); 0.5 ml of the patient's plasma; 0.5 ml of distilled water; 3 drops of 1.0 N hydrochloric acid. This is then extracted with 5 ml of redistilled chloroform by gentle mechanical shaking in the upright position for 10 min. The organic phase is then separated by filtration through phase-separating paper, which has just been rinsed and then moistened with chloroform, into a 15-ml conical tube. When filtration has almost, but not completely ceased, the aqueous phase is returned to the original tube. The filter cone is rinsed a second time with 2 ml of chloroform, which is then also returned to the original tube. The tube is then shaken by hand for 10 sec and carefully poured through the original filter paper. When the organic phase has passed completely through, the filter paper is removed and discarded. Three drops of isoamylacetate are then added to the tube along with a carborundum chip and the chloroform evaporated in a water bath maintained a 65°C, until approximately 20 μl remains. The sample is then reconstituted with chloroform to approximately 50 μl, and 1 μl is injected into the gas-liquid chromatographic unit.

Instrumentation

Two types of gas-liquid chromatographs are utilized by our laboratory for the detection and quantitation of ethosuximide. The original instrument is a Hewlett-Packard Model 402 equipped with a flame ionization detector (FID) and 4-ft U-shaped ¼-in. i.d. glass columns packed with 5% XE-60 on an acid-washed and dimethyldichlorosilane-treated support, 80-100 mesh. Assay conditions are as follows: oven temperature, 155°C; injection port, 185°C; flame ionization detector, 190°C. The carrier gas is nitrogen. Retention times are 3.8 min for the internal standard and 4.8 min for ethosuximide. A typical chromatogram showing the analysis of plasma from a patient receiving ethosuximide along with several other anticonvulsants is shown in Fig. 1.

A Hewlett-Packard Model 5711 gas chromatograph equipped with flame ionization detectors is also employed. The extracted plasma is injected into 6-ft coiled glass columns, 2 mm internal diameter, packed with 3% OV-17 on Gas Chrom Q, 100–120 mesh. The chromatogram run is programmed using

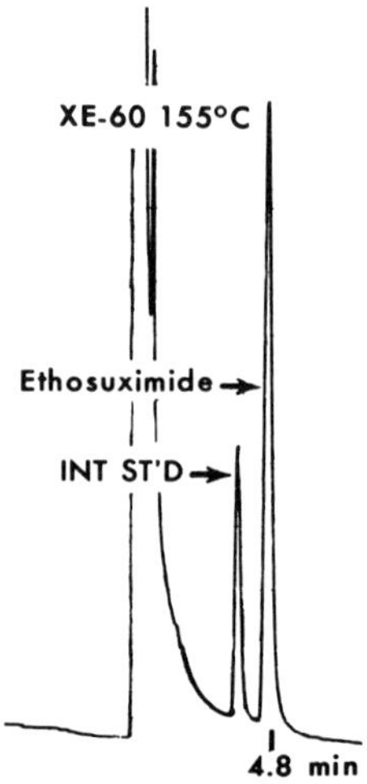

FIG. 1. Gas-liquid chromatogram obtained from a patient receiving ethosuximide showing the drug and the internal standard, α,α-dimethyl-β-methylsuccinimide, which was added to the sample prior to extraction. Column support: 5% XE-60, 80–100 mesh.

the following settings: detector temperature, 300°C; injection port, 300°C; initial column temperature, 100°C. The program is set at oven temperature 100°C for 2 min followed by a rate of increase of 8°C/min to 200°C which is maintained for 16 min. The whole "run" takes approximately 30 min to complete. Figure 2 is a typical chromatogram of internal standard and ethosuximide, the retention times of which were 6.2 and 7.2 min, respectively.

Calibration

A known quantity of drug is added to blank human plasma, which is assayed as described previously. A standard curve is prepared by plotting the peak height ratio, obtained by dividing the peak height of ethosuximide by that of the internal standard, versus the known concentration of drug. The standard curve thus obtained is used to calculate the unknown sample concentration. As can be seen, the chromatographic run on the XE-60 is by far the fastest and most practical. However, when one possesses only one gas-liquid chromatograph for the analysis of antiepileptic drugs, one column, the OV-17, can serve to analyze all the compounds. This eliminates the necessity of cooling down the instrument and changing columns.

The method for the extraction and quantitation of ethosuximide has several areas that must be carefully approached and dealt with. In the extraction step, care must be taken that the shaking is not vigorous, as this results in an emulsion with consequent loss of sample. The phase-separating filter paper should be rinsed well with chloroform. In addition, during the filtration step, the aqueous phase must not be allowed to stand for any length of time in the filter paper. As soon as the organic phase has finished filtering through, the paper is to be discarded immediately. Failure to do this results in impurity

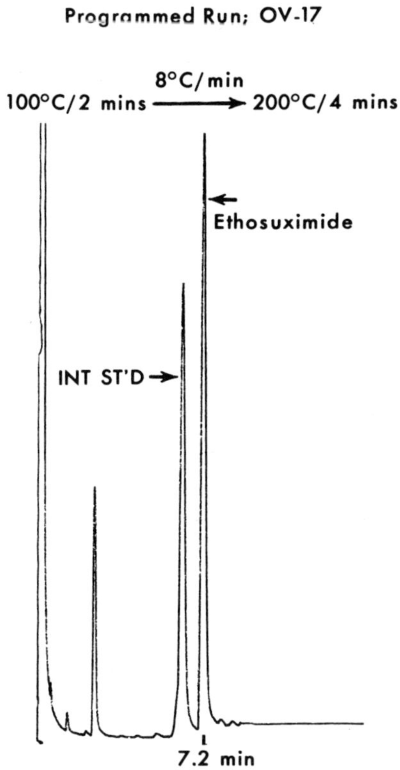

FIG. 2. Typical gas-liquid chromatographic recording of patient's plasma showing ethosuximide and a known concentration of the internal standard. Column packing: 3% OV-17, 80–100 mesh.

peaks in the chromatographic run. As ethosuximide is volatile at room temperature, care must be undertaken to ensure adequate recoveries of the drug from plasma. To accomplish this a few drops of isoamyl acetate are added to the chloroform extract to lower the vapor pressure of ethosuximide. Failure to do this can result in a loss of recovery of approximately 40%. The final crucial step involves the evaporation of chloroform. It is imperative that the samples are not evaporated to dryness. When this occurs accidentally recoveries of ethosuximide are poor, and in addition, a rather large impurity peak follows that of ethosuximide on the chromatographic recording. As a result the run must be allowed to proceed an additional 10 to 15 min before injection of the next sample. When these precautions are observed the assay is rapid, simple, and accurate (coefficient of variation, 1.21%).

In studies done in our laboratory, we found an excellent correlation ($r = 0.97$) between the gas-liquid chromatographic assay of ethosuximide, utilizing the XE-60 column as described above, and the concomitant determination of the drug by means of the EMIT® assay technique (Fig. 3). Eighty-seven patients were studied, with plasma levels ranging from 8 μg/ml to 114 μg/ml.

The cerebrospinal fluid resembles an ultrafiltrate of plasma and, hence, serves as an indicator of the degree of protein binding. We found a significant

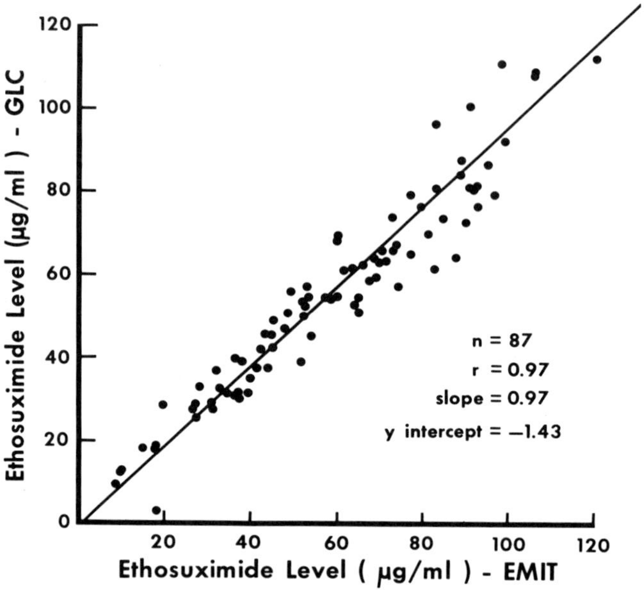

FIG. 3. Correlation between two techniques: Gas-liquid chromatography and the EMIT[R] assay, in the determination of simultaneous triplicate samples obtained from patients receiving ethosuximide for absence (petit mal) seizures. Approximately one-third of the patients were also receiving other anticonvulsants because of a past or present history of generalized tonic-clonic seizures.

correlation between total plasma and cerebrospinal fluid levels of ethosuximide (Fig. 4), with a CSF:plasma ratio of 1.01 ± 0.15 ($\pm$ SD) (9). Salivary levels of ethosuximide were also found to be equivalent to those of plasma (6). Measurements of ethosuximide concentration in saliva may be particularly useful as absence (petit mal) seizures are predominantly a disorder of children. The EMIT® technique can also be adapted to saliva, but standards must be prepared by diluting the drug in pooled saliva obtained from subjects not taking any drugs.

Numerous methods have been developed for monitoring ethosuximide levels in plasma. In view of the need for a rapid and reliable quantitative technique for chemical analysis, we have found the described procedures to be most suitable for routine clinical and research purposes.

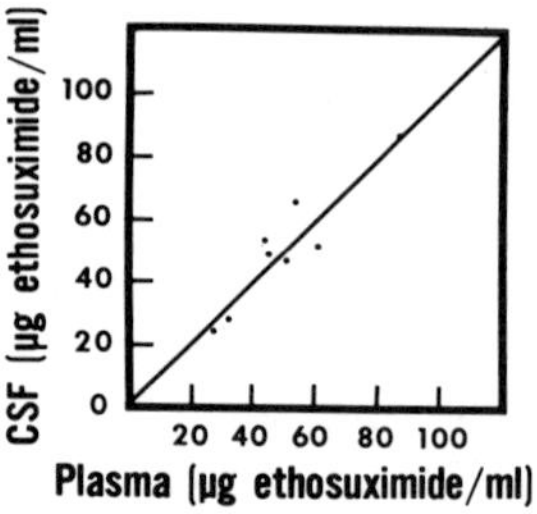

FIG. 4. Correlation between ethosuximide levels in cerebrospinal fluid (CSF) and plasma in 8 patients with epilepsy, obtained during the course of diagnostic lumbar puncture usually prior to pneumoencephalography ($r = 0.99$).

ACKNOWLEDGMENTS

This work was supported by a grant from the Medical Research Council of Canada.

The assistance of Rees Cosgrove in carrying out the comparison of the GLC technique with the EMIT® assay is greatly appreciated. Mrs. E. Cohen kindly reviewed and typed the manuscript.

REFERENCES

1. Browne, T. R., Dreifuss, F. E., Dyken, P. R., Goode, D. J., Penry, J. K., Porter, R. J., White, B. G., and White, P. T. (1974): Ethosuximide in the treatment of absence (petit mal) seizures. *Neurology* (Minneap.), 25:515–524.
2. Buchanan, R. A., Fernandez, L., and Kinkel, A. W. (1969): Absorption and elimination of ethosuximide in children. *J. Clin. Pharmacol.,* 9:393–398.
3. Dill, W. A., Peterson, L., Chang, T., and Glazko, A. J. (1965): Physiological disposition of α-methyl-α-ethylsuccinimide (Ethosuximide; Zarontin®) in animals and man. *Abst. of Papers, 149th Meeting Am. Chem. Soc., Detroit, Mich., April 5–9, 1965,* p. 30N.
4. Glazko, A. J., and Dill, W. A. (1972): Ethosuximide. Chemistry and methods for determination. In *Antiepileptic Drugs,* edited by D. M. Woodbury, J. K. Penry, and R. P. Schmidt, pp. 413–415. Raven Press, New York.
5. Hansen, S. E. (1963): Quantitative determination of ethosuximide (Zarontin®; α-methyl-α-ethylsuccinimide) in serum. *Acta. Pharmacol. Toxicol.* (Kbh.), 20:286–290.
6. McAuliffe, J. J., Sherwin, A. L., Leppik, I. E., Fayle, S. A., and Pippenger, C. E. (1977): Salivary levels of anticonvulsants: A practical approach to drug monitoring. *Neurology* (Minneap.), 27:409–413.
7. Meijer, J. W. A. (1971): Simultaneous quantitative determination of antiepileptic drugs, including carbamazepine, in body fluids. *Epilepsia* (Amst.), 12:341–352.
8. Reidel, E., Krüger, U., Bayer, H., and Horak, H. (1975): Comparison of methods for determination of drugs in serum and plasma. In *Clinical Pharmacology of Anti-Epileptic Drugs,* edited by H. Schneider, D. Janz, C. Gardner-Thorpe, H. Meinardi, and A. L. Sherwin, pp. 312–316. Springer-Verlag, New York.
9. Sherwin, A. L., Robb, J. P., and Lechter, M. (1973): Improved control of epilepsy by monitoring plasma ethosuximide. *Arch. Neurol.,* 28:178–181.
10. Solow, E. B., and Green, J. B. (1971): The determination of ethosuximide in serum by gas chromatography. Preliminary results of clinical application. *Clin. Chim. Acta.,* 33:87–90.
11. Van der Kleijn, E., Collste, P., Norlander, B., Agurell, S., and Sjoqvist, F. (1973): Gas chromatographic determination of ethosuximide and phensuximide in plasma and urine of man. *J. Pharm. Pharmacol.,* 25:324–327.
12. Vedso, S., Rud, C., and Place, J. F. (1969): Determination of phenytoin in serum in the presence of barbiturates, sulthiame and ethosuximide by thin layer chromatography. *Scand. J. Clin. Lab. Invest.,* 23:175–180.
13. Wechselberg, K., and Hubel, G. (1967): Zur Resoption and Verteilung von Methyl-Athyl-Succinimid (MAS) im Serum und Liquor bei Kindern. *Z. Kinderheilkd,* 100:10–19.
14. Zimmerman, F. T., and Burgemeister, B. B. (1958): A new drug for petit mal epilepsy. *Neurology* (Minneap.), 8:769–775.

Antiepileptic Drugs: Quantitative Analysis and Interpretation, edited by C. E. Pippenger, J. K. Penry, and H. Kutt, Raven Press, New York, © 1978.

Chapter 10
Homogeneous Immunoassay System (EMIT) for Quantitation of Antiepileptic Drugs in Biological Fluids

Dorothy D. Schottelius

The usefulness of serum levels of antiepileptic drugs to achieve adequate seizure control in the epileptic patient has been well documented (4,8,26). Several methods have been available for the determination of these drugs, which have utilized spectrophotometric and gas-liquid chromatographic (GLC) equipment for quantitation. This methodology has been reviewed by Rose et al. (15), Meijer et al. (11) and Schneider et al. (19). Determination of antiepileptic drugs by spectrophotometric and GLC methods involves extraction of the compounds from the serum prior to the quantitation—a process that is both time consuming and requires exacting techniques to provide reliable results. In addition, the latter methods require GLC equipment, which is expensive to purchase, maintain, and operate. There existed, therefore, a need for a procedure that would provide rapid, specific, and reliable results for the quantitation of these drugs. One procedure was developed that employed radioimmunoassay and is described elsewhere in this volume. Another method utilizes a homogeneous immunoassay system that has the advantages of radioimmunoassay without the use of radioactive compounds and the specialized training and equipment required for their analysis. A description of this procedure, its theory, practicality, reliability, and pitfalls in the analysis of phenytoin, primidone, phenobarbital, carbamazepine, and ethosuximide in serum and other biological fluids is the subject of this chapter.

IMMUNOASSAYS

In 1959 a new class of assays was used for the measurement of insulin (27) in serum that was based on the use of radiolabeled ligands. This methodological principle was enthusiastically accepted because of the inherent specificity and sensitivity of the technique and has been utilized for the quantitation of many compounds.

Immunoassays are all based on the same principle, that is, the competitive displacement of a labeled substance from an antibody complex by the unlabeled substance in the sample:

$$AB \cdot S^* + S \rightleftharpoons AB \cdot S + S^*$$

where

AB = antibody
S* = labeled substance
S = unlabeled substance in a sample

The amount of substance displaced is related in a simple but nonlinear fashion to the amount of unlabeled substance added. Although antibody specificity for the original substance is high, it must be emphasized that other substances of similar structure may also react so that any positive result from an immunological assay must be confirmed by a nonimmunological technique.

To obtain a curve with optimal sensitivity and accuracy, the antibody should (a) bind the labeled and unlabeled substance equally well, (b) have a binding constant for the substance that is large enough to favor complex formation, and (c) have a 1:1 ratio of binding sites to a labeled substance.

There are four common types of immunoassay systems, which differ in the manner in which the substance is labeled and in the method by which the displaced substance is measured and quantitated. These are radioimmunoassay (labeled with radioactive isotope and quantitated by scintillation counter), free-radical assay technique (labeled with stable free radical and quantitated by electron spin resonance spectrophotometry), enzyme multiplied immunoassay technique (labeled with an enzyme and quantitated by enzyme activity), and hemagglutination inhibition (labeled with red blood cell and observed by human eye). The first three assays yield quantitative results, whereas the last is utilized primarily in a semiquantitative fashion. The radioimmunoassay requires a separation step to remove the displaced labeled substance from the antibody-bound labeled substance prior to quantitation. The other two methods do not require this separation step.

A review by Sunshine (23) presents a more detailed discussion of these four immunological techniques used in the assay of drugs. Two other reviews concerning enzyme immunoassay have recently appeared (17,25).

HOMOGENEOUS ENZYME IMMUNOASSAY

In 1972 Rubenstein et al. (16) employed the homogeneous enzyme immunoassay for the detection of morphine by utilizing morphine antibodies coupled to a conjugate of morphine and lysozyme. This led to a group of assays for detection of drugs of abuse in urine (12) and then the development of the enzyme-mediated immunoassay technique (EMIT®, Syva Company, Palo Alto, Calif.) for the quantitation of the antiepileptic drugs phenytoin, phenobarbital, primidone, carbamazepine, and ethosuximide. The initial report comparing phenytoin and phenobarbital serum levels obtained by gas-liquid chromatography and EMIT was published in 1975 (13). Several laboratories, including the Department of Neurology at the University of Iowa, have been involved in the performance evaluations as the assays have been developed.

Principles of the Homogeneous Enzyme Assay

The term homogeneous enzyme assay is used to distinguish the method from most other immunochemical methods, which are heterogeneous and depend at some stage on the physical separation of antigen bound to antibody from the unbound antibody (2).

The principles involved in the assay system for the quantitation of antiepileptic drugs is presented schematically in Fig. 1. An enzyme (glucose-6-

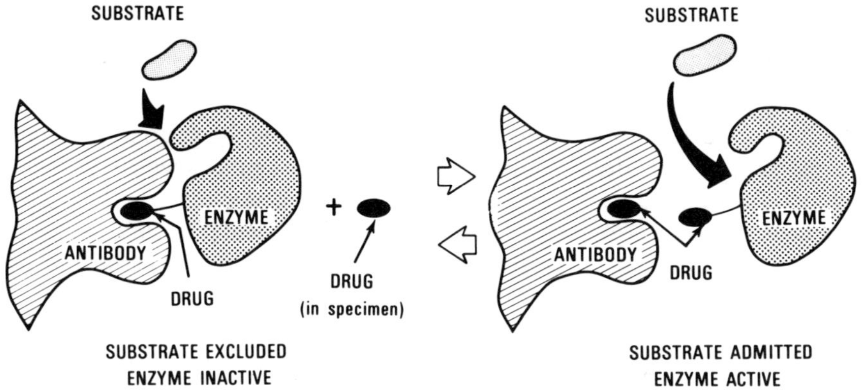

FIG. 1. Homogeneous enzyme immunoassay. Left side shows the antibody bound to the enzyme labeled with drug in a configuration that blocks active enzyme site. Right side illustrates drug in patients' serum bound to the antibody, thus preventing the binding of the drug-labeled enzyme and the enzyme is active.

phosphate dehydrogenase, 1.1.1.49) is conjugated to the drug to be assayed in such a fashion that it does not significantly alter its activity. However, when this drug-enzyme conjugate is bound to the antibody for the drug, the configuration is such that the active site of the enzyme is blocked and thus excludes the substrate and the enzyme activity is reduced. When the complex is not bound, the active site is available to interact with the substrate. If free drug is present in the unknown sample, this will bind to the antibody, thus preventing the binding of the drug-enzyme conjugate. This decreases the antibody-induced inactivation of the enzyme activity in proportion to the drug concentration in the sample.

Performance of an EMIT Assay

The unknown sample is mixed with a reagent that contains antibodies to the particular drug and the necessary enzyme substrate and coenzyme (glucose-6-phosphate and nicotinamide adenine dinucleotide). All drug antibodies have been produced by chemically coupling the drug to a macromolecular carrier and immunizing sheep with the resulting antigen. The second reagent, which contains the drug-enzyme complex, is then added with appropriate buffering. This labeled drug combines with any remaining unfilled antibody binding sites, thus reducing the enzyme activity in proportion to the unknown drug concentration. The unbound drug-enzyme reacts with the substrate and the coenzyme NAD is reduced. This reduction of NAD to NADH is measured spectrophotometrically at 340 nm. The coenzyme NAD utilized in the assay functions only with the glucose-6-phosphate dehydrogenase from bacteria (*Leuconostoc mesenteroides*) and thus is not influenced by the glucose-6-phosphate dehydrogenase activity that may be present in the sample.

Procedure

Our laboratory utilizes the following equipment for the routine determination of antiepileptic drugs: Gilford Stasar microsample spectrophotometer (Gilford Instruments, Oberlin, Ohio), a Syva pipetter-diluter (Syva, Palo Alto, Calif.), and a Tektronix 31 Programmable Calculator with instrument coupler (Tektronix Inc., Beaverton, Ore.). This instrumentation is used solely for the determination of antiepileptic drugs, and the assays are performed on a daily schedule by two technicians. The same individual performs the calibration and unknown assays on a daily basis. All measurements are made in duplicate and readings which differ by more than 4 Δ A units are repeated. Calibration curves are prepared daily for each drug and analyzed by a least-squares program provided on the EMIT antiepileptic drug program tape. Differences of more than 4 Δ A units are not accepted and the calibrator is repeated. Differences usually do not exceed 2 Δ A units. The EMIT antiepileptic drug control is determined immediately after the calibration curves are obtained and is repeated several times throughout the day. In our laboratory the calibration curve is repeated if the control value falls outside the following limits for the various drugs: phenytoin $\pm$0.5 μg/ml; phenobarbital $\pm$1.0 μg/ml; ethosuximide $\pm$3.0 μg/ml; primidone $\pm$0.5 μg/ml and carbamazepine $\pm$0.3 μg/ml. All reagents, samples, and materials are at room temperature prior to determinations. Adequate time has been allowed for the spectrophotometer to stabilize at the 340 nm wavelength setting and the thermal setting to equilibrate at 30°C. The calibrator control or unknown sample is diluted 1:6 Tris hydrochloride buffer pH 7.9 (Syva) utilizing the pipetter-diluter (50 μl of sample + 250 μl of buffer). This provides sufficient material to perform duplicate assays of two drugs; if the patient is taking more than two drugs, a second sample is added to the 2.0-ml disposable beaker. A second dilution is prepared (1:6 with buffer) and delivered into a second beaker. Fifty microliters of reagent A (antibody-substrate) plus 250 μl of buffer are added to the second beaker followed by 50 μl of reagent B (enzyme-labeled drug) + 250 μl of buffer. The sample is immediately aspirated into spectrophotometric flow cell. This automatically activates the timer sequence for a 15-sec delay period, and at this time, with the Tektronix system, an initial 0 reading is made; an absorbance reading is made every second for 30 sec; a linear regression for the change in absorbance is calculated and extrapolated to a measurement time of 80 sec. With the unknown sample the rate measurement, the $\Delta A - \Delta A_0$ and concentration are calculated and available on the tape printout after the instrument has been calibrated. The calibration set contains a zero calibrator and five different concentrations of antiepileptic drugs, which cover different ranges for the five assays. Unknown values that fall outside these ranges can be assayed by omitting the second dilution step in the procedure (samples below the range) or by making the appropriate dilution with blank serum or plasma (samples close to or over the highest calibrator). Appropriate directions for reconstituting reagents, procedures, stability, etc., can be found in each package insert obtained with the Syva reagents (1).

PRECISION AND SPECIFICITY OF ASSAYS FOR PHENYTOIN, PHENOBARBITAL, PRIMIDONE, CARBAMAZEPINE, AND ETHOSUXIMIDE

Precision

The within-day reproducibility has been determined for all five drugs in several laboratories by analyzing 20 replicate analyses of calibrator 3. This contains the following concentrations of drugs: phenytoin, 10.0 μg/ml; phenobarbital, 20.0 μg/ml; primidone, 10.0 μg/ml; carbamazepine, 5.0 μg/ml; and ethosuximide, 50.0 μg/ml. In our laboratory the following coefficients of variation have been obtained: phenytoin, 4.0%; phenobarbital, 5.0%; primidone, 5.0%; carbamazepine, 4.7%; and ethosuximide, 10.4%. Between-day precision values have been obtained in our laboratory by analyzing 25 values from the control GLC calbrator from Syva, which contains the following concentrations: phenytoin, 15.0 μg/ml; phenobarbital, 30.0 μg/ml; primidone, 12.0 μg/ml; carbamazepine, 6.0 μg/ml; and ethosuximide, 75.0 μg/ml. The following results have been obtained (mean ± standard error and coefficient of variation): phenytoin, 15.09 ± 0.15, 4.9%; phenobarbital, 29.5 ± 0.19, 3.2%; primidone, 11.9 ± 0.09, 3.9%; carbamazepine, 6.1 ± 0.06, 5.0%; ethosuximide, 73.3 ± 1.5, 5.5%. All of these values have been obtained utilizing the Tektronic programmable system with the exception of ethosuximide, which was analyzed on the semiautomatic system. Similar coefficients of variation have been obtained with repeated analysis of patient samples containing various quantities of the antiepileptic drugs. It is entirely possible to achieve coefficient of variation values of 3 to 5% both within day and between day with these reagents.

Specificity

The drugs that have been specifically tested for cross-reactivity and the results have been published by Syva (1) for phenytoin, phenobarbital, primidone, and carbamazepine. We have tested several clinical samples along with other laboratories and have not found any variance from these data. In addition ethosuximide has been evaluated in our laboratory and patient samples containing phenytoin, phenobarbital, primidone, clonazepam, and carbamazepine did not vary from the zero calibrator for ethosuximide.

Further work should be done on the cross-reactivities that may be present when very high levels of drugs are present, although we have not encountered any significant problems in this area in our laboratory. No interference in specificity or accuracy has been found with serum samples that were moderately hyperlipidemic or hyperbilirubinemic.

COMPARISON OF EMIT AND GAS-LIQUID CHROMATOGRAPHY ASSAYS OF ANTIEPILEPTIC DRUGS

It is necessary to confirm positive results from any immunological assay by a nonimmunological technique and for the antiepileptic drugs the preferred comparison has been between EMIT and GLC. Figure 2 presents data obtained both in our laboratory and others of such comparisons. In our laboratory we have compared the EMIT values to GLC values obtained using our modification (5) of Kupferberg's method for phenytoin, phenobarbital, and primidone. Carbamazepine was determined by a slight modification of Friel and Green's method (6) and by a modification of Kupferberg's method (7). Figure 2 illustrates results of this comparison obtained in our laboratory for phenytoin, primidone, phenobarbital, and combined results from our laboratory and two others for carbamazepine. These will be compared to other results published in the literature.

The following statistical abbreviations will be utilized: $\bar{x}$, mean; SD, standard deviation; SE, standard error; *a*, intercept of least-squares regression line; *b*, slope; *r*, correlation coefficient; and S*y*, standard error of estimate (24). All values are given in micrograms per milliliter.

Phenytoin

Forty-nine patient samples were compared by GLC and EMIT (utilizing saline reagents) and the regression line in Fig. 2 has an intercept of −0.34, slope 0.99, and $r = 0.95$. The S*y* was 2.7 μg/ml. The $\bar{x} \pm$ SE was as follows: GLC, 16.1 ± 0.42; EMIT, 15.7 ± 0.42. Combined data (109 samples) from two other laboratories utilizing similar techniques were as follows: $\bar{x}$, GLC = 15.49; EMIT = 14.65; $a = 0.26$, $b = 0.93$, $r = 0.985$, and S*y* = 1.89 μg/ml. Booker and Darcey (3) compared the original EMIT reagents and GLC for

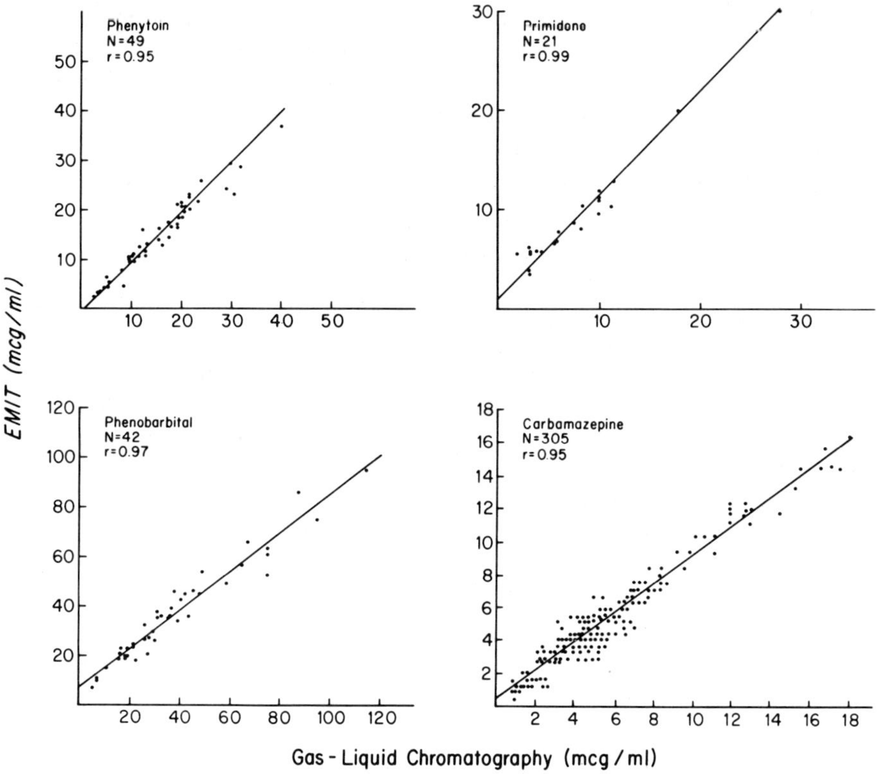

FIG. 2. EMIT versus GLC analyses of phenytoin, primidone, phenobarbital, and carbamazepine. Phenytoin: EMIT value = −0.34 + 0.994 GLC; Primidone: EMIT value = 1.07 + 1.03 GLC; Phenobarbital: EMIT value = 7.45 + 0.778 GLC; Carbamazepine: EMIT value = 0.42 + 0.90 GLC.

197 specimens containing phenytoin and obtained a regression line with an $r = 0.98$, $a = -0.90$, and $b = 1.09$, $Sy = 1.80$. Another study (9) with 90 patients has shown comparable values ($b = 0.97$, $r = 0.9$). Spiehler et al. (21) have published a comparative study on 60 phenytoin samples ($b = 0.786$, $a = 0.976$, $r = 0.957$, and $Sy = 2.04$). Schmidt (18) has compared 88 samples by both techniques: EMIT = 0.97 GLC + 0.35, $r = 0.982$.

A diversity of GLC techniques have been used in these comparisons, and several hundred samples have been compared utilizing the two techniques with good agreement.

Primidone

Twenty-one patient samples were compared in our laboratory by GLC and EMIT for this drug. The $\bar{x} \pm$ SE was as follows: GLC, 8.3 ± 0.52; EMIT, 9.6 ± 0.5. The least-squares values were $a = 1.06$, $b = 1.03$, $r = 0.99$, and

$Sy = 0.92$. Combined data from two other laboratories utilizing a similar GLC procedure gave the following statistics on 37 patients: GLC, $\bar{x} = 10.7$; EMIT, $\bar{x} = 10.4$; $a = 0.02$, $b = 0.971$, $r = 0.989$, and $Sy = 1.15$. Data have also been published an 94 patients (22) comparing GLC and EMIT ($a = 0.51$, $b = 0.97$, $r = 0.967$). Another correlation from 10 patients (9) indicated the following: GLC, $\bar{x} = 9.0$; EMIT, $\bar{x} = 8.5$; $b = 1.00$ and $r = 0.97$.

Phenobarbital

Our comparative results for 42 patients' serum analyzed for this drug were as follows: GLC, $\bar{x} \pm SE = 37.97 \pm 0.78$; EMIT, $\bar{x} \pm SE = 37.01 \pm 0.69$; $a = 7.4$, $b = 0.78$, $r = 0.97$, $Sy = 4.7$. Two other laboratories using similar procedures presented the following statistics on 81 patient samples: GLC, $\bar{x} = 29.61$; EMIT, $\bar{x} = 29.37$; $a = 2.53$, $b = 0.906$, $r = 0.981$, and $Sy = 3.86$. Published data included 197 patients, $a = 2.15$, $b = 0.79$, $r = 0.97$, $Sy = 3.8$ (3); 45 patients, GLC, $\bar{x} = 22.6$; EMIT, $\bar{x} = 22.4$; $b = 0.87$, $r = 0.97$ (9); 32 patients, $a = 0.797$, $b = 0.901$, $r = 0.917$, $Sy = 4.65$ (21). Schmidt (18) has evaluated 28 samples with the following correlation analysis: GLC = 1.16 EMIT + −2.9, $r = 0.983$.

These data indicate larger errors than any of the other comparisons and may reflect the difficulties encountered when analyzing this drug by GLC procedures.

Carbamazepine

The data for this drug were combined from three laboratories and the GLC procedures utilized were not identical (14). The data were analyzed for 305 patient samples with the following statistics: GLC, $\bar{x} = 5.37$; EMIT, $\bar{x} = 5.27$; $a = 0.42$, $b = 0.90$, $r = 0.95$, $Sy = 0.95$. No interference was found in these samples for other anticonvulsant drugs, no false positives were found, and no cross-reactivity was found with various psychotropic drugs.

Ethosuximide

Correlations of GLC and EMIT values have been done on 265 patients (20; Chapter 9, Fig. 3) with the following statistics: GLC, $\bar{x} = 52.3$; EMIT, $\bar{x} = 53.0$; $a = 1.41$, $b = 0.99$, $r = 0.945$, $Sy = 9.32$. The specificity of this assay is equivalent to the others, with no cross-reactivity found with phenytoin, primidone, phenobarbital, clonozepam, or carbamazepine.

Difficulty will be encountered in the determination of samples where the ethosuximide concentration is above 50μg/ml. Currently the enzyme system is loaded to yield $\Delta A - \Delta A_0$ of approximately 0.5 per μg/ml concentration above this concentration. This compares to $\Delta A - \Delta A_0$ of 2 per μg/ml concentration in the 10- to 25-μg/ml concentration range. It will be necessary to dilute samples that have a concentration above 50 μg/ml to achieve a more accurate value. Care must be taken with these dilution procedures to avoid errors.

ANTIEPILEPTIC DRUG QUALITY CONTROL SAMPLES DETERMINED BY EMIT ANALYSIS

We have determined varying numbers of the samples distributed by the Epilepsy Foundation of America Quality Control Program using the EMIT procedure employed daily in our laboratory for clinical samples. The results are presented in Fig. 3. The following statistical data were obtained from the linear regression: phenytoin, AED-QC value = − 0.28 + 0.96 UI value, $r =$ 0.998; primidone, AED-QC value = −0.12 + 0.97 UI value, $r = 0.993$; phenobarbital, AED-QC value = −0.20 + 0.98 UI value, $r = 0.989$; and carbamazepine, AED Q-C value = 0.04 + 0.97 UI value, $r = 0.993$. The

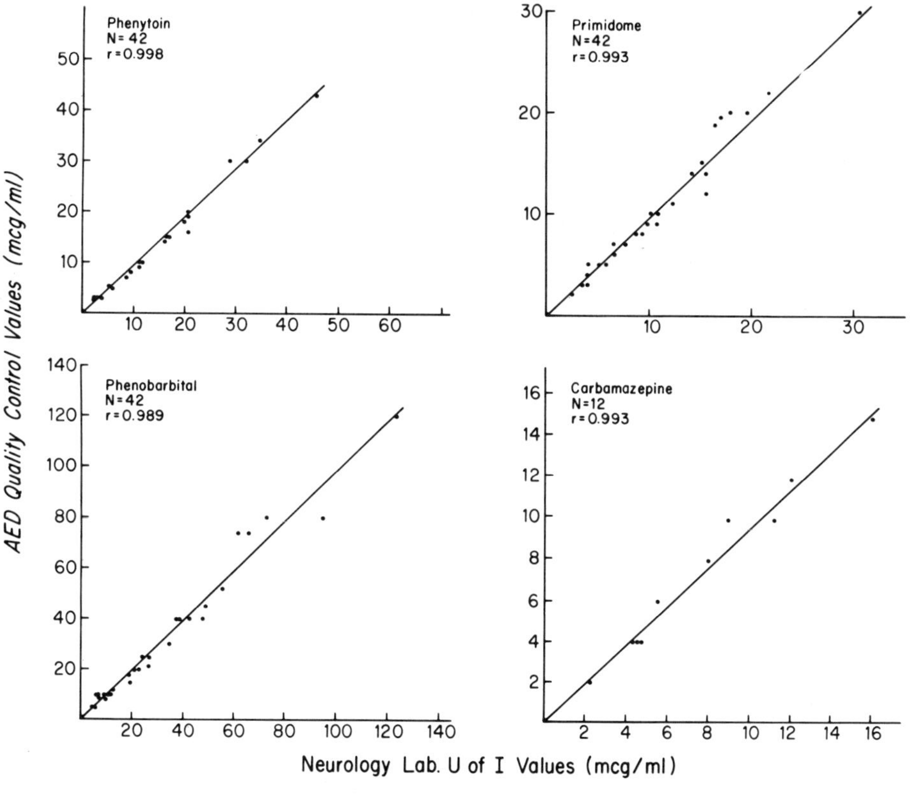

FIG. 3. Comparison of antiepileptic drug Quality Control (AED-QC) samples and Neurology Laboratory University of Iowa (UI). Phenytoin: AED-QC = −0.28 + 0.96 UI value; primidone: AED-QC = −0.12 + 0.97 UI value; phenobarbital: AED-QC = −0.20 + 0.98 UI value; carbamazepine: AED-QC = 0.04 + 0.97 UI value.

accuracy and reliability of this procedure based on the Quality Control Program appears satisfactory.

COMPARATIVE ANALYSIS OF OTHER BODY FLUIDS BY EMIT AND GLC

Saliva

A comparative analysis of salivary drug levels measured by EMIT and GLC has been published by McAuliffe et al. (10) and indicates a good correlation of the two methods (phenytoin: $N = 19$, EMIT $\bar{x} = 1.2$, GLC $\bar{x} = 1.3$, $r = 0.96$; phenobarbital: N = 20, EMIT $\bar{x} = 8.7$, GLC $\bar{x} = 6.8$, $r = 0.87$; and primidone: N = 10, EMIT $\bar{x} = 6.9$, GLC $\bar{x} = 6.1$, $r = 0.90$. Further work is in progress to verify the usefulness of this procedure in the assay of antiepileptic drugs in saliva.

Cerebrospinal Fluid

We have compared the values obtained in cerebrospinal fluid from patients in whom a lumbar puncture was required as part of their neurological examination and who were taking antiepileptic drugs. These results are presented in Table 1. The small sample necessary for the determination of antiepileptic drug concentrations by the EMIT procedure allows the quantitation of all three of these drugs with less than 0.5 ml of cerebrospinal fluid.

Comparative values for carbamazepine and ethosuximide are not available, but the same correlation of these two methods may be anticipated.

TABLE 1. *Cerebrospinal fluid antiepileptic drug values by EMIT and GLC methods (μg/ml)*

Drug	N		x ± SE	a	b	Sy	r
Phenytoin	20	GLC	1.5 ± 0.3	0.345	1.11	0.27	0.99
		EMIT	2.0 ± 0.3				
Primidone	6	GLC	8.2 ± 1.0	0.90	0.91	1.19	0.98
		EMIT	8.4 ± 1.0				
Phenobarbital	13	GLC	15.5 ± 1.0	1.20	0.94	2.56	0.98
		EMIT	15.9 ± 1.0				

x, mean, SE, standard error; *N*, number of patients; *a*, intercept; *b*, slope; Sy, standard error of estimate, *r*, correlation coefficient.

ADVANTAGES AND DISADVANTAGES OF THE EMIT SYSTEM

Advantages

Microsamples: It is possible to assay five drugs from one 50-μl serum sample provided that duplicates are not done or from 100 μl of serum if duplicates are done. We have compared the results for venous (VP) and capillary drug (FS) concentration utilizing the EMIT procedure with the following results $\bar{x} \pm$ SE: phenytoin, VP $= 10.0 \pm 0.65$, FS $= 9.7 \pm 0.65$; phenobarbital, VP $= 24.5 \pm 1.0$, FS $= 25.1 \pm 1.0$; primidone, VP $= 12.0 \pm 0.45$, FS $= 11.6 \pm 0.67$. Therefore, reliable results can be obtained in the pediatric age group utilizing heel or fingerprick procedures. The sample necessary for this system permits the determination of antiepileptic drugs in other biological fluids such as saliva and cerebrospinal fluid.

Speed: Determination of a single drug in a patient sample requires about 8 min from serum to delivered result. These are times required in our laboratory utilizing a Tektronix programmable calculator and doing all determinations in duplicate. The daily calibration curve requires 30 min per drug. Utilizing this system, two technicians have processed 40 patient samples involving 100 drug assays in an 8-hr day. One technician performs all the calibrations and assays during the day whereas the other processes the samples, types the results, and maintains the record-keeping procedures. It would be possible with this system to process 700 to 800 patient samples in a 20-day month with as many as 2,000 drug determinations. Results on emergency samples are available to the physician approximately 10 min after a blood sample is received in our laboratory.

This system allows us to have antiepileptic drug levels available to the physician when he examines an epileptic patient in our outpatient clinic, and he is able to discuss with the patient necessary therapeutic adjustments.

Performance and accuracy: The accuracy of this system has been amply verified by comparison to GLC determination for five drugs—phenytoin, phenobarbital, primidone, carbamazepine and ethosuximide. The reagents used are nonradioactive; therefore, the precautions and equipment necessary for radioimmunoassay are not required. No significant cross-reactivity had been demonstrated in these determinations with a wide variety of drugs. The procedure does demand careful attention to detail, and best results are achieved by well-trained and supervised technicians in a dedicated laboratory. Since no extraction is required prior to analyzing the drugs, there is less of a problem with recovery of the drugs and more consistent values are obtained.

Disadvantages

High or low drug concentrations: the procedure is designed to cover a specified range with the reagents, and patient samples that fall outside of this range must be diluted (high) or redetermined without dilution (low) to obtain a value. In most cases this was unnecessary for determination by GLC procedures. To achieve the best accuracy one must examine the curves for the various drugs to decide the upper limit of concentration before making a dilution, and this should be based on the $\Delta A - \Delta A_0$ differences per μg/ml concentration. The carbamazepine curve provides a good difference even in the upper range with approximately 6 $\Delta A - \Delta A_0$ per μg/ml in the 5- to 10-μg/ml range. The primidone curve is also quite good, with 4 units of difference per μg/ml concentration in the 15- to 20-μg/ml concentration range. The phenytoin presents some difficulties in the 20- to 30-μg/ml range, with only 1.6 difference per μg/ml, and dilution is recommended for samples above 25 μg/ml. The phenobarbital curve presents problems above 35 to 40 μg/ml with a 0.75 difference between 40 to 80 μg/ml and dilutions should be done. The ethosuximide curve presents the most problems; the differences are 0.5 to 0.6 in the 50- to 150-μg/ml range. It would be preferable, therefore, to make appropriate dilutions whenever there is less than a difference of 2 in the $\Delta A - \Delta A_0$ per μg/ml concentration.

Equipment requirements: In order to have a laboratory capable of quantitation of all antiepileptic drugs, it is necessary to have GLC capabilities, so the EMIT system could be considered as a duplication of equipment. The equipment is relatively expensive, as are the reagents. With the EMIT system it is necessary to determine the drugs individually, whereas it is possible to obtain quantitation of several of the antiepileptic drugs with one GLC determination.

Interfering substances: Any compound present in the serum that significantly increases the optical density above the A_0 value of the zero calibrator will influence the determination of the antiepileptic drugs. Therefore excess lipidemia, bilirubinemia, or hemoglobin will result in erroneous values, and these types of samples must be analyzed by GLC.

SUMMARY

The homogenous enzyme immunoassay combines the simplicity and convenience of enzyme measurements with the sensitivity, specificity, and reproducibility of immunoassay for five of the most widely used antiepileptic drugs. It has provided a reliable method for their quantitation utilizing small samples and with rapid availability of the results. Correlation with a variety of GLC techniques and this system has been very satisfactory, therefore, little doubt remains concerning the clinical usefulness of this technique. It has not and should not replace gas-liquid chromatography or GLC-mass spectrophotometric techniques, but provides an additional valuable tool for the routine determination of phenytoin, phenobarbital, primidone, carbamazepine, and ethosuximide.

ACKNOWLEDGMENT

The author gratefully acknowledges the cooperation of Syva for providing reagents used in some of the studies reported and for providing data obtained in comparative studies.

REFERENCES

1. Antiepileptic Drug Assays (1976): Syva Bulletin 6A164–1, Syva, Palo Alto, Calif.
2. Bastiani, R. J., Phillips, R. C., Schneider, R. S. and Ullman, E. F. (1973): Homogeneous immunochemical drug assay. *Am J. Med. Tech.*, 39:211–216.
3. Booker, H. E., and Darcey, B. A. (1975): Enzymatic immunoassay vs. gas-liquid chromatography for determination of phenobarbital and diphenylhydantoin in serum. *Clin. Chem.*, 21:1766–1768.
4. Eadie, M. J., and Tyrer, J. H. (1974): *Anticonvulsant Therapy.* Churchill Livingstone, Edinburg and London.
5. Fincham, R. W., Schottelius, D. D., and Sahs, A. L. (1974): The influence of diphenylhydantoin on primidone metabolism. *Arch. Neurol.*, 30:259–262.
6. Friel, P., and Green, J. R. (1973): Quantitative assay for carbamazepine serum levels by gas-liquid chromatography. *Clin. Chim. Acta,* 43:69–72.
7. Kupferberg, H. J. (1970): Quantitative estimation of diphenylhydantoin, primidone and phenobarbital in plasma by gas-liquid chromatography. *Clin. Chim. Acta,* 29:283–288.
8. Kutt, H., and Penry, J. K. (1974): Usefulness of blood levels of antiepileptic drugs. *Arch. Neurol.*, 31:283–288.
9. Legaz, M., and Raisys, V. A. (1976): Correlation of the "EMIT" antiepileptic drug assay with a gas-liquid chromatographic method. *Clin. Biochem.*, 9:35–38.
10. McAuliffe, J. J., Sherwin, A. L., Leppick, I. E., Fayle, S. A., and Pippenger, C. E. (1977): Salivary levels of anticonvulsants: A practical approach to drug monitoring. *Neurology* (Minneap.) 27:409–413.
11. Meijer, J. W. A., Meinardi, H., Gardner-Thorpe, C., van der Kleijn, E., editors (1973): *Methods of Analysis of Anti-epileptic Drugs.* Excerpta Medica, Amsterdam.
12. Mule, S. J., Sunshine, I., Bruade, M., and Willette, R. E., editors (1974): *Immunoassays for Drugs Subject to Abuse.* CRC Press, Cleveland.
13. Pippenger, C. E., Bastiani, R. J., and Schneider, R. S. (1975): Evaluation of an experimental homogeneous enzyme immunoassay for the quantitation of phenytoin and phenobarbitone in serum or plasma. In *Clinical Pharmacology of Anti-epileptic Drugs,* edited by H. Schneider, D. Janz, C. Gardner-Thorpe, H. Meinardi, and A. L. Sherwin, pp. 331–335. Springer-Verlag, New York, Heidelberg, Berlin.
14. Pippenger, C. E., Kutt, H., and Schottelius, D. D. (1976): EMIT carbamazepine assay, clinical evaluation. (*unpublished data.*)
15. Rose, S. W., Smith, L. D., and Penry, J. K. (1971): Blood level determinations of antiepileptic drugs. Clinical value and methods. National Institutes of Health, Bethesda, Md.
16. Rubenstein, K. E., Schneider, R. S., and Ullman, E. F. (1972): "Homogeneous" enzyme immunoassay. A new immunochemical technique. *Biochem. Biophys. Res. Commun.*, 47:846–851.
17. Scharpe, S. L., Cooreman, W. M., Bloome, W. J., and Laekeman, G. M., (1976): Quantitative enzyme immunoassay: Current status. *Clin. Chem.*, 22:733–738.
18. Schmidt, D. (1976): Measurement of diphenylhydantoin and phenobarbital by enzyme immunoassay and gas-liquid chromatography. *J. Neurol.*, 213:41–6.
19. Schneider, H., Janz, D., Gardner-Thorpe, C., Meinardi, H., and Sherwin, A. L., editors (1975): *Clinical Pharmacology of Anti-epileptic Drugs.* Springer-Verlag, New York, Heidelberg, and Berlin.
20. Sherwin, A. L., Pippenger, C. E., and Kutt, H. (1976): EMIT ethosuximide assay, clinical evaluation. (*Unpublished data*).
21. Spiehler, V., Sun, L., Miyada, D. S., Sarandis, S. G., Walwick, E. R., Klein, M. W., Jordan, D. B., and Jessen, B. (1976): Radioimmunoassay, enzyme immunoassay, spectrophotometry and gas-liquid chromatography compared for determination of phenobarbital and diphenylhydantoin. *Clin. Chem.*, 22:749–753.
22. Sun, L., and Walwick, E. R. (1976): Primidone analyses: Correlation of gas-chromatographic assay with enzyme immunoassay. *Clin. Chem.*, 22:901–902.

23. Sunshine, I. (1974): Immunoassay of drugs. Ciba Foundation Symposium #26, pp. 193–200.
24. Westgard, J. O., and Hunt, M. R. (1973): Use and interpretation of common statistical tests in method-comparison studies. *Clin. Chem.,* 19:49–57.
25. Wisdom, G. B. (1976): Enzyme immunoassay. *Clin. Chem.,* 22:1243–1255.
26. Woodbury, D. M., Penry, J. K., Schmidt, R. P., editors (1972): *Antiepileptic Drugs.* Raven Press, New York.
27. Yalow, P., and Berson, S. (1959): Assay of plasma insulin in human subjects by immunological methods. *Nature,* 184:1648–1649.

SPECIAL ANALYTICAL TECHNIQUES

Antiepileptic Drugs: Quantitative Analysis and Interpretation, edited by C. E. Pippenger, J. K. Penry, and H. Kutt, Raven Press, New York, © 1978.

Chapter 11
Electron Capture-GLC in the Quantitation of 1,4-Benzodiazepines

J. Arthur F. de Silva

The electron capture (EC) detector is one of the most sensitive gas chromatographic detectors in current use (2,18). It has an added advantage of having a higher degree of specificity than other ionization detectors, because only compounds having electron-capturing functional groups, or "electrophores," respond to it. The EC detector is capable of measuring 10^{-12}-g (picogram) amounts of organic compounds that are highly electron capturing. The EC detectors in current use have many types of configurations or geometry and employ either ^{63}Ni (10 to 15 mCi), titanium tritide (tritium $^{3}H_1$), or scandium tritide (200 to 250 mCi) as the β-ionization source to produce thermal "free" electrons by ionization of the carrier gas.

The EC detector is the brainchild of James Lovelock, who designed the first working unit called the "agron ionization detector" (11). It used argon as the carrier gas and a 10-mCi source of ^{90}Sr as the β-ionization source. The principle of its operation was refined and led to its use in functional group analysis of organic molecules separated by gas-liquid chromatography (GLC) by what was termed by Lovelock and Lipsky (13) as "electron affinity spectroscopy," the foundation of modern EC detection.

CHARACTERISTICS OF EC DETECTORS

The early EC detectors were of plane-parallel geometry, since the anode (collector) and the cathode (β-ionization source) were housed in a cell parallel to each other (Fig. 1). The cell was operated in the direct current (DC) mode and used nitrogen as the carrier gas, because it was very pure and inert, and could be ionized readily (13). The cell had a fairly large "dead volume," was difficult to manufacture, and exhibited certain undesirable operational features.

In practice, the carrier gas is charged by an applied (DC) polarization potential sufficient to collect all the "thermal" electrons liberated from the gas by the β-ionizing radiation. The resulting current flow between the anode and cathode (β-ionization source) is called the background or standing current of

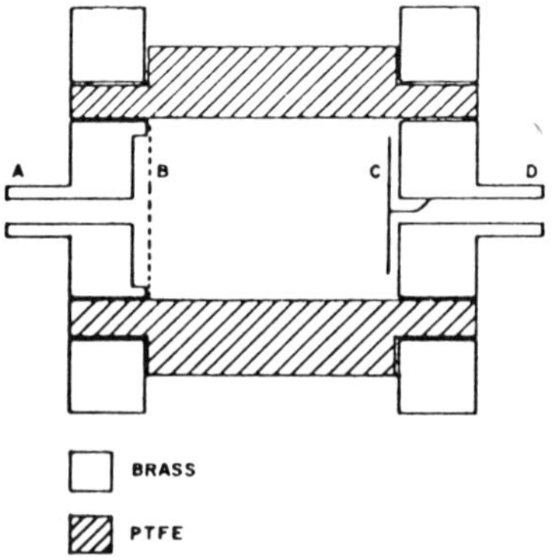

FIG. 1. Plane-parallel design of electron capture detector. A, inlet for carrier gas and anode; B, diffuser made of 100-mesh brass gauge; C, source of ionizing radiation; D, gas outlet and cathode. (Courtesy American Chemical Society.)

the detector. When an electron-capturing species enters the detector, it will absorb (capture) a portion of the electrons (depending on its EC coefficient), which results in a decrease in the standing current proportional to the concentration of the absorbing species. This follows a Beer-Lambert law relationship, but over a narrow range of concentration. The negative signal is electronically presented as a "positive" peak in the chromatogram.

The parallel-plate detector operated in the DC mode, and using N_2 as the carrier gas, manifested certain undesirable effects, chiefly contact potentials (due to the buildup of static electricity) and space charge effects, which gave erratic peak response and poor reproducibility. These effects were overcome

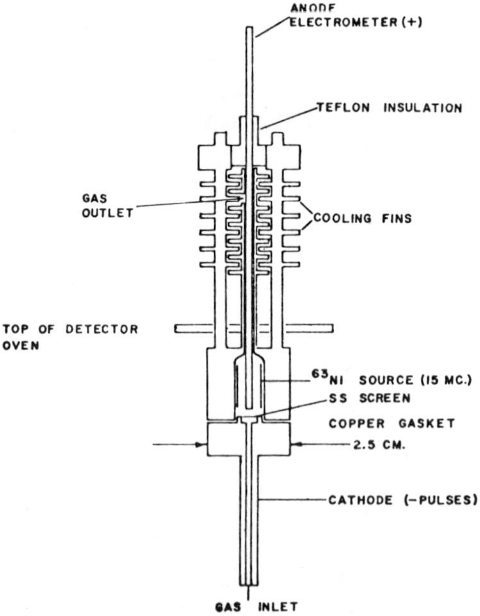

FIG. 2. Pin cup design of electron capture detector. (Courtesy American Chemical Society.)

by using pulse sampling techniques, where the applied DC voltage (30 to 90 V) was pulsed at an optimal pulse rate (150 to 300 μsec) and pulse width ranging from 0.5 to 4 μsec (12).

This modification resulted in improved sensitivity and linearity over a wider dynamic range (3,4). The early EC detectors developed between 1960 and 1965 using a tritium ($^3H_1$) occluded in titanium (as titanium tritide) had source strengths of 100 to 250 mCi but suffered an upper temperature limit of 225°C, above which hazardous amounts of tritium ($^3H_1$) were volatilized off the foil into the carrier gas. These detectors had to be cleaned out frequently and were very easily "poisoned" as a result of column effluent condensing on the foil, which limited the usable upper range of column temperature. The need for high-temperature detectors had long been established; the search for a suitable source led to the selection of ^{63}Ni, a soft β-emitter with an upper temperature limit of 400°C.

The first commercial ^{63}Ni EC detector was the pin cup type (Fig. 2) developed by Yauger et al. (29), which has led the way to significant improvements in commercial EC detectors. Four EC detector geometries were developed, using either titanium or scandium tritide (6) or ^{63}Ni as the β-source:

1. Plane parallel plate design—Lovelock and Lipsky (13)
2. Concentric tube design—Varian Instruments (28)
3. Pin cup design—Yauger et al. (29)
4. Concentric cup design—Tractor Instruments, Inc. (23)

The use of ^{63}Ni is now considered an optimum source material for the following reasons:

1. It is a β-emitter with no other radioactive emission associated with its decay.
2. The β-energy is low (0.06 meV), hence it has a high safety factor.
3. The radionuclide is a metal of high melting point and can be electroplated uniformly onto a stainless steel or gold foil backing, which is also chemically stable for cleaning.
4. The half-life is very long (about 85 years).
5. The detector can be operated at high temperatures (300 to 350°C), permitting the use of high column temperatures, and is not as susceptible to "poisoning" as a result of column effluent condensates.
6. It is easily cleaned by raising the detector temperature to 400°C, which pyrolyzes any condensates off the foil.

INFLUENCE OF OPERATING VARIABLES ON EC DETECTOR PERFORMANCE

Temperature

Since the capture mechanisms are temperature sensitive, their kinetics are significantly influenced by temperature changes. The phenomenon is attributed to change in the density of the carrier gas with temperature, since thermal electrons are collected more easily at higher temperatures because of fewer collisions with gas molecules (26,30).

Detector Noise

The background electrical noise results from the statistical nature of radioactive emissions, i.e., the type of particle emitted (α-, β-, or γ-rays) and its energy (meV). For a given type of particle, the noise is a function of the source activity assuming that detector standing current is proportional to the radioactivity of the source. In practice, the detector noise can be effectively filtered out by electronic circuitry.

Variation of Response with Carrier Gas Flow

Detector response is maximal at an optimal flow rate of the column for a given compound or series of related compounds, since the response depends on concentration and not on *mass* flow rate. However, the other operational parameters of the detector play an even more significant part in performance than flow rate alone. The mathematical relationships of the effect of the above operating variables on EC detector performance have been presented by Devaux and Guiochon (3,4).

Carrier Gas

Nitrogen is used in the DC mode and also more recently in the newer "linearized" EC detectors, which are operated in the constant-current, frequency-modulated mode. Argon-methane (90:10 or 95:5) is preferred for operation in tne pulsed (DC) constant-frequency or constant-current modes. The gas must be of prepurified grade (Matheson or Linde), the carrier gas and scavenger flow rates must be adjusted for optimum response, and the entire system must be kept *scrupulously clean.* Traces of moisture or oil in the gas lines must be removed by "scrubbing" the gas through a Linde molecular sieve before it enters the instrument, and the samples for analysis should be introduced in anhydrous solvent systems.

Column bleed is a severe limitation on detector performance, since even a small bleed rate can seriously "poison" the detector. Columns containing the silicone phases OV-1, OV-17, OV-225, QF-1, XE-60, properly conditioned using "no flow" conditions and operated at 50°C below their bleed limits, would ensure minimization of column bleed (22).

ELECTRON CAPTURE MECHANISMS

Many mechanisms have been postulated from Lovelock's original reports (11,12). Recently, Wentworth and Chen (26) summarized the various mechanisms of electron attachment to molecules. The EC detector was used in the pulsed (DC) mode, because the mathematical analysis of the kinetic model was greatly simplified; also, optimal EC response and sensitivity can be elicited in this operational mode (27).

The kinetic model represents four possible mechanisms summarized as follows:

$$\beta^- + \mathrm{Ar} + \mathrm{CH_4} \xrightarrow{kpR_\beta} e^- + \mathrm{P}\oplus\mathrm{R}\cdot + \beta^*$$

$$e^- + \mathrm{AB} \underset{k_2}{\overset{k_1}{\rightleftharpoons}} [\mathrm{AB}]^- \qquad \text{(Nondissociative)} \qquad \text{(I)}$$

$$e^- + \mathrm{AB} \xrightarrow{k_{12}} A\cdot + \mathrm{B}^- \qquad \text{(Dissociative)} \qquad \text{(II)}$$

$$[\mathrm{AB}]^- \xrightarrow{k_2} \mathrm{A}\cdot + \mathrm{B}^- \qquad \text{(Dissociative)} \qquad \text{(III)}$$

or

$$\searrow \mathrm{A}^- + \mathrm{B}\cdot \qquad \text{(Dissociative)} \qquad \text{(IV)}$$

Thus, ionization of the carrier gas argon-methane (90:10) due to the emission of high-energy electrons from the β-source produces "free" thermal electrons, positively charged species, and free radicals from the ionized gas.

1. Initial electron-methane collisions under free field conditions reduce the electron energy to thermal distribution from a higher energy level when initially emitted.
2. Initial electron attachment may occur nondissociatively (mechanism I) to produce a negatively charged molecular ion. This phenomenon was recently demonstrated using negative ion mass chromatography (9,10).
3. Electron attachment may cause dissociation in a single step to produce a radical and negative ion (mechanism II). This mechanism was identified using plasma chromatography of polychlorinated biphenyls (10).
4. Further dissociative electron attachment may also occur according to mechanisms III and IV.

According to these schemes, simple aromatics, polycyclic aromatics, carbonyl, halogen, amide, nitrile, nitroso, and nitro group-containing compounds have shown nondissociative electron attachment according to mechanism I.

Aliphatic Cl, Br, and I compounds undergo electron attachment by mechanism II and the corresponding aromatic compounds by mechanism III or IV, which are not distinguishable.

An approximation of electron capture response factors for highly electrophilic compounds such as perfluoro derivatives based on their electron capture coefficients was recently reported by Sullivan (20).

MODERN EC DETECTORS

The present generation of EC detectors are operated either in the pulsed (DC) mode, where the polarization voltage (DC) is applied as pulses of a fixed amplitude and variable pulse rate and pulse width (pulsed constant frequency mode), each of which can be adjusted to optimize the detector response for the type of compound being analyzed (5,7,23), or in the linearized pulsed, constant-current, frequency-modulated mode (14,24). This is in contrast to the continuous voltage DC mode, where the polarization voltage was applied at a peak or plateau value at a constant flow rate and detector temperature (3,4,23,29). The DC mode of operation was limited in its sensitivity and linearity because of high background "noise" and space charge effects formed near the radioactive source, which decreased the effective electrical field and opposed electron collection. It was also susceptible to quenching, or detector saturation effects from sample overloading.

The ^{63}Ni EC detectors are operated at high temperature ($>$300°C) and, irrespective of source geometry (plane parallel, pin cup, concentric tube, or cylindrical cup), are operated optimally in the pulsed (DC) mode, using argon-methane (90:10 or 95:5) as the carrier gas.

An EC detector of current design (1969) that provides all-round excellent performance is that manufactured by Tracor Instruments (Austin, Tex.), which is fitted to their Micro Tek series of GLC instruments. A sectional view of this detector is shown in Fig. 3. It will be noted that its geometry is neither plane parallel nor pin cup, but a hybrid that possesses some of the best features of each. Its geometry is best described as a concentric cylindrical cup,

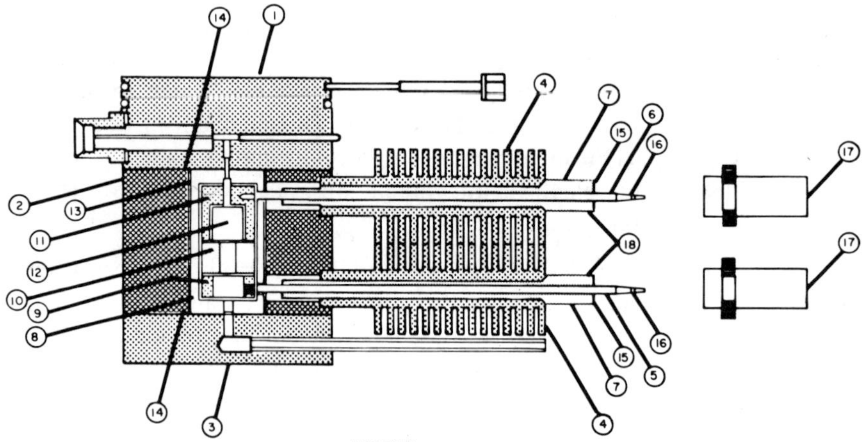

LEGEND

1 TOP BISCUIT - 439360
2 CELL BODY - 430360
3 BOTTOM BISCUIT - 430361
4 ELECTRODE TUBE - 430367
5 ANODE CONNECTOR ROD - 430365
6 CATHODE CONNECTOR ROD - 430366
7 ELECTRODE TUBE INSULATOR - 430371
8 ANODE INSULATOR - 430369
9 ANODE - 430364
10 WINDOW - 430370
11 CATHODE - 430363
12 NICKEL 63 SOURCE
13 CATHODE INSULATOR - 430368
14 RING SEAL - 430362
15 "O" RING - .093 I.D. X .218 O.D. X .062 THK.
16 AMPHENOL ELECTRODE CONNECTOR
17 AMPHENOL CONNECTOR
18 "O" RING - .187 I.D. X .312 O.D. X .062 THK.

FIG. 3. Cross-section of concentric cup design of high temperature ^{63}Ni electron capture detector. (Courtesy Tracor Instruments, Inc., Austin, Texas.)

since both the foil (cathode) and collector (anode) are cylindrical cups positioned in a concentric geometry of low dead volume. Many of the design features of this detector, summarized below, are not particularly unique by themselves, but together they provide the proper combination of features for excellent performance:

1. A high-temperature radionuclide (^{63}Ni) of high specific activity (15mCi), which is a soft β-emitter, is used.
2. The high operational temperature (>330°C) keeps the foil clean and free of contamination, since it can be "baked" out at 400°C for cleaning purposes.
3. Boron nitride is used as the insulator, which ensures proper electrical isolation, especially at high temperatures.
4. A pulsed (DC) voltage is used, which maximizes the time of encounter between an electron and a capturing molecule.
5. Asymmetric design (geometry) circumvents the normal space charge problems associated with DC operation.
6. The path length from anode to cathode has been maximized to increase the time of encounter between electrons and capturing molecules even longer.
7. The geometry and path length of the detector ensure a more uniform mean free energy of the electron, hence a more reproducible response and low background noise level.
8. The detector is leak tight and unaffected by small changes in carrier gas flow rate.
9. The detector is operated in conjunction with a power supply in the nonlinearized version, which gives the operator the capability of varying (a) applied polarization (DC) voltage amplitude from 0 to 90 V, (b) operation in either DC or pulsed DC codes, (c) variable pulse rate control, and (d) variable pulse width control.

Standard performance data for this detector as published by the manufacturer (23) were determined in the normal DC and pulsed DC modes on two new detectors equivalent with respect to the ^{63}Ni source strengths and standing (background) current obtained with pure carrier gas. The test compound was the insecticide lindane (benzene hexachloride), a strong electron-capturing compound, which was chromatographed on a 6-ft × ¼-in. borosilicate glass column containing 3% SE-30 coated on Chromosorb WHP (100-120 mesh) operated at 180°C, the detector temperature was 286°C, and the flash heater was at 227°C. The carrier gas used in the DC mode was nitrogen at a column flow rate of 60 ml/min and a purge flow of 20 ml/min, whereas argon-methane (90:10) was the carrier gas in the pulsed (DC) mode at a total flow rate of 76 ml/min. Performance curves of the detector operated in the DC mode and in the pulsed (DC) mode are shown in Figs. 4A and 4B respectively.

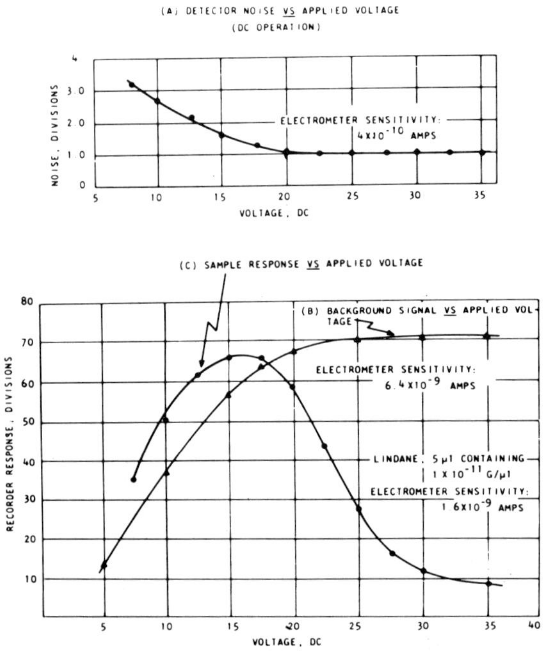

Performance Curves for DC Operation

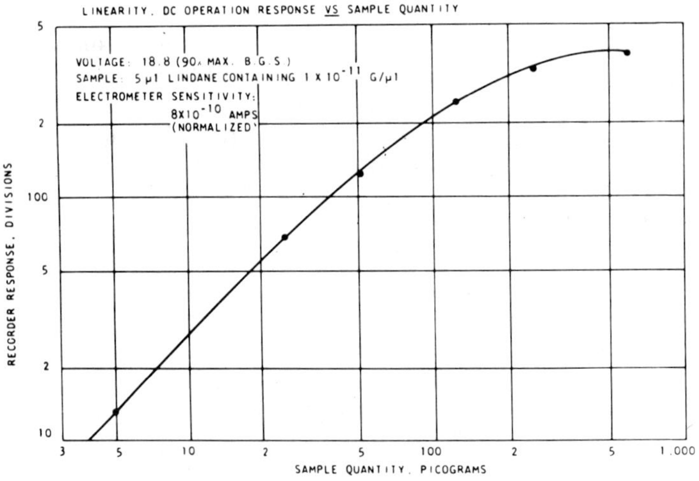

Sample Quantity Response Linearity, DC Operation

FIG. 4A. Performance characteristics of the EC dectector operated in the DC mode. (Courtesy Tracor Instruments, Inc., Austin, Texas.)

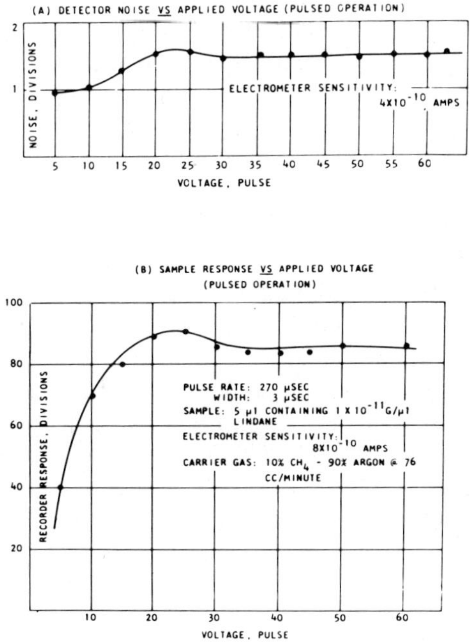

Performance Curves for Pulsed Voltage Operation

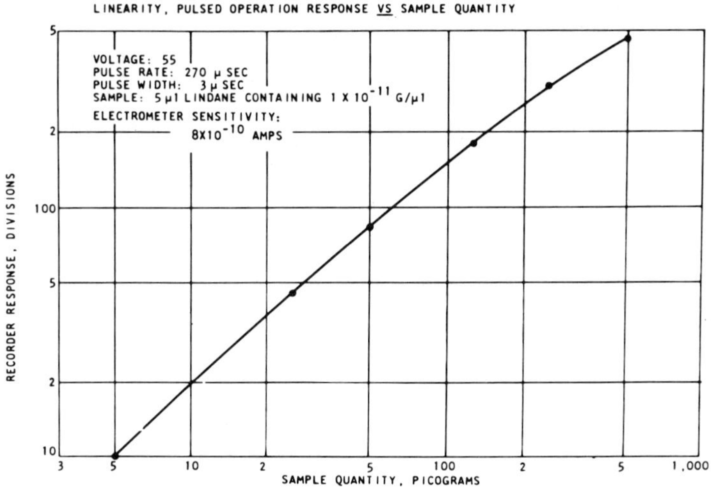

Sample Quantity Response Linearity, Pulsed Voltage Operation

FIG. 4B. Performance characteristics of the EC detector operated in the pulsed DC mode. (Courtesy Tracor Instruments, Inc., Austin, Texas.)

In both modes of operation, the polarization (DC) voltage applied affects the performance of the detector significantly. The detector noise due to the radioactive emission from the foil is stabilized at a constant level above 20 V in the DC mode and above 30 V in the pulsed mode (see top panels in Figs. 4A and 4B).

The standing current (background current) of the detector increases linearly up to 20 V in the DC mode (see middle panels in Figs. 4A and 4B) and plateaus beyond 25 V as a result of the accelerated collection of the electrons emitted from the cathode. The sample response curve, on the other hand, increases rapidly with applied voltage, reaching a peak at 15 V followed by a gradual decrease between 20 and 35 V, producing a typical bell-shaped response curve with optimal response occurring between 15 and 17 V. The optimum voltage changes with each compound and has to be determined for each compound analyzed. In the pulsed mode the response rises sharply with increasing voltage up to 20 to 25 V and reaches a plateau between 30 and 60 V using a pulse rate of 270 μsec and a pulse width of 3 μsec.

The linearity of the detector operated in the DC mode is narrow and ranges from 5 to 50 pg, deviating significantly from linearity at 100 pg. In the pulsed mode, however, the linearity is greatly improved and ranges from 5 to 250 pg (see bottom panels in Figs. 4A and 4B).

Variation of Response with Pulse Period (Rate) and Pulse Width (Interval)

In the pulsed (DC) mode, polarization (DC) voltage is usually applied at or near its plateau value (approximately 25 to 30 V), the optimal pulse rate lies between 150 and 300 μsec and the pulse width between 2 to 5 μsec, under which conditions optimal detector standing current is established. Generalized conditions for optimized sensitivity for strongly electron-capturing compounds are as follows: applied voltage (pulsed) ~ 50 V DC, pulse period (rate) ~ 150 μsec, pulse width ~ 3 μsec. In practice, the final values depend on the geometry of the detector used, the source strength, the specific type of compound analyzed, and the absence of interfering background in the system. This flexibility enables the operator to "fine tune" the detector for optimal response to a given series of compounds, usually also with suppression of the background, especially from biological materials.

Linearity of EC Detectors

The relatively small linear dynamic range of the EC detector is a serious handicap in quantitative analysis, especially in automated systems. The normal linear range is about two orders of magnitude when operated in the DC mode using N_2 as the carrier gas and improves to three orders in the pulsed (DC) mode. Quantitation is based on the fact that the decrease in detector standing current is proportional to the concentration of an electron capturing species and follows a Beer's law relationship over a narrow concentration range. The capture of electrons by compounds volatilized within an EC detector is described by the expression:

$$N = N_0 e^{kcb} \tag{1}$$

where N_0 = number of electrons reaching the anode in the presence of carrier gas only (standing current), N = number of electrons reaching the anode in the presence of an electron-capturing species at concentration c, k = electron capture (absorption cross-section) coefficient for a given species, and b = constant for the cell geometry used. The expression is analogous to that derived for radioactive decay. This expression was modified by Wentworth et al. (27) in terms of the currents measured under these conditions. Thus:

$$\frac{I_b - I_e}{I_e} = kc \tag{2}$$

where I_b = detector standing (background) current, that is, a constant applied current of magnitude equal to I_e when only carrier gas is flowing, where $(I_b - I_e) = 0$ when no electron-capturing species is present, I_e = decrease in detector standing current due to the presence of an electron-capturing species, k = electron capture coefficient of the compound, c = concentration in grams per milliliter per second flowing through the detector.

An EC compound lowers the standing current below baseline, resulting in a negative signal that is electronically converted into a positive signal for display as a positive peak on the chromatogram.

The problem of linearity was reviewed by Fenimore et al. (5,7), who devised a linearization process by analogue conversion to process the signals obtained in accordance with Eq. 2 using the pulsed (constant-frequency) mode of operation. The ^{63}Ni detector was operated in the pulsed (DC) mode at a pulse amplitude of −60 V, with a high-frequency pulse rate (2,000 μsec) and a narrow pulse width (1 μsec) using argon-methane (90:10) as the carrier as described by Simmonds et al. (19). This represented a significant advance in linearity and reliable quantitation over a wider dynamic range of three to four orders of magnitude. The main advantage of this mode of operation was higher sensitivity as a result of optimized electron collection by adjusting the essential detector parameters, i.e., pulse amplitude (−60 V DC), pulse frequency, and pulse width to "fine tune" the detector for maximum optimized sensitivity to a given compound or a series of compounds.

However, in order to fully utilize the potential of "totally automated GC analysis," it was necessary to extend the linear dynamic range of the EC detector even further to cover five to six orders of magnitude without sacrificing its inherent high sensitivity. Since detector geometry and β-ionization source strength have been almost fully optimized, the next step required a significant change in electronics to accommodate this requirement. To this end, the new pulsed (constant-current) mode of operation was developed by Maggs et al. (14). The EC detector geometry and its operating principle remain unchanged. However, processing the EC signal from the detector is significantly changed using sophisticated electronics. The circuitry for this mode is quite different from that used in the constant-frequency mode, since now the pulse frequency must be adjusted automatically, as it is the change in pulse frequency and not the cell current that is proportional to concentration. The constant current mode also uses brief voltage pulses (−60 V DC) for electron collection, as does the constant frequency mode. In the "constant-current" mode, the standing current of the cell is maintained at a constant value by modulating the pulse frequency. In actuality, a baseline is established by a "standing frequency" value rather than a standing current.

A simplified circuit diagram of a ^{63}Ni EC detector and linearizer is shown in Fig. 5. The standing current of the detector is balanced by a reference current equal to the standing current fed into the integrating electrometer (comparing amplifier), which drives the frequency pulser through a voltage/frequency converter. When the standing current of the detector and reference current are matched, baseline is established. However, when a sample enters the cell and captures electrons, the cell current drops below the reference current, the change in current being proportional to concentration.

The comparing amplifier responds to this change in cell current by increasing its output voltage, which is fed simultaneously to the recorder to begin drawing the leading edge of the chromatographic peak and to the V/F converter to increase the frequency to the pulser. As the sample leaves the cell, its standing current begins to rise back to its normal value, the amplifier decreasing its output voltage to the recorder, which draws the trailing edge of the peak, and to the V/F converter, which reduces the frequency to the pulser and reestablishes the baseline. The resultant recorder plot is linear with sample concentration over a wide dynamic range. Thus the information from

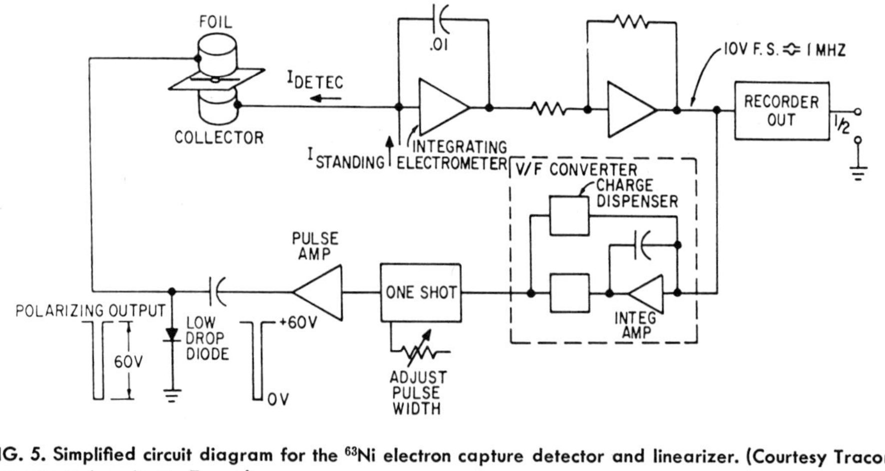

FIG. 5. Simplified circuit diagram for the ^{63}Ni electron capture detector and linearizer. (Courtesy Tracor Instruments, Inc., Austin, Texas.)

the EC detector is processed as a frequency change (which is proportional to concentration) while attempting to maintain the cell standing current constant. Operation in the constant-current mode sets a few limitations on instrumental parameters that are preset by the manufacturer and whose specifications are determined using a pesticide (lindane) as the test sample. These preset parameters are then assumed to be applicable to most EC substances, hence represent a compromise set of conditions.

The important fixed parameters for the Tracor EC detector and linearizer (24) are shown in Figs. 6 through 8. The preferred carrier gas is argon-methane (95:5) for the widest dynamic range, although nitrogen is also usable over a somewhat narrower range (Fig. 6). The polarizing voltage is preset at −60 V DC, which is also the output of the pulser used. The detector standing current appears to be critical, a value of 0.5×10^{-9} A giving the best results. Values much above or below this value deviate significantly from linearity (Fig. 7). Hence detector standing current has to be carefully preset by judicious selection of a foil having the correct source strength, that is, 15 mCi ^{63}Ni and carrier gas ionizing characteristics. Consequently a very "hot" foil or a contaminated one will not perform satisfactorily to provide a wide linear dynamic range.

The pulse width is also important with respect to linearity. A short pulse width of duration of 0.7 μsec was found to be optimal, with pulse widths much above or below this value deviating from linearity. Optimal detector operating temperature was found to be between 300 and 325°C, and should

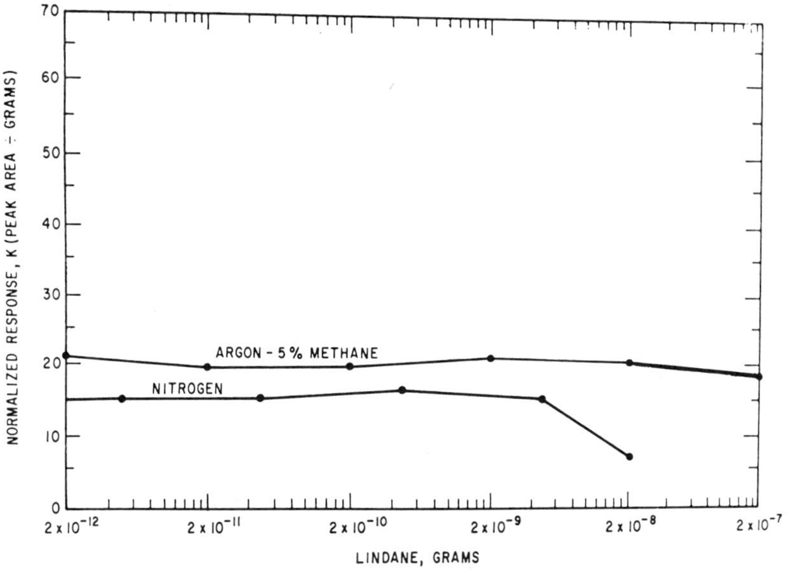

FIG. 6. Influence of carrier gas in the EC detector operated in the constant-current, frequency-modulated "linearized" mode. (Courtesy Tracor Instruments, Inc., Austin, Texas.)

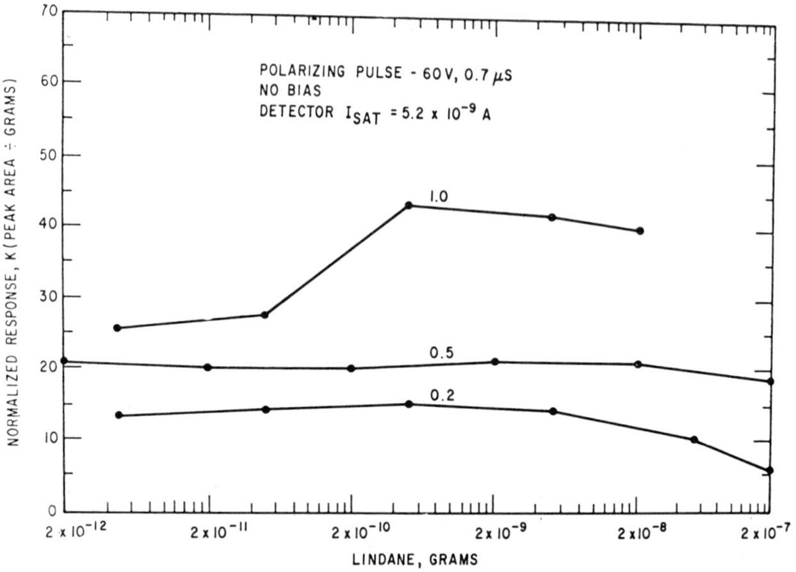

FIG. 7. Influence of standing current on detector linearity. (Courtesy Tracor Instruments, Inc., Austin, Texas.)

be carefully preset for the analysis in question and the column temperature used. The detector standing current profiles comparing argon-methane (95:5) versus nitrogen are shown in Fig. 8. The detector standing current increases in large increments by stepwise increase of the polarizing pulse voltage from 1 through 200 × 10^3 HZ using argon-methane (95:5), whereas with nitrogen the profile is not so dramatic (left panel). The differences in carrier gas performance is even more dramatic with a slightly dirty detector (right panel) where argon-methane still provides a very usable standing current profile, whereas with nitrogen the standing current drops off drastically and is not usable for quantitation.

Notwithstanding these fixed parameters, the constant-current pulsed mode of operation is heavily favored by manufacturers, since it preserves the sensitivity and specificity of EC detection with a wide linear dynamic range of 10,000:1, which is necessary for fully automated computer controlled EC-GLC analysis. All the major instrument manufacturers (Hewlett-Packard, Tracor, Varian, and Perkin-Elmer) have developed individualized EC detectors of different cell geometry, using 10 to 15 mCi ^{63}Ni foils as the β-ionization source and argon:methane or nitrogen as the carrier gas, the latter being cheaper, all the detectors being operated in the pulsed constant-current linearized mode. Factors resulting in nonlinearity in constant-current electron capture detection have recently been discussed (21). A recently published manual entitled *Electron Capture Handbook,* by Rowland and Burgett (17), is recommended reading.

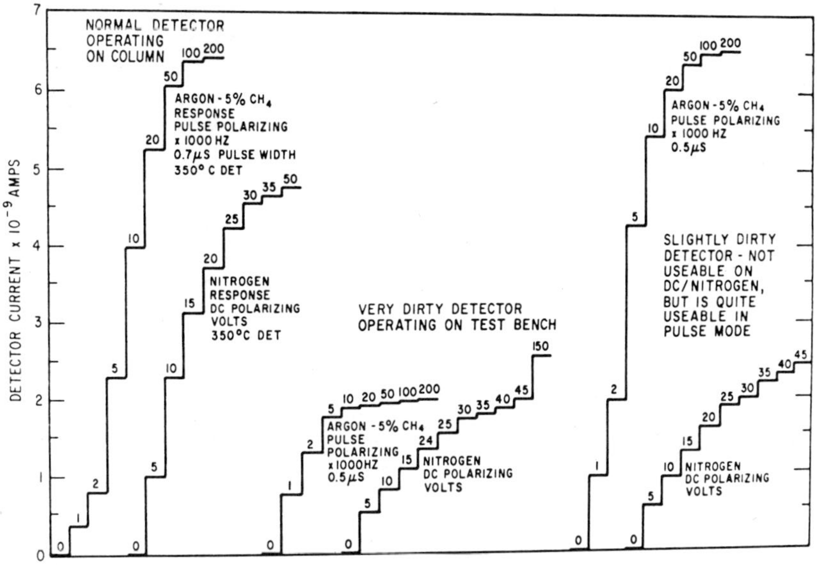

FIG. 8. Detector response profile comparison for different carrier gases. (Courtesy Tracor Instruments, Inc. Austin, Texas.)

MOLECULAR STRUCTURE AND EC RESPONSE

The ability of organic compounds to capture thermal electrons depends on the presence of certain functional groups in the molecule called "electrophores." Compounds containing halogens, nitro, carbonyl, amido, thio, and nitrile functional groups, especially in a conjugated resonance form, have shown high EC properties. The resonance of the carbonyl and amide group is believed to be a primary electrophore in the initial capture of electrons, hence its presence in the molecule can significantly affect the sensitivity of the compound to EC detection (15).

The 1,4-benzodiazepin-2-ones and their *o*-aminobenzophenone derivatives (Fig. 9) possess not only the required electrophores in the molecule but are also highly conjugated aromatic systems with high resonance energy in the molecule. They tend to exhibit resonance readily, thus enhancing their EC sensitivity. Drug compounds that do not contain electrophores, but that contain highly polar functional groups, such as hydroxyl, carboxyl, amines, and alcohols, can be derivatized to yield compounds more amenable for GLC assay with enhanced sensitivity for EC detection (1,8). Thus the silylation of phenols, alcohols to produce silyl ethers (16), the esterification of carboxylic acids to produce pentafluorobenzyl esters and trichloroethyl esters, and the acylation of amines with the appropriate acid anhydride to produce trifluoroacetamides, pentafluoroproprionamides, or heptafluorobutyramide derivatives have enabled the EC-GLC analysis of many types of drugs, such

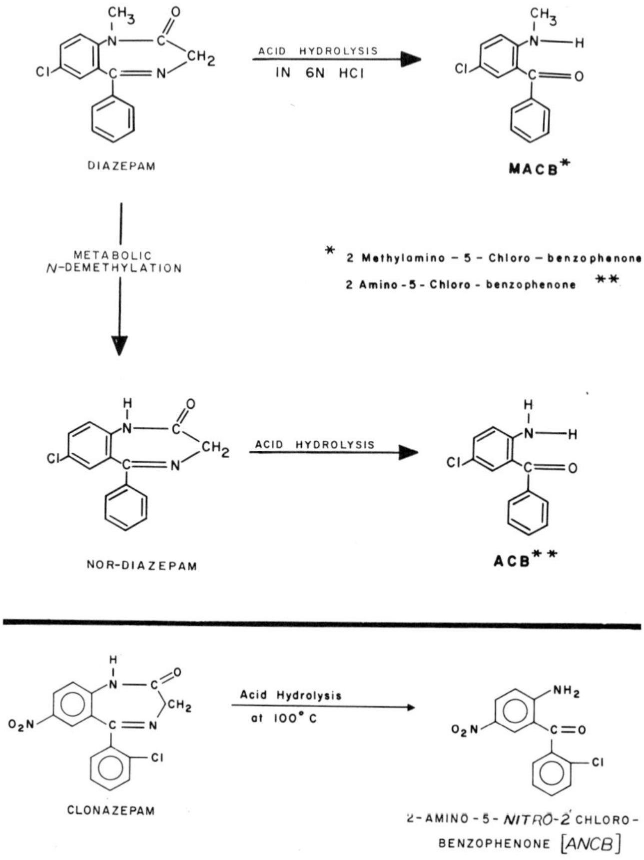

FIG. 9. Chemical structures and reactions of diazepam, nordiazepam, and clonazepam.

as barbiturates and phenytoin (25). Such derivatization reactions are readily adaptable for routine analysis, because they produce quantitative yields at nanogram levels.

EC-GLC ANALYSIS OF 1,4-BENZODIAZEPINES

The 1,4-benzodiazepine class of compounds has yielded several important drugs that are widely used in clinical practice as antianxiety agents or mild tranquilizers, muscle relaxants, hypnotics, and anticonvulsant agents (48,53). Of these, diazepam (Valium) and clonazepam (Clonopin) are used as anticonvulsant agents (51). Diazepam, which is widely used as an antianxiety agent, is also effective against recurrent convulsions produced by status epilepticus (31,46,50), whereas clonazepam is effective against petit mal seizures (33,43,45,49,55).

The benzodiazepines undergo extensive biotransformation in man and other animal species (51,61), resulting usually in the presence of one or more metabolites that have to be resolved from the parent drug for accurate quantitation in biological fluids. The chemistry and pharmacology of the 1,4-benzodiazepines have been reported (60).

Diazepam undergoes N-demethylation to yield nordiazepam, the major metabolite in blood, which then undergoes hydroxylation to yield oxazepam, which is eliminated mainly as a glucuronide. Diazepam can also undergo hydroxylation first to yield 3-hydroxydiazepam (temazepam), which is then N-demethylated to yield oxazepam (61). Clonazepam is metabolized mainly by reduction of the nitro group to yield 7-amino-clonazepam, which is then acetylated to yield 7-acetamido-clonazepam (44). The metabolites of diazepam are all pharmacologically active, whereas those of clonazepam are inactive (60). Hence the determination of the metabolite profile in man following diazepam administration is necessary to correlate its pharmacokinetics with clinical effectiveness.

Although the benzodiazepines are amenable to analysis by a number of different methods (35), their determination in blood or plasma is best accomplished using GLC (21) in combination with specific detectors. The numerous GLC assays that have been reported for the determination of specific 1,4-benzodiazepines in biological fluids are the subject of two excellent reviews (34,54). The majority of these methods use electron capture detection due to the presence of an electronegative group in the 7-position of the molecule (usually a halogen or nitro group), a halogen in the 2′-position of the 5-phenyl ring, and a carbonyl group in position 2 of the 1,4-benzodiazepine ring (Fig. 9). Conversion of diazepam, nordiazepam (38,41), and clonazepam (40) by hydrolysis in strong acids to their respective benzophenones (Fig. 9), which are also very sensitive to EC-GLC, is advantageous where the parent drug is the major component present in blood, as with clonazepam (40).

Most of the previously published assays (34,54) required extensive "cleanup" of the sample extract (usually diethyl ether) prior to EC-GLC analysis, making them time consuming and not readily amenable to rapid routine analysis. Alternative extraction, cleanup, and derivatization procedures were investigated in order to take advantage of GLC assay automation and to accommodate the large numbers of specimens generated for analysis from large-scale clinical studies.

A simplified procedure for the systematic analysis of a number of clinically active benzodiazepines both currently marketed and others under development was reported recently (37). It is based on their optimal extractability into benzene-methylene chloride (90:10) at specific pH values and requires a minimal amount of sample "cleanup" prior to EC-GLC analysis. The procedures are rapid, quantitative, and readily automated, and the sensitivity and specificity fulfills the requirements for its use in clinical pharmacokinetic evaluation (Fig. 10).

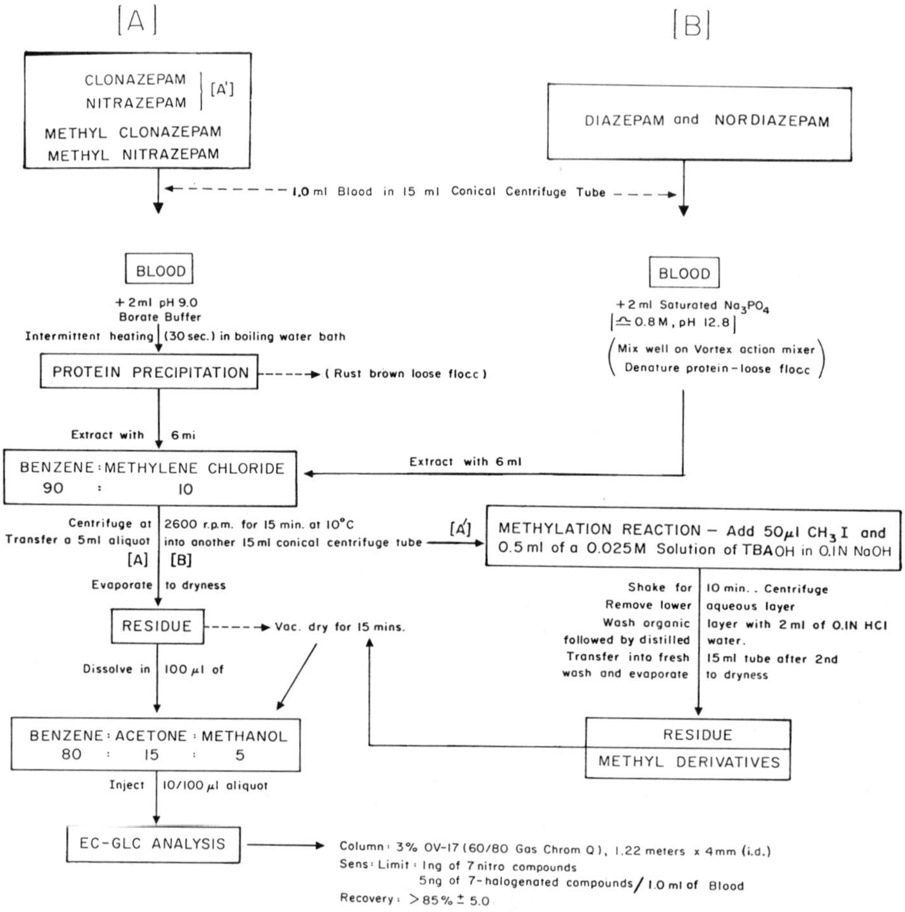

FIG. 10. Flow diagram for the analysis of diazepam, nordiazepam, clonazepam, and nitrazepam from whole blood.

EXPERIMENTAL CONDITIONS FOR EC-GLC ANALYSIS

Column

The column was a U-shaped 4-ft, 4-mm-i.d. borosilicate glass column, containing 3% OV-17 on 60–80 mesh Gas Chrom Q (Applied Science Labs, State Park, Pa.). The column was conditioned using a "no flow" procedure as previously described (39).

Instrumental Parameters

A Micro Tek MT-220 gas chromatograph (Tracor Instruments, Inc., Austin, Tex.) equipped with 15-mCi ^{63}Ni electron capture detector was used. All other operational parameters are given in Table 1.

TABLE 1. *Parameters for EC-GLC analysis of 1,4-Benzodiazepine-2-ones in blood*

Instrument:	Micro-Tek Model MT-220 equipped with a ^{63}Ni electron capture detector (15 mCi-^{63}Ni-β ionization source)
Column:	4 ft (1.22 m), 4 mm i.d. borosilicate glass column containing 3% OV-17on 60/80 mesh Gas-Chrom Q (Applied Science Labs., State Park, Pa.)
Carrier gas:	Argon-methane (90:10)—Matheson Column head pressure = 40 psig Flow rate = 75 ml/min (detector purge = 20 ml/min); total flow $\simeq$ 100 ml/min
Operational temp.:	Injection port = 290°C Oven (column) = 220–260°C (variable) Detector = 325°C
Electrometer (model 8169):	Input = 10^2, output = 32; response = 3.2×10^{-9} A—f.s.d.
E. C. detector:	Operated in pulsed (DC) mode at 45 to 60 V (DC); pulse rate = 270 μsec Pulse Width = 4 μsec.
Sensitivity:	1 ng of 7-nitro compounds or 5 ng of 7-halogenated compounds/10 μl injected $\simeq$ full scale (> 95%) response

General Extraction Procedure

The flow diagram of the extraction procedures is outlined in Fig. 10. The compounds to be analyzed are divided into two groups, depending on the pH and method of optimal extractability. Clonazepam, nitrazepam, and their N-1-methyl derivatives are classified in group A, whereas diazepam, nordiazepam, and the reference standard, 7-iodo-2′-fluoro analogue of diazepam (Ro 7–9957), are classified in group B. They are extracted into benzene-methylene chloride (90:10) from blood following mild protein precipitation at pH 9.0 and 13.0, respectively.

The benzene-methylene chloride extracts containing diazepam and nordiazepam, or methyl clonazepam and methyl nitrazepam *per se* can be analyzed directly by EC-GLC without any derivatization (Fig. 10). Compounds in group A′ (clonazepam and nitrazepam) are first converted to their N-1-methyl derivatives using CH_3I as the alkylating agent and tetrabutylammonium hydroxide (TBAOH) (Eastman Chemicals) or tetrabutylammonium hydrogen sulfate (TBAHS) (Aldrich Chemicals) in 0.1 N NaOH as the counter ion for their quantitative extraction and methylation in the solvent (36). The hydroxide (TBAOH) in either methanol or in 0.1 N NaOH is preferred,[1] since it is very pure and results in more reproducible and higher methylation yields than does TBAHS, which also has to be recrystallized twice from methanol prior to use. The excess reagents must be removed by successive washing of the organic phase with 0.1 N HCl followed by distilled water.

The rapid extraction procedures described above for the compounds in

[1] R. E. Weinfeld and I. Bekersky, *personal communication* (1976), Hoffmann-La Roche, Inc.

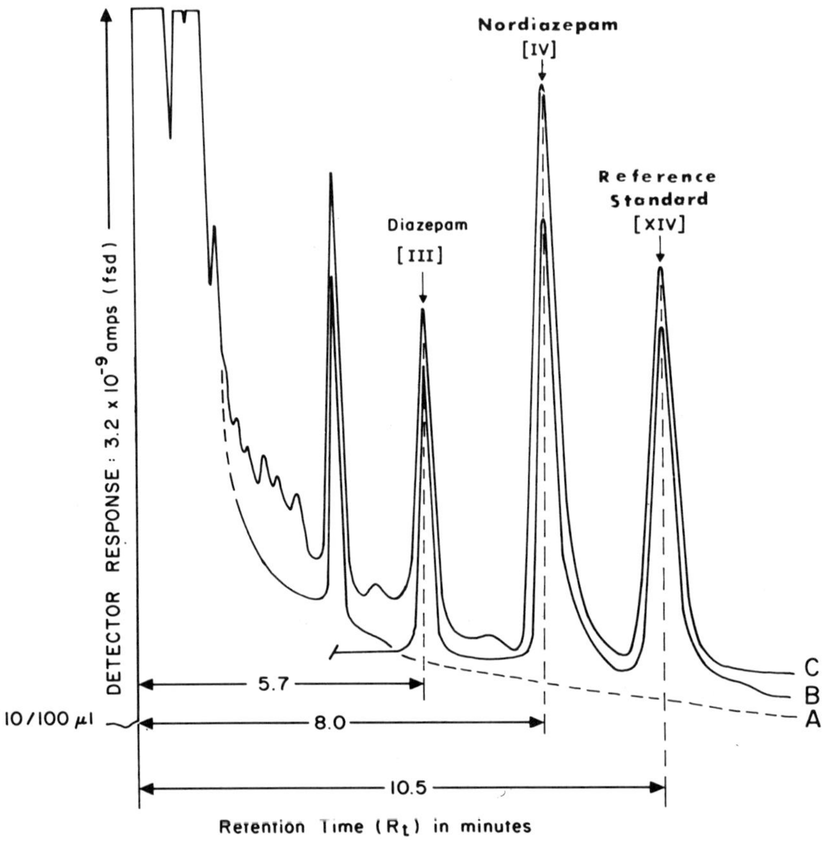

FIG. 11. Chromatogram for the analysis of diazepam from whole blood. A, control blood extract; B, authentic standards; C, authentic standards recovered from blood.

groups A and B are limited to the analysis of only 1.0 ml or less of whole blood by this simplified assay procedure. The analysis of larger sample volumes of whole blood or plasma (up to 4 ml) requires more rigorous "cleanup" prior to EC-GLC analysis and permits the analysis of diazepam and nordiazepam, either as the intact moiety (39) or as their benzophenone derivatives following acid hydrolysis (41) (Fig. 9). Similarly, clonazepam can also be analyzed as its benzophenone derivative (ANCB), the details of which have been previously published (40).

The residues of biological specimens processed by the simplified method yield chromatograms devoid of extraneous impurities in the retention areas of interest for the respective compounds (Figs. 11, 12) resulting in baseline resolution of the peaks for accurate quantitation by fully automated computer controlled techniques (63).

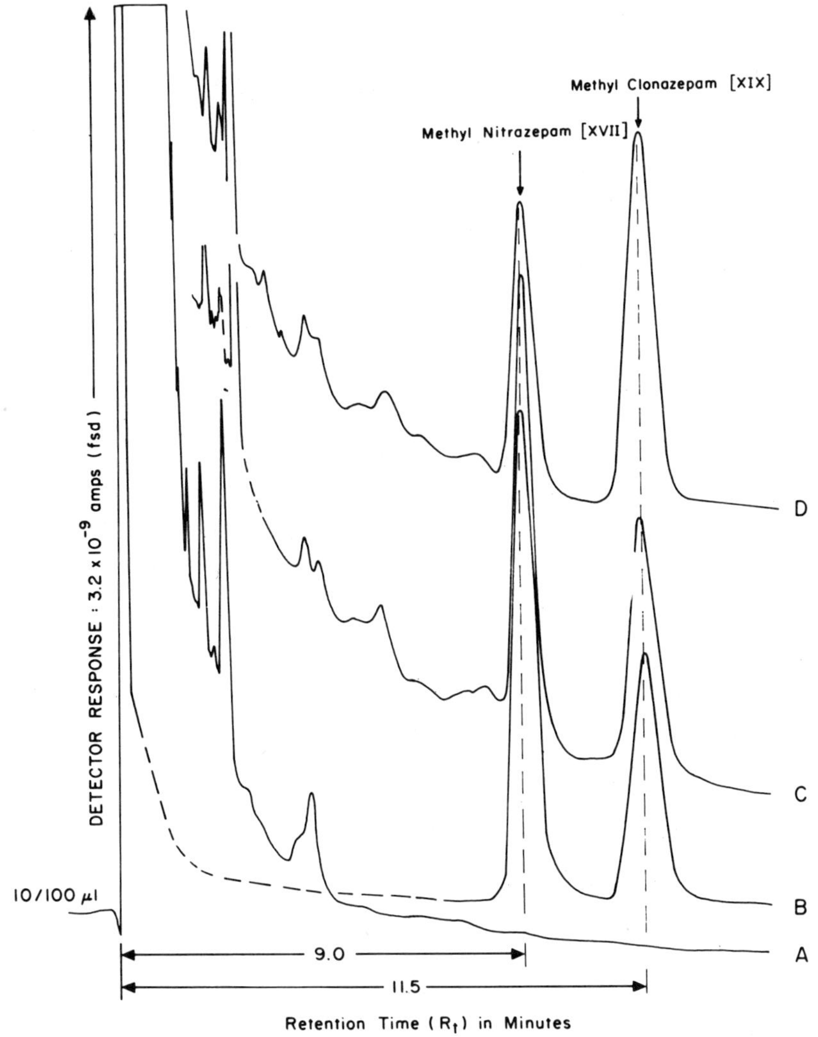

FIG. 12. Chromatograms for the analysis of clonazepam from whole blood. A, control blood extract; B, authentic standards; C, authentic standards recovered from blood; D, blood extract 2 hr after 2-mg oral dose of clonazepam. (Courtesy American Chemical Society.)

RECOVERY

The overall recovery of diazepam, nordiazepam, clonazepam, and nitrazepam is of the order of 90% ± 5.0 (SD) or better. The accuracy of the chemical assay was also verified by scintillation radiometry using ^{14}C-labeled drug (diazepam and clonazepam), and both gave recovery values of 90% ± 5.0 attesting to the accuracy and reproducibility of EC-GLC analysis. The

N-1-desalkyl compounds, nordiazepam, clonazepam, and nitrazepam, when chromatographed as authentic standards in the absence of a blood extract, show considerable "tailing." This "tailing" effect is diminished in the presence of a blood extract and results in more symmetrical Gaussian-shaped peaks, which improves peak area integration. This behavior is probably due to the formation of an "adsorption complex" of the extracted lipids with active sites on the column, thereby reducing adsorption losses during EC-GLC analysis, resulting in enhanced recovery and more symmetrical peaks for these compounds albeit at relatively high column temperatures ($> 280°C$), especially for the nitro compounds, clonazepam and nitrazepam. It is, therefore, necessary to prime the column (daily) with the control blood extract prior to EC-GLC analysis. Alternatively, a solution of either cholesterol, methylcholate, or lecithin (a phospholipid) in acetone can be used, since they also are excellent "column conditioners" for deactivating adsorption sites on the column (58).

The N-desalkyl-1,4-benzodiazepin-2-ones can also be derivatized to improve not only their volatility and peak shape but also to reduce adsorption losses. Therefore, compounds such as nitrazepam and clonazepam should be converted to their respective N-1-methyl derivatives using CH_3I as the alkylating agent, with TBAOH in 0.1 N NaOH as the counter ion for quantitative ion-pair extraction and methylation (36). Although the analysis of clonazepam and nitrazepam as their trimethylsilyl (TMS) derivatives using *bis*-trimethylsilyl acetamide (BSA) in pyridine has been reported (52), the methyl derivatives are preferred because of their chemical stability, reproducibility, enhanced sensitivity to EC detection, and minimized adsorption losses.

SPECIFICITY OF THE ASSAY

The EC-GLC conditions used enable the specific quantitation of the parent drug and its major metabolites only when each drug alone is administered to the subject in carefully controlled clinical studies. It is not specific when multiple benzodiazepine drug therapy or ingestion is involved, because of the similar or overlapping retention times of different metabolites, which would interfere. The general method is of clinical utility in monitoring blood levels following individual drug administration of single or chronic oral dosing and for biochemical, pharmacological, toxicological, and pharmacokinetic evaluation of the correlation of blood drug levels with clinical effect of benzodiazepines in man and other animal species (47).

APPLICATION IN PHARMACOKINETIC STUDIES

Diazepam

The pharmacokinetic profile of diazepam following intravenous and oral administration is well defined. According to Kaplan et al. (57), intravenous administration of a single 10 mg dose resulted in a triphasic blood concentration versus time profile with peak concentration of about 300 ng/ml, declining to a concentration of about 30 ng/ml at 48 hr. The half-life (β) of elimination was of the order of 27 to 37 hr. Diazepam is rapidly and completely absorbed as the intact drug following oral administration (10 mg) with peak blood concentrations of about 200 ng/ml attained within 1 to 1.5 hr, declining to about 40 ng/ml at 48 hr. The major blood metabolite, nordiazepam, showed a similar profile following both i.v. and oral dosing of diazepam, a maximum concentration of about 35 ng/ml between 26 to 48 hr, suggesting a slow rate of formation and elimination of this component. The analysis of these blood concentrations requires 0.5 to 1.0 ml of whole blood, especially at 48 hr after dosing. The simplified procedure has sufficient sensitivity and recovery of drug to be more than adequate to the task in these studies.

Administration of multiple 10-mg oral doses every 24 hr for 14 days resulted in steady-state (plateau) diazepam blood levels by the seventh day, which ranged from a mean maximum of about 225 ng/ml and a mean minimum of about 100 ng/ml. The relatively constant steady-state diazepam blood levels substantiates the constancy and reproducibility of the absorption, distribution, metabolism, and excretion of each administration of the drug, with all the processes following apparent first-order kinetics. The steady-state profile also indicates no enzyme induction of diazepam metabolism and no unpredicted drug accumulation (57).

The blood-level profile of nordiazepam formed under the above multiple drug regimen revealed apparent steady-state levels ranging from 90 to 160 ng/ml from day 6 to 14. The relatively constant nordiazepam blood levels reflect the slow rates of formation and elimination of this metabolite. Consequently the apparent half-life (β) of elimination of nordiazepam ($\sim$ 72 hr) is slower than might be anticipated when it is administered *per se,* due to the continued formation of this metabolite from diazepam released from "deep" storage depots in the body. Steady-state blood concentrations of diazepam and nordiazepam are sufficiently high so that a substantially smaller sample volume (0.1 to 0.5 ml) can be used for analysis. Endogenous impurities are also significantly reduced in the extract residue, which can be readily analyzed by computer-controlled automated EC-GLC analysis (63).

Clonazepam

The pharmacokinetics of the recently introduced anticonvulsant agent Clonopin have been the subject of intensive investigation (32,56,62). Since the compound is clinically effective at very low doses (0.5 to 2.0 mg), monitoring blood levels in the low nanogram range resulting from these doses requires the high sensitivity of EC-GLC. Clonazepam undergoes metabolism mainly by NO_2 group reduction, resulting in the 7-amino and 7-acetamido metabolites (44), which are pharmacologically inactive (60). The parent drug is the active anticonvulsant moiety and can be determined in whole blood or plasma either as the benzophenone derivative (40) or as the N-1-methyl derivative of clonazepam (36) without any interference from metabolites with the same degree of sensitivity and specificity of analysis. Peak blood concentrations of clonazepam following single 2-mg oral doses in normal volunteer adults (0.027 mg/kg) ranging from 6.0 to 10.0 ng/ml were obtained 1.5 to 2.0 hr after dosing, and declined to concentrations of about 1.0 ng/ml at 48 hr. The apparent half-life (β) of elimination ranged from 19 to 39 hr in these subjects (56).

Pharmacokinetic studies following single 2-mg intravenous and oral administrations in healthy adult volunteers were also reported by Berlin and Dahlstrom (32). The disposition curves following i.v. dosing showed a biexponential decline with apparent half-lives ranging from 24 to 60 hr. Absorption of orally administered 2-mg doses was rapid, with peak plasma concentrations ranging from 7.0 to 22.1 ng/ml seen at 1 to 4 hr after dosing. The apparent half-life (β) of elimination ranged from 19 to 42 hr in these subjects. The pharmacokinetics and side effects of clonazepam and its 7-amino metabolite following multiple oral administration in man were also reported (62). The relatively low peak plasma concentrations of 6 to 20 ng/ml and the long half-life of the drug, ranging from 19 to 60 hr, require the high sensitivity of EC-GLC. The two methods described have sensitivity limits of about 0.5 ng/ml using 1 ml of blood or plasma per assay. The sensitivity of the hydrolysis method (40) can be increased by extracting up to 4 ml of blood or plasma, in which event the sensitivity is about 0.15 ng/ml, equivalent to about 50 pg of benzophenone injected. The high sensitivity for clonazepam or its benzophenone is possibly due to the fortuitous presence of a nitro, halogen (Cl), and carbonyl group in the respective molecules present in a conjugated aromatic system, making them excellent electrophores.

CONCLUSIONS

Electron capture GLC is one of the most sensitive techniques available for quantitative analysis of drugs in biological fluids. It is also more specific than the flame ionization detector, since it responds only to those compounds that contain strong electronegative functional groups (i.e., electrophores, such as —NO_2, Cl, Br, F, I, >C═O, CH_3S—) in the molecule, or those that can be easily derivatized to yield electronegative groups, such as the perflurophenyl or mono or dinitrophenyl derivatives. Recently developed detection techniques, such as the nitrogen-specific flame ionization detector, gas chromatography-mass spectroscopy (GC-MS) using chemical ionization, or atmospheric pressure ionization (API), have challenged EC-GLC in sensitivity, specificity, and linearity of detection.

EC-GLC is the method of choice in the analysis of 1,4-benzodiazepines in biological fluids, and its utility in the quantitation of these compounds either as the intact moiety (36,37,39) or its corresponding benzophenone derivative (38,40,41) is well documented by chromatographic and other techniques (34,35,54). Recently developed radioimmunoassay techniques for diazepam (59) and clonazepam (42) have proved useful in clinical therapeutic monitoring of these anticonvulsant agents in man. The sensitivity, specificity, simplicity, and ease of analysis by radioimmunoassay have challenged EC-GLC as an alternative means of analysis. Their major limitation is that they do not always differentiate metabolites present that may be pharmacologically active.

The new generation of highly sensitive "linearized" EC detectors that operate in the constant-current, frequency-modulated mode have a wide linear dynamic range, covering five to six orders of magnitude, and are well suited for totally automated computer-controlled EC-GLC analysis (63).

ACKNOWLEDGMENTS

The author thanks Mrs. A. Szilagyi for the preparation of the manuscript, and Mr. R. McGlynn for the drawings of Figs. 9 through 12.

REFERENCES

Electron Capture Detection

1. Ahuja, S. (1976): Derivatization in gas chromatography. *J. Pharm. Sci.,* 65:163–182.
2. David, D. J. (1974): *Gas Chromatographic Detectors,* pp. 76–113. Wiley–Interscience, New York.
3. Devaux, P., and Guiochon, G. (1967): The variations of the response factors of the electron capture detector with various parameters. *J. Gas. Chromatogr.,* 5:341–352.
4. Devaux, P., and Guiochon, G. (1970): Determinations of optimum operating conditions of the electron capture detector. *J. Chromatogr. Sci.,* 8:502–508.
5. Fenimore, D. C., and Davis, C. M. (1970): Linear electron capture detection. *J. Chromatogr. Sci.,* 8:519–523.
6. Fenimore, D. C., Loy, P. R, and Zlatkis, A. (1971): High temperature tritium source for electron capture detectors—applications to a low volume detector. *Anal. Chem.,* 43:1972–1975.
7. Fenimore, D. C., Zlatkis, A., and Wentworth, W. E. (1968): Linearization of electron capture detector response by analog conversion. *Anal. Chem.,* 40:1594–1596.
8. Hammerstrand, K., and Bonelli, E. J. (1968): *Derivative Formation in Gas Chromatography,* Bulletin #6/68-A-1006, Varian Aerograph, Walnut Creek, Calif.
9. Horning, E. C., Horning, M. G., Carroll, D. I., Dzidic, I., and Stillwell, R. N. (1973): New picogram detection system based on a mass spectrometer with an external ionization source at atmospheric pressure. *Anal. Chem.,* 45:936–943.
10. Karasek, F. W. (1971): Plasma chromatography of the polychlorinated biphenyls. *Anal. Chem.,* 43:1982–1986.
11. Lovelock, J. E. (1961): Ionization methods for the analysis of gases and vapors. *Anal. Chem.,* 33:162–178.

12. Lovelock, J. E. (1963): Electron absorption detectors and technique for use in quantitative and qualitative analysis by gas chromatography. *Anal. Chem.,* 35:474–481.
13. Lovelock, J. E., and Lipsky, S. (1960): Electron affinity spectroscopy—a new method for the identification of functional groups in chemical compounds separated by gas chromatography. *J. Am. Chem. Soc.,* 82:431–433.
14. Maggs, R. J., Joynes, P. L., Davies, A. J., and Lovelock, J. E. (1971): The electron capture detector—a new mode of operation. *Anal. Chem.,* 43:1966–1971.
15. Matin, S. B., and Rowland, M. (1972): Electron capture sensitivity comparison of various derivatives of primary and secondary amines. *J. Pharm Sci.,* 61:1235–1240.
16. Pierce, A. E. (1968): *Silylation of Organic Compounds.* Pierce Chemical Co., Rockford, Ill.
17. Rowland, F. W., and Burgett, C. A. (1975): *Electron Capture Handbook,* Cat. #5950–3529 (Fiche P/N–5950–3530). Hewlett-Packard Instruments, Inc. (Analytical Division), Avondale, Pa.
18. Sevcik, J. (1976): *Detectors in Gas Chromatography,* Journal of Chromatography Library Sciences, Vol. 4, pp. 72–86. Elsevier Scientific Publishing Co., Amsterdam.
19. Simmonds, P. G., Fenimore, D. C., Pettitt, B. C., Lovelock, J E., and Zlatkis, A. (1967): Design of a nickel-63 electron absorption detector and analytical significance of high temperature operation. *Anal. Chem.,* 39:1428–1433.
20. Sullivan, J. J. (1973): Approximation of electron capture response factors for highly electrophilic compounds. *J. Chromatogr.,* 87:9–16.
21. Sullivan, J. J., and Burgett, C. A. (1975): Nonlinearity in constant current electron capture detection. *Chromatographia,* 8:176–179.
22. Supina, W. R. (1974): *The Packed Column in Gas Chromatography.* Supelco, Inc., Bellefonte, Pa.
23. Tracor Instruments, Inc. (1969): *Operation and Service Manual—Nickel-63 High Temperature Electron Capture Detector,* Bulletin #12002-A, pp. 42–50. Tracor, Inc., Austin, Tex.
24. Tracor Instruments, Inc. (1975): *Electron Capture Linearizer Operation Manual,* Bulletin #114556-E, pp. 15–30. Tracor, Inc., Austin, Tex.
25. Walle, T. (1975): Electron capture gas chromatography of barbituric acids and diphenylhydantoin after pentafluorobenzylation. *J. Chromatogr.,* 114:345–350.
26. Wentworth, W. E., and Chen, E. J. (1967): Electron attachment mechanisms, analytical importance of temperature and concentration variables. *J. Gas Chromatogr.,* 5:170–179.
27. Wentworth, W. E., Chen, E. J., and Lovelock, J. E. (1966): The pulse sampling technique for the study of electron attachment phenomena. *J. Phys. Chem.,* 70: 445–458.
28. Wilkens Instruments and Research, Inc. (Varian Instruments, Inc.) (1965): *Electron Capture Detector for Aerograph Hy-Fi Gas Chromatographs—Instruction Manual.*
29. Yauger, W. L., Addison, L. M., and Stevens, R. K. (1966): Response characteristics of a new high temperature electron capture detector. *J. Assoc. Off. Anal. Chem.,* 49:1053–1057.
30. Zlatkis, A. and Pettitt, B. C. (1969): Effect of detector temperature on the sensitivity of some electron absorbing derivatives. *Chromatographia,* 2:484–492.

EC-GLC Analysis of 1,4-Benzodiazepines

31. Barbeau, A. (1968): Le diazepam (Valium) intraveineux dans le traitement des etats de mal epileptique-une etude a double insu. *Int. J. Clin. Pharmacol.,* 1(6): 550–557.
32. Berlin, A., and Dahlstrom, H. (1975): Pharmacokinetics of the anticonvulsant drug clonazepam evaluated from single oral and intraveneous doses and by repeated oral administration. *Eur. J. Clin. Pharmacol.,* 9:155–159.
33. Browne, T. R. (1976): Clonazepam—a review of a new anticonvulsant drug. *Arch. Neurol.,* 33:326–332.

34. Clifford, J. M., and Smyth, W. F. (1974): The determination of some 1,4-benzodiazepines and their metabolites in body fluids, a review. *Analyst,* 99:241 272.
35. de Silva, J. A. F. (1976): Choice of sensitivity and specificity in the analysis of drugs in biological fluids; use of electron capture-GLC, spectrophotofluorometry, differential pulse polarography, and radioimmunoassay in the analysis of 1,4-benzodiazepines. In *Quantitative Analytic Studies in Epilepsy,* edited by P. Kellaway and I. Peterson, pp. 11–38. Raven Press, New York.
36. de Silva, J. A. F., and Bekersky, I. (1974): Determination of clonazepam and flunitrazepam in blood by electron capture gas liquid chromatography. *J. Chromatogr.,* 99:447–460.
37. de Silva, J. A. F., Bekersky, I., Puglisi, C. V., Brooks, M. A., and Weinfeld, R. E. (1976): Determination of 1,4-benzodiazepines and diazepin-2-ones in blood by electron capture gas liquid chromatography. *Anal. Chem.,* 48:10–19.
38. de Silva, J. A. F., Koechlin, B. A., and Bader, G. (1966): Blood level distribution patterns of diazepam and its major metabolite in man. *J. Pharm. Sci.,* 55:692–702.
39. de Silva, J. A. F., and Puglisi, C. V. (1970): Determination of medazepam (Nobrium), diazepam (Valium) and their major biotransformation products in blood and urine by electron capture GLC. *Anal. Chem.,* 42:1725–1736.
40. de Silva, J. A. F., Puglisi, C. V., and Munno, N. (1974): Determination of clonazepam and flunitrazepam in blood and urine by electron capture GLC. *J. Pharm. Sci.,* 63:520–527.
41. de Silva, J. A. F., Schwartz, M. A., Stefanovic, V., Kaplan, J., and D'Arconte, L. (1964): Determination of diazepam (Valium) in blood by gas liquid chromatography. *Anal. Chem.,* 36:2099–2105.
42. Dixon, W. R., Young, R. L., Ning, R., and Liebman, A. (1977): Radioimmunoassay of the anticonvulsant agent clonazepam. *J. Pharm. Sci.,* 66:235–237.
43. Dreifuss, F. E., Penry, J. K., Rose, S. W., Kupferberg, H. J., Dyken, P., and Sato, S. (1975): Serum clonazepam concentrations in children with absence seizures. *Neurology* (Minneap.), 25:255–258.
44. Eschenhoff, E. (1973): Metabolism of the anticonvulsant clonazepam in the rat, dog, and man. *Arzneim. Forsch.,* 23:390–400.
45. Fazio, C., Manfredi, M., and Piccinelli, A. (1975): Treatment of epileptic seizures with clonazepam—a reappraisal. *Arch. Neurol.,* 32:304–307.
46. Ferngren, H. G. (1974): Diazepam treatment for acute convulsions in children. *Epilepsia,* 15:27–37.
47. Garattini, S., Marcucci, F., Morselli, P. L., and Mussini, E. (1973): In *Biological Effects of Drugs in Relation to Their Plasma Concentrations,* edited by D. S. Davies and B. N. C. Prichard, pp. 211–225. Macmillan Publishers, London.
48. Garattini, S., Mussini, E., and Randall, L. O., editors (1973): *The Benzodiazepines.* Raven Press, New York.
49. Gaustaut, H., Courjon, R., Poire, R., and Weber, M. (1971): Treatment of status epilepticus with a new benzodiazepine more active than diazepam. *Epilepsia,* 12: 197–214.
50. Gastaut, H., Naquet, R., Poire, R., and Tassinari, C. A. (1965): Treatment of status epilepticus with diazepam (Valium). *Epilepsia,* 6:167–182.
51. Glasson, B., and Benakis, A. (1973): In *International Encyclopedia of Pharmacology and Therapeutics* (*IEPT*), Section 19, "Anticonvulsant Drugs," edited by J. Mercier, Vol. 1, pp. 273–292.
52. Greaves, M. S. (1974): Quantitative determination of medazepam, diazepam, and nitrazepam in whole blood by flame ionization gas liquid chromatography. *Clin. Chem.,* 20:141–147.
53. Greenblatt, D. J., and Shader, R. I. (1974): *Benzodiazepines in Clinical Practice.* Raven Press, New York.
54. Hailey, D. M. (1974): Chromatography of the 1,4-benzodiazepines. *J. Chromatogr.,* 98:527–568.
55. Howard, F. M., Seybold, M. E., and Reiber, J. (1968): The treatment of recurrent convulsions with intravenous injections of clonazepam. In *Medical Clinics of North*

America—Neurological Diseases, edited by R. E. Sickert, Vol. 52 (No. 4), pp. 977–987. W. B. Saunders Co., Philadelphia.
56. Kaplan, S. A., Alexander, K., Jack, M. L., Puglisi, C. V., de Silva, J. A. F., Lee, T. L., and Weinfeld, R. E. (1974): Pharmacokinetic profiles of clonazepam in dog and humans and of flunitrazepam in dog. *J. Pharm. Sci.,* 63:527–532.
57. Kaplan, S. A., Jack, M. L., Alexander, K., and Weinfeld, R. E. (1973): Pharmacokinetic profile of diazepam in man following single intravenous and oral and chronic oral administrations. *J. Pharm. Sci.,* 62:1789–1796.
58. Leitch, W. E., Stuart, L. P., and Forchielli, E. (1973): The use of lecithin as a priming agent in gas liquid chromatography with electron capture detection at the picogram level. *Anal. Biochem.,* 56:580–583.
59. Peskar, B., and Spector, S. (1973): Quantitative determination of diazepam in blood by radioimmunoassay. *J. Pharmacol. Exp. Ther.,* 186:167–172.
60. Randall, L. O., Schallek, W., Sternbach, L. H., and Ning, R. Y. (1974): Chemistry and pharmacology of the 1,4-benzodiazepines. *Med. Chem., A Ser. Monogr. (Psychopharmacological Agents, III),* 4:175–281.
61. Schwartz, M. A. (1973): Pathways of metabolism of the benzodiazepines. In *The Benzodiazepines,* edited by S. Garattini, E. Mussini, and L. O. Randall, pp. 53–74. Raven Press, New York.
62. Sjo, O., Hvidberg, E. F., Naestoft, J., and Lund, M. (1975): Pharmacokinetics and side effects of clonazepam and its 7-amino metabolite in man. *Eur. J. Clin. Pharmacol.,* 8:249–254.
63. Weinfeld, R. E., Posmanter, H., Koo, K.-C., and Puglisi, C. V. (1977): Rapid determination of diazepam and nordiazepam in plasma by EC-GLC: Application in clinical pharmacokinetic studies. *J. Chromatogr.* 143:581–595.

Antiepileptic Drugs: Quantitative Analysis and Interpretation, edited by C. E. Pippenger, J. K. Penry, and H. Kutt, Raven Press, New York, © 1978.

Chapter 12

Nitrogen-Selective Detectors: Application to Quantitation of Antiepileptic Drugs

H. Bryan Bente

Gas-liquid chromatography (GLC) has found many applications to therapeutic drug monitoring because it is a versatile technique that allows qualitative and quantitative analysis of a wide range of drugs. For some analyses, however, GLC techniques have been limited by insufficient detector sensitivity and selectivity. Most GLC procedures for therapeutic monitoring have involved the use of the flame ionization detector (FID). Such procedures have called for sample sizes of 1 to 2 ml in order to assure adequate detection limits, and the analysis of drugs for which the therapeutic levels are less than 1 mg/liter may not be feasible with this detector. In addition, extensive cleanup procedures may be required to avoid interference by other sample constituents. Other detectors having greater sensitivity and selectivity for the drugs of interest have been investigated. These include the electron capture (EC) detector and the nitrogen-phosphorus (N-P) detector.

Because most drugs are nitrogen-containing compounds, the nitrogen-phosphorus-selective detector has demonstrated potential in the field of therapeutic monitoring. The N-P detector uses the thermionic emission of alkali metal ions from a hot alkali metal salt to ionize nitrogen or phosphorus containing compounds. A detector that utilized this ionization method for nitrogen-containing compounds was first described and used in 1966 (2,16). Commercial detectors based on this principle followed. These detectors were modifications of the flame ionization detector in which the flame was used to heat an alkali halide salt. Because the flame temperature and geometry were too variable to provide a constant and uniform salt temperature, these early detectors were unstable and not suitable for routine work. Abel et al. (1) suggested electrically heating the alkali source, and this method has recently been used in commercial detectors (13). In addition, other alkali materials (13,15) have been substituted for the halide salts and have been found to give improved detector performance. These changes have made the detectors reliable, easy to use, and suitable for routine analyses.

A schematic diagram of the N-P detector is shown in Fig. 1. Basically this detector is a flame ionization detector modified by the addition of an electrically heated alkali source. Conversion from the N-P mode of operation to the standard FID mode may be accomplished by removing the alkali

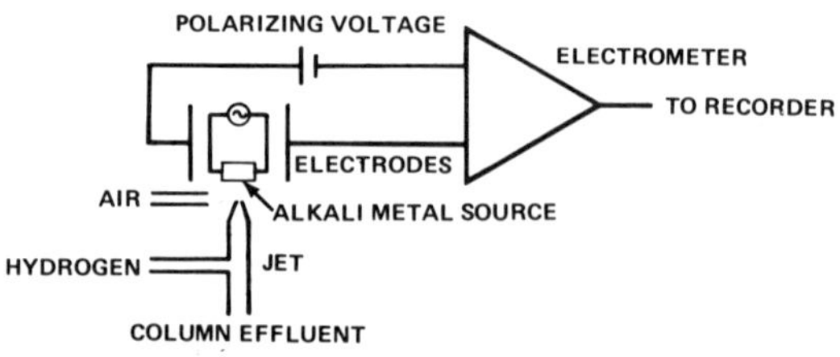

FIG. 1. Schematic diagram of the nitrogen-phosphorus detector. Thermionic emission from the electrically heated alkali source ionizes nitrogen- or phosphorus-containing sample molecules. Ions are collected at the electrodes, and the ion current is amplified by the electrometer.

source and adjusting the gas flows. Hydrogen and air are necessary for nitrogen detection, but the flows required are much lower in this mode (H_2 between 1 and 5 ml/min and air between 40 and 100 ml/min) than those required for flame ionization operation. The combustion and ionization reactions that normally occur in the flame do not proceed as efficiently in the N-P mode, and the response to organic molecules not containing nitrogen or phosphorus is greatly reduced. The N-P detector provides greater sensitivity to nitrogenous compounds than the FID, and it is selective in its response.

The sensitivity and selectivity of the N-P detector frequently make it possible to reduce sample size and to eliminate clean up steps. Least et al. (14), in adapting their FID procedure for theophylline (12) to an N-P detector, were able to reduce the sample size from 1 ml to 20 μl and to eliminate a back-extraction step. Micro methods have also been developed for many of the antiepileptic drugs (17,18). The chromatograms in Fig. 2 demonstrate the advantages provided by the N-P detector for the analysis of phenobarbital, primidone, and phenytoin. A 50-μl aliquot of an internal standard solution containing 20 mg/liter of 5-(*p*-methylphenyl)-5-ethylbarbituric acid (MPB) and 16 mg/liter of 5-(*p*-methylphenyl)-5-phenylhydantoin (MPPH) was added to 50 μl of plasma spiked with phenobarbital (5 mg/liter), primidone (2 mg/liter), and phenytoin (4 mg/liter). The plasma was buffered with 0.1 ml of 1 M phosphate buffer (pH 6.8) and the drugs extracted into 1 ml of methylene chloride. The methylene chloride was evaporated to dryness and the residue dissolved in 50 μl of 0.01M trimethylphenylammonium hydroxide (TMPAH) in methanol. A 2-μl sample was then injected into the chromatograph. The first chromatogram was run using an N-P detector; the second chromatogram was run under identical conditions with the detector in the flame ionization mode. These chromatograms show the enhanced sensitivity of the N-P detector and demonstrate the advantages of the selective detector in minimizing interfering peaks from the plasma.

The N-P detector has also been used to monitor drugs that have a therapeutic range too low for detection by a conventional FID. Bailey and Jatlow

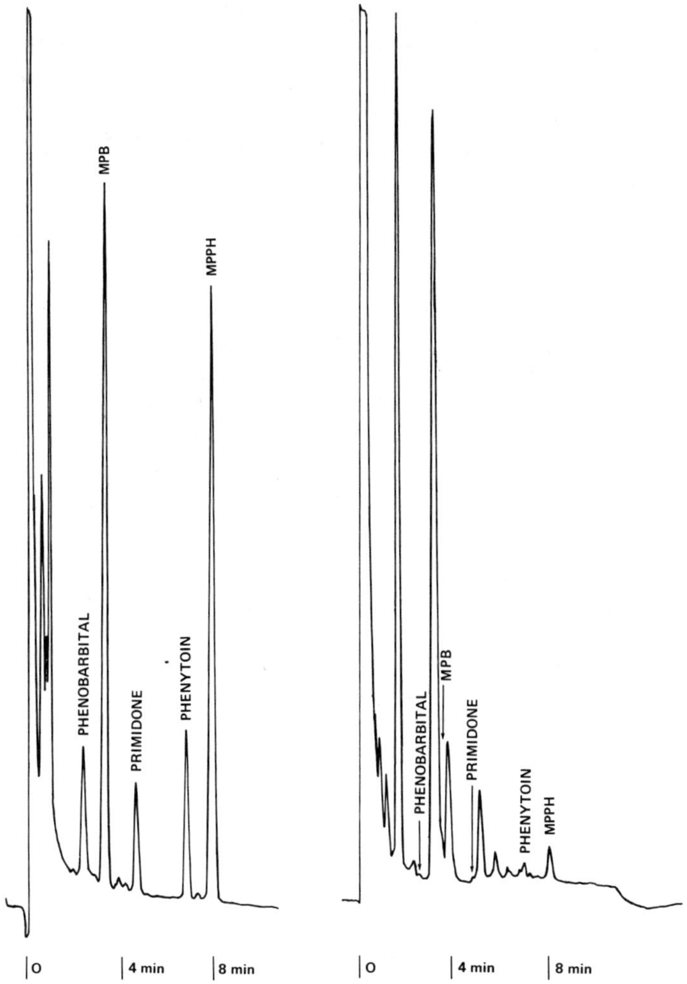

FIG. 2. Left: N-P detector range 1 attenuation 64. (32×10^{-10}; a full scale). Right: FID range 1 attenuation 64. Methyl derivatives of phenobarbital, primidone, and phenytoin extracted from 50 μl of plasma and analyzed with both an N-P detector and an FID. The conditions were identical for each chromatogram: 4-ft $\times$ 2-mm-i.d. glass column packed with 2% OV-17 on Chromosorb W-HP, 80–100 mesh; injection port at 250°C; detector at 300°C; He carrier gas at 30 ml/min; oven at 200°C for 2 min, then programmed to 240°C at 8°C/min. Hewlett-Packard Model 5730 gas chromatograph.

(3,4) have measured plasma levels of the tricyclic antidepressant drugs as low as 5 μg/liter using an N-P detector. Another class of drugs for which this detector shows potential is the 1,4-benzodiazepines. Sensitive analytical methods using GLC with EC detection have been developed for these drugs (6–11). These procedures may also be followed for use with the N-P detector.

Figure 3 shows the application of the N-P detector to the analysis of clonazepam in plasma. Nitrazepam was added to the spiked plasma as an internal standard and the drugs were extracted by the procedure of de Silva et al. (7). The derivatization procedure was modified to use 0.025 M tetrabutylammonium hydrogen sulfate (TBAHS) and 0.1 M TMPAH in methanol in place of the TBAHS-sodium hydroxide solution. The methanolic reagent

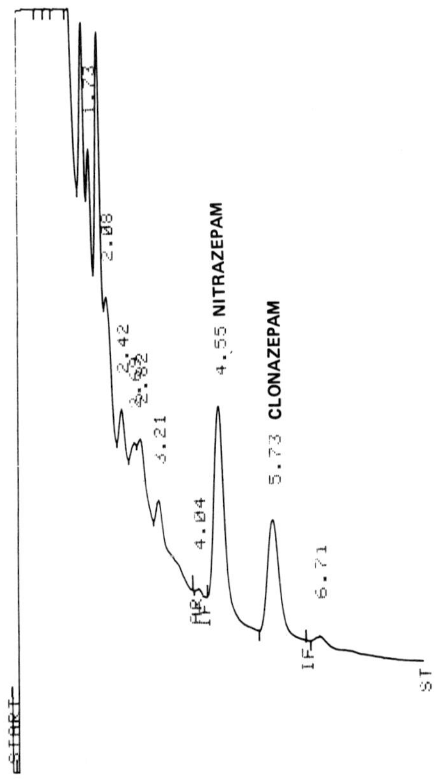

SERUM CLONAZEPAM CONCENTRATION: 25 μg/l
NITRAZEPAM INTERNAL STANDARD: 40 μg/l

HP RUN # 16 OCT/31/76 TIME 20:01:18
ISTD

RT	EXP RT	AREA	CAL #	AMT
4.55	4.56	15920	(R) 1	
5.73	5.71	11280	2	25.363

DIL FACTOR: 1.0000 E+ 0 ISTD AMT: 4.0000 E+ 1

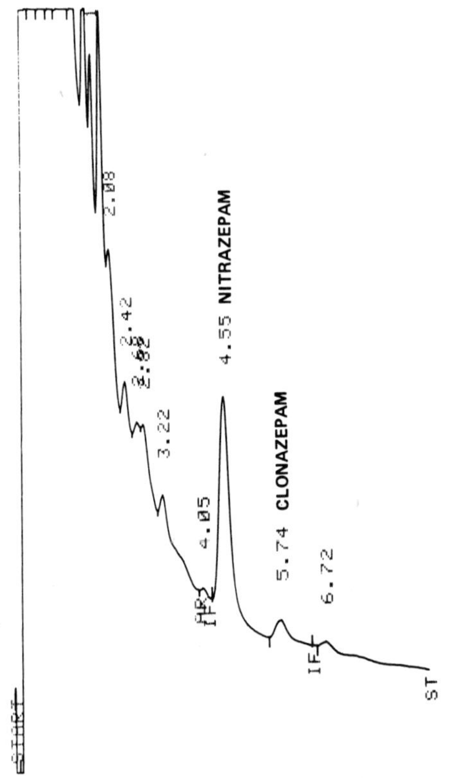

SERUM CLONAZEPAM CONCENTRATION: 5 μg/l
NITRAZEPAM INTERNAL STANDARD: 40 μg/l

HP RUN # 14 OCT/31/76 TIME 19:19:35
ISTD

RT	EXP RT	AREA	CAL #	AMT
4.55	4.56	17510	(R) 1	
5.74	5.71	2168	2	4.432

DIL FACTOR: 1.0000 E+ 0 ISTD AMT: 4.0000 E+ 1

FIG. 3. Serum extracts of clonazepam and nitrazepam as the methylderivatives. N-P detector response to the methyl derivatives of clonazepam and nitrazepam (internal standard) extracted from 1 ml of plasma. Chromatographic conditions: 4-ft × 2-mm-i.d. glass column packed with 2% OV-101 on Chromosorb W-HP, 100–120 mesh; injection port at 300°C; detector at 300°C; oven isothermal at 230°C; He carrier gas at 30 ml/min. Hewlett-Packard Model 5730 gas chromatograph. A Hewlett-Packard 3385 Automation System was used to record the chromatograms and to calculate the amount of clonazepam by the internal standard method.

was miscible in the benzene-methylene chloride phase, so the alkylation was not an extractive procedure. The methylation reaction mixture was heated to 65°C for 15 min to assure complete reaction. Spiked plasmas (5, 15, 25, 35, 45, 55, 65, and 75 μg/liter) were extracted and derivatized by this procedure and then were analyzed with both an N-P detector and an EC detector. The two methods were in good agreement, with a correlation coefficient of 0.996. Thus, the N-P detector is a viable alternative to the EC detector for the analysis of clonazepam.

Other benzodiazepines that have been analyzed by the N-P detector include diazepam and its N-desmethyl metabolite, flurazepam and its metabolites, and flurnitrazepam and metabolites (5). Benzodiazepines having a nitro group in the 7-position often have 7-amino metabolites (6). These metabolites do not give good EC response, but may be detected with the N-P detector. This capability should make the N-P detector an important addition to the EC detector for metabolic studies of the benzodiazepines.

The N-P detector should find many such applications in the field of therapeutic drug monitoring. Its sensitivity to most nitrogen-containing drugs is from 10 to 100 times greater than the sensitivity of the flame ionization detector.[1] The selectivity of the N-P detector frequently makes elaborate cleanup procedures unnecessary (see Fig. 2). Recent changes in detector design have made them easy to use and stable enough for routine use. However, there are still problems, usually chemical in origin, in the use of these detectors, which should be recognized and avoided.

Column adsorption can be a serious problem, especially when the detector is used with low sample concentrations. Solvents must be very pure, and each new lot should be checked. Chlorinated solvents may cause some loss of sensitivity and stability and are not recommended. Phosphate-containing laboratory detergents should be avoided; glassware should be acid washed, then rinsed with distilled water and a suitable solvent. Because the N-P detector is very sensitive to bleed from liquid phases containing cyano groups (OV-225, XE-60) or other nitrogen-containing groups, these should be avoided, as should columns and glass wool treated with phosphoric acid. The detector sensitivity is a strong function of carrier gas flow rate, which needs to be carefully regulated. Septums should be changed regularly. Bleed from heavily loaded ($> 5\%$) silicone columns and silanizing agents can contaminate the alkali material and decrease its useful lifetime. If silanization reactions are necessary, they should be carried out "off column" and the excess reagent removed prior to sample injection. "Ghost" peaks can arise from nicotine, for example, when cigarette smoke in the laboratory is adsorbed on the syringe needle. It has also been reported (14) that the stoppers used in some sample collection tubes contain a phosphate plasticizer, which

[1] Not all nitrogenous compounds give N-P detector response: Nitroglycerin is an example of a class of compounds that give no detector response.

may be extracted and then interfere with an analysis. These are some areas where analytical problems may arise, but with care and forethought they may be avoided and the N-P detector used for many kinds of routine analyses.

The N-P detector has been found to have many applications to therapeutic monitoring. For drugs such as phenobarbital and phenytoin, it is possible to use this detector to develop methods for micro samples. For drugs with lower therapeutic levels, such as the tricyclic antidepressants and the benzodiazepines, the detector has sufficient sensitivity for blood-level monitoring. The detector is very selective, and cleanup procedures can often be shortened when it is used. There are precautions that must be observed in using this detector, but with care, it may be used with success on a routine basis.

REFERENCES

1. Abel, K., Lanneau, K., and Stevens, R. K. (1966): Response characteristics of a new "stacked" flame ionization detector. *J. Assoc. Off. Anal. Chem.,* 49:1022–1027.
2. Aue, W. A., Gehrke, C. W., Tindle, R. C., Stalling, D. L., and Ruyle, C. D. (1967): Application of the alkali-flame detector to nitrogen containing compounds. *J. Gas Chromatogr.,* 5:381–382.
3. Bailey, D. N., and Jatlow, P. I. (1976): Gas-chromatographic analysis for therapeutic concentrations of amitriptyline and nortriptyline in plasma, with use of a nitrogen detector. *Clin. Chem.,* 22:777–781.
4. Bailey, D. N., and Jatlow, P. I. (1976): Gas-chromatographic analysis for therapeutic concentrations of imipramine and desipramine in plasma, with use of a nitrogen detector. *Clin. Chem.,* 22:1697–1701.
5. Bente, H. B. (1977): Application of the nitrogen-phosphorus detector to the analysis of 1,4-benzodiazepine drugs. Application Note ANGC 1-77, Hewlett-Packard Co., Avondale, Pa. (*unpublished data*).
6. de Silva, J. A. F., and Bekersky, I. (1974): Determination of clonazepam and flunitrazepam in blood by electron-capture gas-liquid chromatography. *J. Chromatogr.,* 99:447–460.
7. de Silva, J. A. F., Bekersky, I., Puglisi, C. V., Brooks, M. A., and Weinfeld, R. E. (1976): Determination of 1,4-benzodiazepines and -diazepin-2-ones in blood by electron-capture gas-liquid chromatography. *Anal. Chem.,* 48:10–19.
8. de Silva, J. A. F., and Puglisi, C. V. (1970): Determination of medazepam (Nobrium), diazepam (Valium) and their major biotransformation products in blood and urine by electron capture gas-liquid chromatography. *Anal. Chem.,* 42:1725–1736.
9. de Silva, J. A. F., Puglisi, C. V., Brooks, M. A., and Hackman, M. R. (1974): Determination of flurazepam (Dalmane®) and its major metabolites in blood by electron-capture gas-liquid chromatography and in urine by differential pulse polarography. *J. Chromatogr.,* 99:461–483.
10. Ehrsson, M., and Tilly, A. (1973): Electron capture gas chromatography of nitrazepam in human plasma as methyl derivatives. *Anal. Lett.,* 6:197–210.
11. Gerna, M., and Morselli, P. L. (1976): A simple and sensitive gas chromatographic method for the determination of clonazepam in human plasma. *J. Chromatogr.,* 116:445–450.
12. Johnson, G. F., Dechtiaruk, W. A., and Solomon, H. M. (1975): Gas-chromatographic determination of theophylline in human serum and saliva. *Clin. Chem.,* 21:144–147.
13. Kolb, B., and Bischoff, J. (1974): A new design of a thermionic nitrogen and phosphorus detector for GC. *J. Chromatogr. Sci.,* 12:625–629.

14. Least, C. J., Jr., Johnson, G. F., and Solomon, H. M. (1976): Gas-chromatographic micro-scale procedure for theophylline with use of a nitrogen-sensitive detector. *Clin. Chem.*, 22:765–768.
15. Prager, M. J., and Deblinger, B. (1967): Continuous monitoring of organophosphorus compounds in air with an alkali metal-dual flame ionization detector. *Environ. Sci. Tech.*, 1:1008–1010.
16. Ruyle, C. D., Aue, W. A., Gehrke, C. W., Stalling, D. L., and Tindle, R. C. (1966): Improved detection of nitrogen compounds. Presented at the 5th National Meeting, Society for Applied Spectroscopy, Chicago, Ill.
17. Toseland, P. A., Albani, M., and Gauchel, F. D. (1975): Organic nitrogen-selective detector used in gas-chromatographic determination of some anticonvulsant and barbiturate drugs in plasma and tissues. *Clin. Chem.*, 21:98–103.
18. Vandemark, F. L., and Adams, R. F. (1976): Ultramicro gas-chromatographic analysis for anticonvulsants, with use of a nitrogen-selective detector. *Clin. Chem.*, 22:1062–1065.

Antiepileptic Drugs: Quantitative Analysis and Interpretation, edited by C. E. Pippenger, J. K. Penry, and H. Kutt, Raven Press, New York, © 1978.

Chapter 13
Gas-Liquid Chromatographic Quantitation of Valproic Acid

Harvey J. Kupferberg

Valproic acid (2-propylpentanoic acid, Depakene) was synthesized almost a century ago, but it was not until 1963 that Meunier and co-workers (3) discovered its anticonvulsant activity. Its structure is radically different from that of other commonly used antiepileptic drugs. Over the last decade, valproic acid has gained wide popularity in Europe for the treatment of absence and generalized seizures, and it is now being evaluated for efficacy in the United States in phase III clinical studies. The drug is usually administered as valproate sodium, although valproate magnesium or valproic acid amide are also used. The valproate sodium is hydroscopic and must be kept free from moisture. The free acid is a clear liquid with a pK_a of 4.5.

Pharmacokinetic studies have shown that valproate sodium is rapidly absorbed following oral administration, usually reaching peak blood levels within 2 hr. The serum half-life ranges from 7 to 15 hr in adults and is slightly shorter in children. A dose of 20 mg/kg in adults results in a blood level of 60 to 130 μg/ml, depending on the frequency of administration and the time of sampling (5). The therapeutic range has not been determined, but it appears to be above 60 μg/ml in some types of seizures.

Only a small amount of unchanged valproate is excreted in the urine, and the major metabolites are a glucuronide of the acid or products of side-chain oxidation.

Methods of analysis for valproic acid do not differ from those used for short-chain fatty acids. Meijer and Hessing-Brand (2), using a microdiffusion technique, were the first to quantitate valproic acid in patients. A 5% FFAP column and 3,3,5-trimethylcaproic acid used as the internal standard were the basis of this quantitative gas chromatographic method. Dijkhuis and Vervloet (1) simplified the analysis by extracting valproic acid from acidified plasma into a small volume of chloroform and injecting 1 to 2 μl of the organic solvent into the gas chromatograph. Naphthenic acid (cyclohexane carboxylic acid) was used as the internal standard. Schobben and van der Kleijn (7) modified this method, using acetophenone as the internal standard.

Recently, Schmidt and colleagues (6) studied the interlaboratory variability of valproate determinations in plasma in 13 research laboratories.

Only 4 of the 13 laboratories had a majority of their results within the 95% confidence limits for each sample. The overall variability of the values was 15.8%. This value is within the range for the determination of phenytoin and phenobarbital in five reference laboratories used in a study of interlaboratory variability by Pippenger et al. (4). The method outlined below gave excellent results for determination of valproic acid in the interlaboratory variability study.

MATERIALS

Column packing was 10% SP-1000 on Chromosorb W 100/120 or 10% D.E.G.S.-SP on Chromosorb W 100/120 (Supelco, Inc., Bellefonte, Pa.). Perchloric acid was made 10% from 70% reagent-grade acid. Chloroform, reagent grade, was used without further purification. Cyclohexane carboxylic acid, 25 μl dissolved in chloroform, was used as an internal standard (Aldrich Chemical Co., Milwaukee, Wi.). Isoamyl acetate was obtained from Fisher Scientific (Fair Lawn, N.J.).

EQUIPMENT

A Hewlett-Packard model 5830 or 5700 gas chromatograph was equipped with flame ionization detectors. Four-foot coiled columns were packed with either 10% D.E.G.S. or 10% SP-1000. The phases were conditioned at 225°C with carrier gas flow for 24 hr. The gas chromatographic conditions were as follows: injection port temperature, 200°C, detector temperature, 300°C; oven temperature, 155°C (D.E.G.S.) or 190°C (SP-1000); nitrogen as a carrier, 25 ml/min; hydrogen, 30 ml/min; air, 240 ml/min. Care must be taken not to exceed the temperature limitations of these two phases.

EXTRACTION PROCEDURE

One-half milliliter of plasma, 25 μl of internal standard solution, and 0.1 ml of 10% perchloric acid were combined with 8 ml of chloroform in a glass-stoppered 13-ml centrifuge tube. The mixture was placed in a shaker for 10 min at 160 cycles/min. The tubes were then centrifuged at 2,000 rpm and the upper, aqueous phase was removed by aspiration. Approximately 7 ml of the remaining organic phase were transferred to a new centrifuge tube and 75 to 100 μl of isoamyl acetate were then added. The chloroform was then removed under water vacuum with the aid of a Buchler Rotary Evapomix. The temperature of the evaporator's water bath can be raised to 30°C without evaporation loss of drug or internal standard. One to two microliters of the residual isoamyl acetate were used for the analysis.

DISCUSSION

Several reports have recently described the gas chromatographic analysis of valproic acid. Most of these methods use a liquid phase traditionally used for the analysis of fatty acids. In the method reported here, both D.E.G.S. and SP-1000 were found to be suitable, but D.E.G.S. appears to be a better choice because of the lower oven temperatures required to accomplish the analysis. A 35°C difference (155°C for D.E.G.S. and 190°C for SP-1000) was found to give equivalent retention times for valproic acid and its internal standard. SP-1000 has the advantage of allowing valproic acid and ethosuximide to be determined simultaneously within 9 min. The same analysis using D.E.G.S. requires approximately 16 min. We have used SP-1000 in a study comparing the efficacy of valproic acid and ethosuximide. A chromatogram of a plasma extract from a patient receiving both valproic acid and ethosuximide is shown in Fig. 1A. Figure 1B is a chromatogram from a patient receiving only ethosuximide.

The relationship between the peak areas of valproic acid and the internal standard is linear between 5 and 60 μg of valproic acid added to plasma and then extracted (Fig. 2). More than 95% of valproic acid is recovered from plasma.

The choice of internal standard is important. It should have physical properties similar to those of valproic acid. Cyclohexane carboxylic acid,

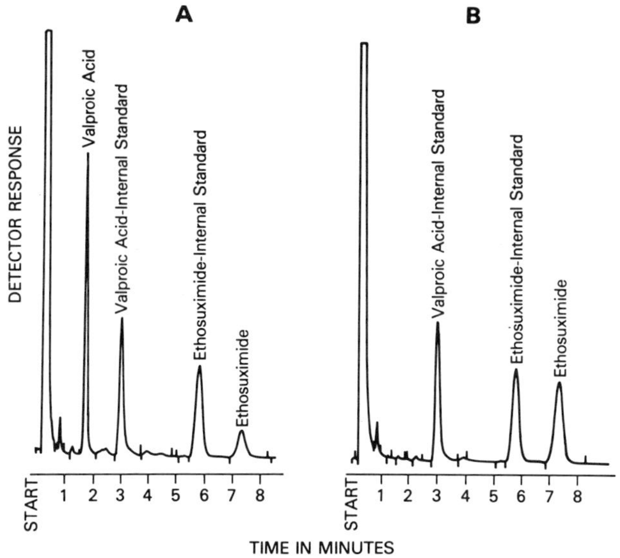

FIG. 1. A chromatogram of a plasma extract from a patient receiving (A) valproic acid and ethosuximide, and from a patient receiving (B) ethosuximide only.

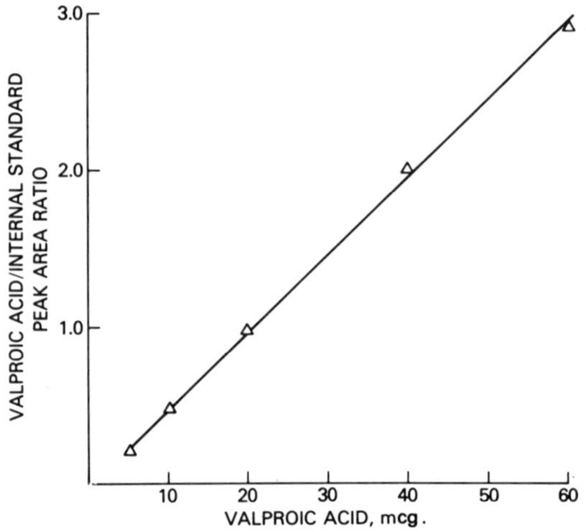

FIG. 2. Peak area ratio of valproic acid to internal standard as a function of valproic acid added to 1 ml of plasma and then extracted. Each dot represents the mean of four determinations (mcg = μg).

3,3,5-trimethylcaproic acid, or other analogs of valproic acid may be used.

Several other phases, such as FFAP (carbowax mixed with 2-nitroterephthalic acid), ethylene glycol adipate, or diethylene glycol adipate can also be used, but they suffer from temperature instability. Silicon phases have been used but tend to give nonsymmetrical peak shape. Alterations in peak shape and loss of sensitivity do occur with D.E.G.S. and SP-1000. These result from destruction in front of the column by plasma constituents extracted by chloroform. Replacement of the front 3 in. of the column packing quickly brings the column back to its original efficiency.

SUMMARY

The method described for the gas-liquid chromatographic quantitation of valproic acid has been found to give precise results in a study of interlaboratory variability among 13 laboratories. The method is rapid, and 30 samples can easily be analyzed daily. A variety of liquid phases and internal standards can be used. SP-1000 was found to be useful for the simultaneous determination of valproic acid and ethosuximide, two agents used in the treatment of absence seizures.

REFERENCES

1. Dijkhuis, I. C., and Vervloet, E. (1974): Rapid determination of the antiepileptic drug di-*n*-propylacetic acid in serum. *Pharm. Weekbl.,* 109:1–4.
2. Meijer, J. W. A., and Hessing-Brand, L. (1973): Determination of lower fatty acids, particularly of the antiepileptic dipropylacetic acid, in biological materials by means of micro-diffusion and gas chromatography. *Clin. Chim. Acta,* 43:215.

3. Meunier, G., Carraz, G., Meunier, Y., Eymard, P., and Aimard, M. (1963): Proprietes pharmacodynamiques de l'acide *n*-dipropylacetique. *Therapie,* 18:435.
4. Pippenger, C. E., Penry, J. K., White, B. G., Daly, D. D., and Buddington, R. (1976): Interlaboratory variability in determination of plasma antiepileptic drug concentrations. *Arch. Neurol.,* 33:351–355.
5. Redenbaugh, J. E., Sato, S., Dreifuss, F. E., and Penry, J. K. (1977): Sodium valproate: Pharmacokinetics and efficacy in patients with intractable seizures. Unpublished data.
6. Schmidt, D., Ferrandes, B., Grandjean, D., Gugler, R., Jakobs, C., Johannessen, S., Klotz, U., Kochen, W., Kupferberg, H. J., Meijer, J. W. A., Richens, A., Schafer, H., Schulz, H. U., and Windorfer, A. (1977): Interlaboratory variability of valproic acid determinations. *Arzneim. Forsch.,* 27:1078–1081.
7. Schobben, F., and van der Kleijn, E. (1974): Determination of sodium di-*n*-propylacetate in plasma by gas-liquid chromatography. *Pharm. Weekbl.,* 109:30–33.

Antiepileptic Drugs: Quantitative Analysis and Interpretation, edited by C. E. Pippenger, J. K. Penry, and H. Kutt, Raven Press, New York, © 1978.

Chapter 14

High-Pressure Liquid Chromatography in Quantitation of Antiepileptic Drugs

Gerald L. Hawk and Louis C. Franconi

The drug metabolism rate of a patient on long-term chemotherapy can change radically over the period of time during which the drug is administered. This change can cause corresponding changes in the concentration of the drug in the patient's blood, resulting in, among other things, a toxic condition or a recurrence of the disease symptoms. To prevent these effects, serum or plasma levels of a drug are measured periodically. The dosage can then be adjusted to compensate for changes in the observed metabolism.

Commonly used methods of measuring drug levels include infrared (IR) and ultraviolet (UV) spectrophotometry, radioimmunoassay (RIA), enzyme immunoassay (EMIT), gas-liquid chromatography (GLC), thin-layer chromatography (TLC) and, more recently, high-performance liquid chromatography (LC). The ideal procedure for determining anticonvulsant drug levels would be one that provides for a rapid, reliable, economical quantitation, in a micro-scale sample, of all of the commonly used drugs. As evidenced by the frequency of publication of new methods for these assays, the desired goal has not yet been reached.

ANTICONVULSANT DRUG LEVELS

Serum or plasma levels of anticonvulsant drugs are valuable in clinical management of epilepsy to determine adequacy of therapy as well as to determine toxicity. It is not feasible to estimate a patient's drug level by prescribed dosage or clinical observation alone, since extremely high levels may be well tolerated by some individuals without signs of toxicity, whereas others develop very high, even toxic levels on low dosage. In some instances, the toxic state may reinduce seizure activity. Kutt and Penry (18) recently reviewed a number of publications that emphasize the usefulness of determining blood levels of antiepileptic drugs in the clinical management of patients with epilepsy. The data from several studies indicated that therapy guided by monitoring the blood levels decreased, by as much as 50%, the number of patients whose seizures were poorly controlled, as compared with empirical treatment periods (5,8,21). However, it has been stated: "Clearly, the best therapeutic results will be obtained when clinical judgement is combined with laboratory information" (18). Several review articles and books (20,25) deal further with the therapeutic drug levels as well as absorption and metabolism of the various drugs, and these topics are not pursued here.

IMMUNOASSAYS

Radioimmunoassays and enzyme immunoassays are rapid and applicable to micro-scale samples, but have the disadvantage of relatively high cost and the limitation of requiring separate assay systems for each anticonvulsant drug (7). Brunk et al. (6) reported the adaptation of the "EMIT" technique for serum phenobarbital and phenytoin assays to the miniature centrifugal analyzer. McClean et al. (19) reported the use of a fully mechanized enzyme analyzer for determining serum levels of primidone, phenobarbital, and phenytoin.

Some researchers have indicated that immunoassays could replace gas-liquid chromatography as the reference procedure for anticonvulsants. However, McClean et al. (19) stated, "We do not agree. The poorer precision relative to gas-liquid chromatography for all three drugs (those indicated in preceding paragraph) and the susceptibility of the phenobarbital assay to interferences would seem to preclude its use as a reference method." However, more data are needed on the use of the immunoassay techniques before any final conclusions can be made.

GAS-LIQUID CHROMATOGRAPHY

There has been an almost continuous evolution of the improvement of GLC procedures for the analysis of anticonvulsant drugs. Solow et al. (23) recently reviewed the methods of using GLC on-column methylation for simultaneous determination of multiple drug therapy. The alkylation techniques discussed in most instances were preferable to direct injection of the underivatized sample extracts, since the later compounds can produce asymmetric peaks and frequently exhibit less stability at the high temperatures required for separation. Most of the anticonvulsants give greater detector response as methyl esters than when the underivatized samples are injected into the GLC. Other investigators (13) have based their analytical procedures on the use of a selective ion detection method that uses gas chromatograph-mass spectrometer-computer systems to enhance sensitivity and specificity of detection. More recently, some researchers (1,9) have described a rapid method for precisely measuring concentrations of phenobarbital, phenytoin, carbamazepine, primidone, and/or ethosuximide. The percentage of drug recovered varied depending on the extraction method employed, but the method of Abraham and Joslin (1) exhibited excellent GLC results for the first four drugs listed above. For pediatric cases, only 0.2 ml of serum was required and the analyses were completed in less than

30 min. Almost monthly, new strategies using GLC to quantify anticonvulsants are reported and, during the last few years, some investigators have started to use another form of chromatography—high-pressure liquid chromatography (HPLC).

LIQUID CHROMATOGRAPHY VERSUS GAS CHROMATOGRAPHY

What are the similarities and differences between these two forms of chromatography? What analogies of gas and liquid chromatography are there?

Both techniques are chromatographic separation processes in which the fundamental concepts and the relationships are the same. Although the chromatographic process is exceedingly complex, it is possible to devise simple models and equations that closely approximate the separation. An understanding of these simple equations or relationships can be of importance to the practitioner (17).

If insufficient resolution is obtained in a given chromatogram, a worker needs to select a new set of conditions to improve the separation. He can select from an infinite variety and, if given sufficient time, should be able to pick a reasonable set of conditions to obtain a satisfactory separation. However, with some knowledge of the fundamentals of separation in chromatography, logic can be used, and a new set of conditions can be chosen that will significantly decrease the amount of time and effort required to find the best of better separation conditions.

Chromatography basically involves separations due to differences in the equilibrium distribution of sample components between two different phases. One of these phases is a moving or mobile phase and the other is a stationary phase.

The sample components migrate through the chromatographic system only when they are in the mobile phase. The velocity of migration of a component is a function of equilibrium distribution. The components having distributions favoring the stationary phase migrate slower than those having distributions favoring the mobile phase. Separation then results from different velocities of migration as a consequence of difference in equilibrium distributions.

Gas and liquid chromatography are both separation processes governed to the first approximation by the same general rules. Gas chromatography separations are based on vapor pressure. Liquid chromatography separations are based on solubility. The choice of the carrier gas used as the mobile phase in gas chromatography is dictated mainly by the type of detector or sensor being used to monitor the effluent from the column. The separation will be similar whether one uses hydrogen, helium, or nitrogen as the carrier. With liquid chromatography, the mobile phase or the composition of the

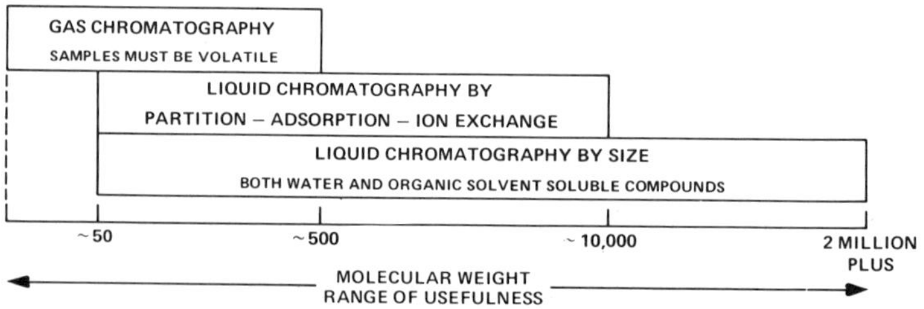

	GAS	LIQUID
MOVING PHASE	COMPRESSIBLE	NON COMPRESSIBLE
DIFFUSION	FAST	SLOW
MASS TRANSFER RESISTANCE	SMALL	LARGE
TEMPERATURE	PRIMARY	SECONDARY
VAPOR PRESSURE	PRIMARY	SECONDARY
SOLUBILITY (STA. PHASE)	PRIMARY	SECONDARY
SOL. IN MOVING PHASE	UNIMPORTANT	PRIMARY
SOLUTE VOLUME LITERS/MOL	22.4	0.2 → 2.0

2569

FIG. 1. Gas-liquid properties affecting chromatography.

mobile phase is of prime importance in the separation. It makes a great deal of difference whether one uses normal hexane, acetonitrile, or water as the moving phase.

In liquid chromatography the mobile phase is relatively noncompressible. Diffusion in the mobile phase is extremely low. Because of this low diffusion in the mobile phase, high-speed liquid chromatography is possible. In addition, the effects of temperature are only of secondary importance, and resistance to mass transfer in a liquid is very high. The various properties affecting gas-liquid chromatography are summarized in Fig. 1.

ELEMENTS OF MODERN LIQUID CHROMATOGRAPHS

A complete liquid chromatographic system with certain optional components is shown schematically in Fig. 2. The basic liquid chromatograph consists of a source of solvent, a single pump system to deliver solvent continuously at selected flow rates through the system, provision for injecting the sample into the system (either manually or automatically), columns, detectors for monitoring the separation, and some device for permanently recording the nature and degree of the separation. The detectors employed, either singly or in series, are UV and/or visible spectrophotometers, fluorescence monitor, electrochemical detector, and a differential refractometer.

In many instances it is necessary to change operating conditions during the course of the separation in order to refine the separation or provide selective separation of specific components. In these circumstances, it is necessary to employ programming. Programming is a method in which a separate external device controls the rate at which the solvent is pumped or, with the addition of a second pumping system, as shown in Fig. 2, regulates the composition of the moving solvent according to a specified program

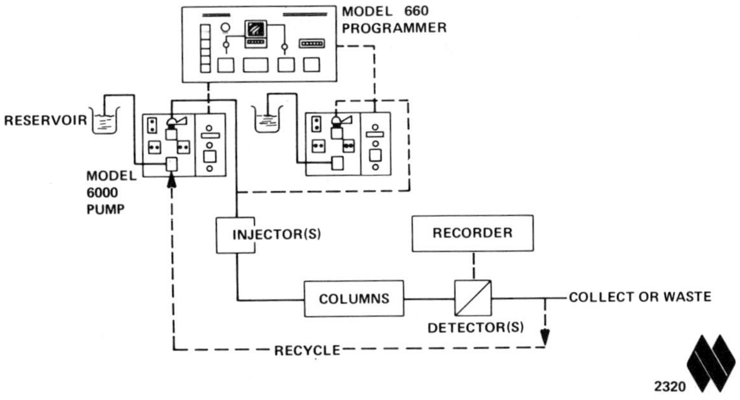

FIG. 2. Schematic diagram of a complete liquid chromatography system.

during the separation. Solvent composition or pH can be varied over preselected time intervals and concentration ranges.

The most advanced pumping systems used in modern liquid chromatographs deliver solvent at a constant flow rate regardless of changes in system back-pressure. This ensures reproducibility and permits the identification of components based on the volume of solvent required to elute a specific component, once a standard has been established. A high-performance solvent delivery system that provides the necessary capabilities is diagrammed in Fig. 2. It delivers flow rates up to 9.9 ml/min, the flow rate being adjustable in 0.1-ml/min increments, has high-pressure capability to a maximum of 6,000 psi, and has a very small positive displacement volume with provision for external solvent supply. These latter factors ensure rapid solvent change-over plus other efficiencies such as use of the recycle technique. Recycling is a method for increasing the effective length of columns to improve the degree of separation without actually using more lengths of column. The newer high-performance liquid chromatographic components described herein are designed to allow use of the recycling technique. Operating flexibility of the components ensures that much of the time spent on nonoperating support activities, such as adding columns, changing solvents, mixing solvent, evaluating various solvent ratios in the course of refining the separation, and other related operations, can now be reduced or virtually eliminated.

Lastly, the separated compounds of a mixture can be recovered intact via a fraction collector for subsequent chemical, physical, and/or biological analysis since LC separations are virtually nondestructive.

WHAT IS LIQUID CHROMATOGRAPHY?

Basically, liquid chromatography is a means of separating mixtures into their individual components. Any sample that can be dissolved in a suitable liquid can be separated by liquid chromatography. There are no requirements of volatility and no limitations on molecular weight.

Dissolved samples are carried by a solvent through a packed bed (a column) of separating medium (the column packing material) at flow rates regulated by a high-pressure, constant-flow pumping system. Chemical or mechanical interactions among the sample, solvent, and column packing material differ for each sample component. These differences result in separation of the sample components as they pass through the packed column.

On emerging from the column, the eluent flows through a detector(s), which monitors the difference (usually in absorbance or refractive index) between the solvent and the eluting sample component. A permanent record of the detector(s) output is provided by a strip-chart recorder that plots detector response versus time. Since this response is linearly related to the concentration of the particular compound eluting, the chromatogram obtained can be used to provide quantitative information on the sample components.

As mentioned earlier, the interactions among sample, solvent, and column packing material are the basis of every LC separation. The nature of these interactions determines the type of liquid chromatography used. Three different LC modes—ion exchange, normal phase, and reverse phase chromatography—have been used to determine serum anticonvulsant concentrations.

In ion exchange chromatography, the ionic sample components are attracted to charged column packing material particles. Changes in the solvent ionic strength or pH during the course of the chromatographic run are usually necessary to effect complete separations. Separation depends on differences in the pK_a's of the sample components.

In normal phase chromatography, the separating medium is highly polar (e.g., silica) and the solvent is nonpolar. Differences in the adsorption and desorption rates of the various sample components cause separations. Elution in this type of chromatography is in order of increasing polarity.

In reverse phase chromatography, a nonpolar separating medium (e.g., μ Bondapak C_{18}) is employed with a polar solvent. Most reverse phase systems operate by a mixture of adsorption and partitioning mechanisms, with partitioning of the sample components between the solvent and the packing material surface being most important. Elution is in order of decreasing polarity. Of the three types of liquid chromatography mentioned here, reverse phase LC is the most versatile and most widely used.

The next section briefly describes an LC determination of serum anticonvulsant levels and lists some of the advantages of this technique.

LC OF ANTICONVULSANT DRUGS

A number of recent publications have reported the use of LC for the analysis of anticonvulsant drugs. Anders and LaTorre (3) used high-speed ion exchange chromatography to separate barbiturates, phenytoin, and metabolites of these compounds. Normal phase chromatography (porous small particle silica) was used in the LC method of Atwell et al. (4) and Evans (11), but the procedure required extensive sample preparation before injecting the sample into the LC. A similar rapid LC method was reported by Westenberg and De Zeeuw (24) and Gauchel et al. (12) but was used to assay carbamazepine only. Another normal phase method was also used for the simultaneous determination of carbamazepine and its active metabolite (carbamazepine 10,11-epoxide) in plasma with the lower limit of sensitivity about 4 ng and 40 ng for the drug and its metabolite, respectively (10).

Kabra et al. (14) more recently reported a μPorasil separation for the simultaneous determination of phenobarbital, phenytoin, and primidone in whole blood and plasma. After preparing the sample by extraction, the three drugs were separated in less than 10 min and the lower limits of detection were 100 ng for primidone, 200 ng for phenytoin, and 300 ng for phenobarbital when monitored at 254 nm. The LC method, when compared to the GLC method, reported a correlation coefficient of >0.98. The LC method was also found to be applicable for pediatric samples of 100 to 500 μl of whole blood or plasma.

Several reverse phase methods have also been reported for the measurement of anticonvulsant levels. Adams and Vandemark (2) developed a procedure that, including the extraction steps, required only 20 min to monitor simultaneously phenobarbital, phenytoin, primidone, ethosuximide, methsuximide, and carbamazepine. The eluted drugs were monitored at 195 nm and sensitivities of 0.1 mg/liter were routinely attained for 0.5-ml serum samples for all drugs except ethosuximide (0.5 mg/liter). Using reverse phase chromatography, Kabra and Martin also reported the LC determination of carbamazepine in blood or plasma (15) and a method to monitor

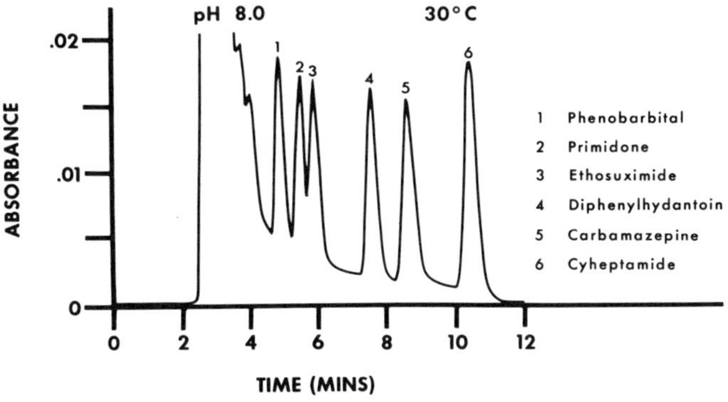

FIG. 3. Chromatogram showing typical anticonvulsant separation on Waters Associates ALC/GPC 204 equipped with variable wavelength detector (200 nm), μ Bondapak C_{18} column, flow rate 0.8 ml/min of 0.01 M KH_2PO_4 (pH 8.0)/CH_3CN (1:1) at 30°C. (Contributed by Steven J. Soldin, Ph.D., The Hospital for Sick Children, Toronto, Ontario, Canada.)

TABLE 1. *Between-day precision by replicate analysis*

Compound	*n*	concentration (mg/liter)	CV%
Phenobarbital	10	15	7.7
	14	33	4.3
Primidone	10	11	7.5
	14	24	4.3
Ethosuximide	10	33	5.0
	14	69	4.9
Phenytoin	10	11	4.4
	14	23	2.4
Carbamazepine	10	7	6.6
	14	15	6.2

Contributed by Steven J. Soldin, Ph.D., The Hospital for Sick Children, Toronto, Ontario, Canada.

the main metabolite of phenytoin [5-(4-hydroxyphenyl)-5 phenylhydantoin] in human urine (16).

The reverse phase method of Soldin and Hill (22) has been in use at the Hospital for Sick Children in Toronto for over 14 months, and over 6,500 drug analyses have been performed. A typical anticonvulsant separation is shown in Fig. 3. The between-day precision by replicate analysis for the five anticonvulsants is shown in Table 1. The total analysis time, including sample preparation, is approximately 10 min, and this method only requires 25 μl of serum or plasma.

Clinically, the differences in the results obtained with GC and LC are insignificant. The LC method, however, has several advantages over other currently used methods. These advantages include faster separation, lack of derivatization, better sample stability, and smaller sample size.

The advantages of LC also apply to monitoring other drugs in plasma and other body fluids. In addition, liquid chromatography permits rapid determinations of many endogenous compounds. Such rapid and reliable analyses will play an increasingly important role in clinical chemistry.

ACKNOWLEDGMENTS

The authors express their appreciation to Dr. J. G. Hill and Dr. S. J. Soldin of the Hospital for Sick Children, Toronto, Canada, for providing previously unpublished data. Also, special thanks go to our secretary, Cecile Jennings, for typing this manuscript.

REFERENCES

1. Abraham, C. V., and Joslin, H. D. (1976): Simultaneous gas-chromatographic analysis for phenobarbital, diphenylhydantoin, carbamazepine, and primidone in serum. *Clin. Chem.*, 22:769–771.

2. Adams, R. F., and Vandemark, F. L. (1976): Simultaneous high-pressure liquid-chromatographic determination of some anticonvulsants in serum. *Clin. Chem.*, 22:25–31.
3. Anders, M. W., and LaTorre, J. P. (1970): High speed ion exchange chromatography of barbiturates, diphenylhydantoin, and their hydroxylated metabolites. *Anal. Chem.*, 42:1430–1432.
4. Atwell, S. H., Green, V. A., and Haney, W. G. (1975): Development and evaluation of method for simultaneous determination of phenobarbital and diphenylhydantoin in plasma by high pressure liquid chromatography. *J. Pharm. Sci.*, 64:806–809.
5. Borofsky, L. G., Louis, S., and Kutt, H. (1973): Diphenylhydantoin in children: Pharmacology and efficacy. *Neurology* (Minneap.), 23:967–972.
6. Brunk, S. D., Hadjiioannou, T. P., and Malmstadt, H. V. (1976): Adaptation of "EMIT" technique for serum phenobarbital and diphenylhydantoin assays to the miniature centrifugal analyzer. *Clin. Chem.*, 22:905–907.
7. Cleeland, R., Christenson, J., Usategui-Gomez, J., Heveran, J., Davis, R., and Grunberg, E. (1976): Detection of drugs, of abuse, by radioimmunoassay: A summary of published data and some new information. *Clin. Chem.*, 22:712–725.
8. Dawson, K. P., and Jamieson, A. (1971): Value of blood phenytoin estimation in management of childhood epilepsy. *Arch. Dis. Child.*, 46:386–388.
9. Dorrity, F., Jr., and Linnoila, M. (1976): Rapid gas-chromatographic measurement of anticonvulsant drugs in serum. *Clin. Chem.*, 22:860–862.
10. Eichelbaum, M., and Bertilsson, L. (1975): Determination of carbamazepine and its epoxide metabolite in plasma by high-speed liquid chromatography. *J. Chromatogr.*, 103:135–140.
11. Evans, J. E. (1973): Simultaneous measurement of diphenylhydantoin and phenobarbital in serum by high performance liquid chromatography. *Anal. Chem.*, 45:2428–2429.
12. Gauchel, G., Gauchel, F. D., and Birkofer, L. (1973): A micromethod for the determination of carbamazepine in blood by high speed liquid chromatography. *Z. Klin. Chem. Klin. Biochem.*, 11:459–460.
13. Horning, M. G., Lertratanang Koon, K., Nowlin, J., Stilwell, W. G., Stilwell, R. N., Zion, T. E., Kellaway, P., and Hill, R. M. (1974): Anticonvulsant drug monitoring by GC-MS-COM techniques. *J. Chromatogr. Sci.*, 12:630–635.
14. Kabra, P. K., Gotelli, G., Stanfill, R., and Marton, L. J. (1976): Simultaneous measurement of phenobarbital, diphenylhydantoin, and primidone in blood by high-pressure liquid chromatography. *Clin. Chem.*, 22:824–827.
15. Kabra, P. K., and Marton, L. J. (1976): Determination of carbamazepine in blood or plasma by high-pressure liquid chromatography. *Clin. Chem.*, 22:1070–1072.
16. Kabra, P. K., and Marton, L. J. (1976): High-pressure liquid chromatographic determination of 5-(4-hydroxyphenyl)-5-phenylhydantoin in human urine. *Clin. Chem.*, 22:1672–1674.
17. Kirkland, J. J., editor (1971): *Modern Practice of Liquid Chromatography.* Wiley-Interscience, New York.
18. Kutt, H., and Penry, K. (1974): Usefulness of blood levels of antiepileptic drugs. *Arch. Neurol.*, 31:283–288.
19. McClean, S. W., Young, D. S., and Yonekawa, W. (1977): Anticonvulsants in serum, determined with a fully mechanized enzyme analyzer. *Clin. Chem.*, 23:116–118.
20. Penry, J. K., Smith, L. D., and White, B. G. (1972): *Blood Level Determinations of Antiepileptic Drugs: Clinical Value and Methods.* NINDS Bibliography Series No. 2. DHEW Publication No. (NIH) 73–396. U.S. Government Printing Office, Washington, D.C.
21. Sherwin, A. L., Robb, J. P., and Lechter, M. (1973): Improved control of epilepsy by monitoring plasma ethosuximide. *Arch. Neurol.*, 28:178–181.
22. Soldin, S. J., and Hill, J. G. (1976): Rapid micromethod for measuring anticonvulsant drugs in serum by high-performance liquid chromatography. *Clin. Chem.*, 22:856–859.
23. Solow, E. B., Metaxas, J. M., and Summers, T. R. (1974): Antiepileptic drugs: A

current assessment of simultaneous determination of multiple drug therapy by gas-liquid chromatography on column methylation. *J. Chromatogr. Sci.*, 12:256–260.
24. Westenberg, H. G. M., and De Zeeuw, R. A. (1976): Rapid and sensitive liquid chromatographic determination of carbamazepine suitable for use in monitoring multiple-drug anticonvulsant therapy. *J. Chromatogr.*, 118:217–224.
25. Woodbury, D. M., Penry, J. K., and Schmidt, R. P., editors (1972): *Antiepileptic Drugs*. Raven Press, New York.

Antiepileptic Drugs: Quantitative Analysis and Interpretation, edited by C. E. Pippenger, J. K. Penry, and H. Kutt, Raven Press, New York, © 1978.

Chapter 15
Radioimmunoassay

C. E. Cook

Radioimmunoassay (RIA) was introduced as an analytical technique in 1959 (35). Since then it has played an increasingly important role in the quantitative analysis of hormones and drugs. Much of the recent rapid progress in endocrinology may in fact be attributed to the availability of this sensitive and accurate method for quantitation of steroidal and protein/peptide hormones. A number of recent books and review articles on RIA are now available (2,15,17,22,25,31,32). Their emphasis is often on steroids, but the techniques are readily applicable to drugs. Immunoassay is still a rapidly growing field, with new techniques being put forward and disagreement about old ones. The analyst should therefore examine immunoassay literature and manufacturers' claims with a critical eye.

The basic premise of RIA is simple (see Fig. 1). A radiolabeled substance (antigen, radioligand) binds to an antibody. Addition of unlabeled antigen results in a competition with the radioligand for binding sites, thus reducing the fraction of radioligand bound. By measuring either the free or bound radioactivity and establishing a standard curve, one can then determine the amount of antigen present in an unknown sample.

Development of an RIA procedure includes preparation of an immuno-

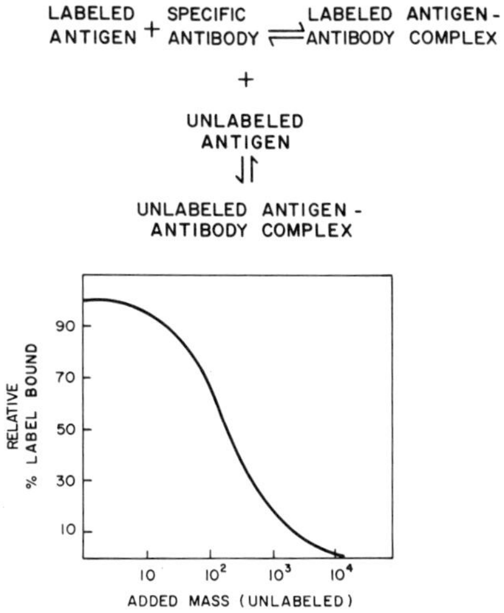

FIG. 1. Basic premise of RIA. From Cook et al. (4).

genic drug-protein conjugate to stimulate formation of antibodies, synthesis of radioligand, and development of an assay procedure. This chapter is not intended to be a comprehensive review but attempts to illustrate these steps and point out requirements for successful RIA.

STEPS IN ASSAY DEVELOPMENT

Immunogen Formation

Small molecules such as the antiepileptic drugs are not in general immunogenic; that is, they are incapable of stimulating the formation of antibodies. However, in the early 1900s, Landsteiner showed that if small molecules were covalently bonded to a large molecule such as a protein, the resulting substance (conjugate) was immunogenic. Antibodies formed by injection of animals with this hapten-protein conjugate could selectively bind the original small molecule. The antibodies had the greatest selectivity for those portions of the small molecule that were not directly involved in the linkage to protein (20). Thus in developing antisera to a drug, if the immunogen is formed by linking the drug to a protein through a site on the drug that is metabolically reactive, the resulting antibody may not be capable of readily distinguishing between the drug and its metabolite. A variety of techniques for conjugate preparation have been described by Erlanger (11).

Immunization

Rabbits, sheep, and goats are the favored animals for production of antisera. The species used is based mainly on considerations of convenience and amounts of serum required and need be of concern to the clinical chemist only if he is using a double antibody RIA procedure. A variety of immunization procedures have been reported (19). Because of variability in antibody formation, several animals are immunized and the antiserum from each bleeding must be characterized. Fortunately the concentration of antibodies (titer) is frequently such that relatively small amounts of serum will suffice for a very large number of assays and antisera are quite stable when stored cold with protection from microbiological contamination.

Radioligands

Since the sensitivity of an RIA procedure (10) and the effective titer of the antiserum are related to the specific radioactivity of the radioligand used, there are significant advantages in using high-specific-activity radiolabeled drug. For this reason the favored isotopes are tritium and ^{125}I. A tritium-labeled drug will have binding properties very similar to those of the unlabeled drug, although isotope effects on binding have been reported (18). Under proper storage conditions (e.g., benzene-ethanol solution at low temperature), tritium-labeled compounds normally exhibit good stability. The greatest disadvantage of tritium is the fact that it is a β-emitter, analyzed by liquid scintillation techniques that require relatively expensive reagents and form an inconvenient step in attempts to automate RIA procedures.

For the above reason, the present trend is to the use of ^{125}I as the radioisotope. ^{125}I has a much shorter half-life than tritium (60 days versus 12.3 years) and thus a much higher theoretical specific activity. (Even higher specific activities are theoretically attainable with ^{131}I, but the very short half-life—8 days—of this isotope requires too frequent preparation of radioligand.) ^{125}I can be measured in a gamma counter, and solutions, precipitates, coated tubes, and so forth can be counted directly if this isotope is used. It is also possible to use liquid scintillation methods for ^{125}I.

Since iodine is a very large atom, its substitution directly on a drug molecule inhibits binding to the antibody. Therefore an iodohistamine or iodophenol derivative (14) may be linked to the derivative of the drug used for the original immunogen preparation. However, this may introduce other problems. The resulting substance may have a structure in which the linkage between drug and iodinated moiety is similar to that for the original drug-protein conjugate. Thus it may exhibit an increased binding versus the parent drug or may select a population of antibodies that has a greater recognition for the link than the drug itself. Large quantities of the drug may then be required to displace the radioligand, and the assay may actually be less sensitive than is the case with the tritium-labeled radioligand (8,14).

Separation of Bound and Free Fractions

Since either the bound or free radioligand must be measured, it becomes necessary to find a method for separating these two entities. Failure to achieve complete separation will impair precision and sensitivity of the assay (10). The factors involved in choosing a separation system have been described (16). Suitability for automation may be an important consideration. Ratcliffe (26) has summarized a large number of separation techniques, of which double antibody, adsorption, precipitation, and solid-phase methods are most common.

The double antibody method employs a second antibody that precipitates the soluble antigen/antibody complexes formed initially. Although a very general method, it is often time consuming.

Adsorption methods, usually those in which the free fraction is removed by adsorption, are widely used because of their simplicity, speed, and large sample capacity when used in a batch procedure. They are also adaptable to automation (1,12). Since most small molecules are readily adsorbed by charcoal, this is perhaps the favorite substance. Dextran is often used to coat the charcoal to exclude the larger bound complexes. Other adsorbants that have been used include silicates (talcum powder, fullers earth, florisil) and anion exchange resin (26). Since removal of the free fraction from solution should result in a displacement of equilibrium and eventual stripping of the radioligand from the antibody, experimental approaches that will minimize this possibility must be followed. These may include carrying out the procedure at low temperature and control of the time intervals during which adsorbant is mixed with the solution.

Precipitation of the immunoglobulin (bound) fraction can be achieved by addition of salts or organic solvents. Many drugs will remain soluble in concentrated ammonium sulfate solutions—a favorite precipitant. A globulin fraction may be added to the incubation tube in order to facilitate precipitation and centrifugation of the antibody/antigen complex. Alternatively, use of a suspension of calcium sulfate in ammonium sulfate solution (34) yields a very compact pellet from which the supernatant can be readily removed. Polyethylene glycol has been shown to be satisfactory for a number of low-molecular-weight substances (30). Precipitation methods may give a different assay profile than adsorption methods. In adsorption methods, stripping will usually occur from antibodies having a lower affinity (assuming a negative correlation between affinity and dissociation rate), whereas precipitation methods will generally bring down all of the immunoglobulin fraction.

The convenience of separation when the antibody is already bound to a solid phase has led to the development of a large number of such methods (26). Antibodies may be adsorbed to polystyrene or polypropylene tubes or disks. They may also be covalently bonded to solid surfaces such as dextran, cellulose, or glass. Solid phase techniques have the advantage of relatively brief incubation periods and are susceptible to automation.

Characterization of Antiserum

The titer is the dilution of antiserum that binds a specific percent of a given amount of radioligand. If an antiserum is diluted 1:10,000 and 0.1 ml of the resulting solution is used in a total incubation volume of 1 ml to obtain a binding of 40%, then the antiserum titer for 40% binding is 1:10,000 (initial dilution) or 1:100,000 (final dilution). Generally, a titer will be used that results in 30 to 50% binding. However, under certain conditions maximum sensitivity may be obtained by initially binding only a very small fraction of the radioligand (9).

The affinity constant (K_a) for an antibody is the equilibrium constant for the reaction: antibody + antigen $\rightleftharpoons$ complex. If other factors are held constant, the minimum detectable concentration of drug has been shown (10) to be proportional to $1/\sqrt{K_a}$. Thus a high affinity constant is required to achieve a sensitive assay. Antisera contain a heterogeneous collection of antibodies and the affinity constant is usually an estimate of an average value (23).

Specificity (selectivity) has been defined (23) as the degree to which an antiserum reacts only to the substance in question under the particular set of radioimmunoassay conditions. Since antisera generally do not bind one compound to the exclusion of all others, we prefer selectivity to describe this property of an antibody (6). Selectivity is usually determined by comparison of the concentrations of various compounds required to displace 50% of the initially bound radioligand. For a homogeneous antibody this type of calculation does not reflect the exact ratio of binding constants of the two compounds. It varies with the bound/free ratio of radioligand in the assay system, and the response curves for two different compounds can never be exactly parallel (7). In many instances, however, comparison of 50% displacement values is a reasonable means for estimating the selectivity of an antiserum for a drug versus potential cross reactants (6).

Selective antisera should then be subjected to more intensive study. Comparison of cross-reactions at 10 to 20% and 80% displacement of radioligand is useful. One can also run a series of standard curves containing increasing amounts of a potentially interfering compound.

ASSAY INTERFERENCE

The most obvious source of interference with an RIA is the presence of metabolites in the sample to be analyzed. The degree of interference is a function both of the cross-reaction (see above) and the concentration of the interfering substance. In instances where metabolite concentration is normally a small fraction that of the drug, even quite nonspecific antisera may prove useful. Thus a good correlation was achieved between RIA for phenytoin and other methods of analysis of this compound in plasma despite the fact that the antiserum used had a 75% cross-reaction with the major metabolite of phenytoin (33). Such an antiserum might be less useful for the analysis of serum from uremic patients in whose serum the concentration of both free and conjugated metabolite increases over that found in nonuremic patients (24). However, the use of a highly selective antiserum for phenytoin (5) results in an excellent correlation between RIA and gas chromatographic analysis of samples from patients with impaired renal function (24). The presence of other closely related drugs may also present a problem. Although reasonable correlation with other methods was found when RIA was carried out using an antiserum that is reactive to barbiturates as a class (33), for the general population one would prefer the use of a more selective antiserum (4). In general, more selective antisera should present fewer problems because of an individual patient's drug history or physical condition.

There may also be less specific, but nonetheless real, interferences from the presence of plasma constituents. If the drug is present in sufficient concentration, simple dilution of the sample (for example, 1:1000) may effectively eliminate such interferences. Plasma interference may arise from protein binding of the drug. Thus in the assay for phenytoin, which is highly bound to plasma protein, the presence of more than 1 μl of plasma in the assay tube may affect the analysis (5), whereas in the case of caffeine, which is very poorly protein bound, the assay can tolerate up to 15% plasma without any need to correct for its presence (6). If plasma interference is corrected for by adding plasma to the standard curve tubes, it is necessary to demonstrate that the plasma interference variation from patient to patient is not sufficient to invalidate the assay. Other interferences can arise from solvents used in extraction procedures (if these are required) or binding of radioligand or drug to the glass or plastic tubes. The pH of the buffer can have a significant effect on binding and adsorption, thereby influencing cross-reactions and interference. Standard and cross-reaction curves should be run at varied pH in order to ascertain the pH best suited for a particular antiserum. Finally, the possibility of interference by common drugs (caffeine, aspirin, diazepam), although unexpected, should be checked.

DATA PROCESSING

Even without automation, an efficient technician may assay hundreds of tubes in a single run, thereby producing a mass of data that must be analyzed. The simplest procedure is to plot cpm versus log of concentration of standards and interpolate graphically. However, this method is liable to subjective bias, and with the proliferation of programmable calculators and minicomputers it is less used now.

Fitting a curve to RIA data is complicated by the nonlinear relationship between concentration of drug and response (cpm bound, etc.). Several ways to overcome this problem have been proposed (3,27). The most popular has been the logit-log transformation (27). Among its advantages are (a) linearization of the concentration-response curve, resulting in the need to fit only two parameters by well-known linear regression methods, (b) the ease of fixing 95% confidence limits for an observation, and (c) its adaptability to programmable desktop calculators. Logit-log graph paper is available for graphic interpretation of the data.

The major disadvantage of the logit-log method is that the transformation results in nonuniformity of variance with a large increase at the ends of the regression line. Thus some means of weighted regression should be used. However, Rodbard and colleagues (27,29) claim that almost all RIA response variables showed nonuniformity of variance, even before logit transformation, so that weighted regressions should always be used. The simplest form of weighting is truncation; that is, only the portion of the curve between 20% and 80% is used for the assay. This has the disadvantage of increasing the minimum concentration which can be analyzed. Logit-log computer programs by Rodbard and Faden (28), which include weighting, are now available. Failure to use weighted regression in the logit-log method will not necessarily result in serious error in the estimate of the curve, but invalidates attempts to calculate 95% confidence limits or the coefficient of variation for the potency estimate based on the scatter of points around the standard curve (29). Rodbard and co-workers (29) point out that some commercial logit-log methods that use "weighting" may actually seriously degrade the performance of the curve-fitting procedure. These workers emphasize that the availability of a canned software program does not relieve the user of the necessity of determining its applicability.

By simplifying theoretical equations (10) it has been shown that a plot of total counts divided by counts bound versus ligand concentration is linear over most of its course and can be used for a variety of assays (13).

In contrast to these linearization techniques are methods for fitting a smooth curve to the data by, for example, the use of polynomials. The use of polynomials suffers from multiple parameters to be fitted and the difficulty of estimating confidence limits (27). However, curve fitting by means of smoothing spline functions has been shown to have certain advantages (21). It may be particularly useful when the logit-log transformation is not linear. There is considerable disagreement about how often this occurs, with estimates ranging from 10 to 50% of the time (21).

Recently, a four-parameter logistic approach has been modified to include weighting and computerization (27,28). This approach is stated to have enormous generality and to be applicable to RIA's that measure either free or bound fraction of ligand, to labeled antibody assays, and to "two-site labeled antibody assays."

QUALITY CONTROL

Regardless of the analytical method or the procedure for curve fitting, a good quality control system is indispensable. One can then combine results from different assays and obtain information on reproducibility. This may permit, in some instances, reduction of the number of replicate tubes in an assay with savings in cost. A running quality control chart also makes it possible to evaluate the stability of the assay system and may help in trouble shooting should problems arise (27).

Figure 2 presents a rudimentary quality control chart (see 27). Total cpm (top line of figure) should be maintained within fairly constant limits if other parameters of the assay are to remain stable. Nonspecific cpm in this case refers to radioactivity not adsorbed in the separation procedure. An increase in this number often reflects decomposition of the radioligand. The fraction of radioligand bound at zero cold concentration $[(B_0 - N)/T]$ will have an effect on sensitivity and selectivity of the assay. A decrease may reflect decomposition of the radioligand or antiserum or changes in the buffer.

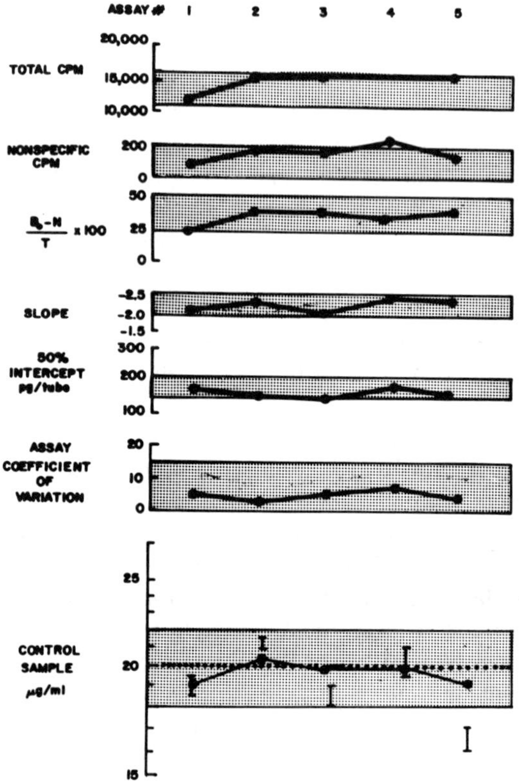

FIG. 2. Sample quality control chart. For explanation see text.

The slope refers to the least-squares regression line. Because of the influence of errors, the intuitively appealing notion that an increase in slope of the response curve means an increase in assay precision is not always correct. If investigator A, who plots B/F versus amount, finds that a change in assay procedure increases the slope of his curve, he may not thereby claim increased precision, since investigator B, who plots F/B, will find that the same change decreases the slope of his curve (9). The 50% intercept is the concentration of unlabeled ligand that results in 50% displacement of the radioligand.

Control samples containing known amounts of the drug should be run with each assay. Ideally, control samples should cover a range of values to be expected in the unknown samples. Thus, for the analysis of phenytoin, one might select plasma samples containing 7.5, 15, and 30 μg/ml of the drug. Control samples should resemble the unknowns as closely as possible. The best control serum would be a large pool from individuals taking the drug (thus containing metabolites, etc.) which has been carefully analyzed by a reliable reference method such as gas chromatography-mass fragmentography. In Fig. 2 the control sample is analyzed in duplicate. The individual results are shown by the small horizontal bars that are connected by vertical lines corresponding to the range. The cumulative average value is shown by the closed circles connected by line segments. The expected value is shown by a dotted horizontal line. Use of a logarithmic ordinate scale is convenient for showing a large range of values. The "contrast" between one day's value and the cumulative result of preceeding assays may be calculated (27).

Both the within- and between-assay variance are of importance and the coefficient of variation within assays and between assays should be recorded. A clear and simple explanation of these terms and their calculation is given by Rodbard (27). It is useful to remember that for fewer than 30 samples it is better to estimate the standard deviation from the range (corrected for outliers) multiplied by a factor that depends on sample size (27).

Quality control is more than a record of variations in the assay. It is also checking on the precision and accuracy of apparatus used and proper training and supervision of personnel. The most rigorous test of pipet accuracy involves weighing aqueous samples delivered. Since sample delivery may be influenced by viscosity, viscous solutions may require separate calibration. For routine practice and checking, radioactive solutions may be used if correction is made for quenching. Pipetting is very important and personnel should clearly understand when *precision* is of major concern (e.g., in addition of radioligand) and when *accuracy* is also required (e.g., sample aliquots).

ADVANTAGES AND DISADVANTAGES OF RIA

RIA has the advantage of excellent sensitivity—amounts of drug down to a few picograms can be measured in rather impure samples of blood or saliva. The analysis of many anticonvulsant drugs is carried out well above the assay limits. Antisera can be prepared to most compounds, radioligands are well characterized and can be reproducibly made, and large numbers of samples may be processed. The skills required to run routine assays are easily learned. On the other hand, meticulous attention to detail and precise pipetting are required for good precision and accuracy, but the repetitive and boring nature of the technique makes human error likely. In the case of the anticonvulsant drugs, no single company has made a concerted effort to market a system, such as has been done for the enzyme immunoassays, so that the user must now go to many sources for assay materials and instruments. Also, insufficient attention has been paid to decreasing turnaround time, and batch processing is still the most efficient procedure. Many of the problems could be solved by automation. Recent reports concerning automated "batch-type" RIA systems that offer high throughput (e.g., 12) and "flow-type" systems with exceptional flexibility (1) are encouraging in this regard.

ACKNOWLEDGMENTS

Support from the National Institute of General Medical Sciences (grant no. 1 RO1 GM23197) is gratefully acknowledged, as is the typing of the manuscript by Mrs. Polli Elliott.

REFERENCES

1. Brooker, G., Terasaki, W. L., and Price, M. G. (1976): Gammaflow: A completely automated radioimmunoassay system. *Science,* 194:270–276.
2. Cameron, E. H. D., Hillier, S. G., and Griffiths, K., editors (1975): *Steroid Immunoassay.* Alpha Omega Publishing, Cardiff, Wales, U.K.
3. Cook, B. (1975): Automation and data processing for radioimmunoassays. In *Steroid Immunoassay,* edited by E. H. D. Cameron, S. G. Hillier, and K. Griffiths, pp. 293–310. Alpha Omega Publishing, Cardiff, Wales, U.K.
4. Cook, C. E., Christensen, H. D., Amerson, E. W., Kepler, J. A., Tallent, C. R., and Taylor, G. F. (1976): Radioimmunoassay of anticonvulsant drugs: Phenytoin, phenobarbital and primidone. In *Quantitative Analytic Studies in Epilepsy,* edited by P. Kellaway and I. Petersén. Raven Press, New York.
5. Cook, C. E., Kepler, J. A., and Christensen, H. D. (1973): Antiserum to diphenylhydantoin: Preparation and characterization. *Res. Commun. Chem. Pathol. Pharmacol.,* 5:767–774.
6. Cook, C. E., Tallent, C. R., Amerson, E. W., Myers, M. W., Kepler, J. A., Taylor, G. F., and Christensen, H. D. (1976): Caffeine in plasma and saliva by a radioimmunoassay procedure. *J. Pharmacol. Exp. Ther.,* 199:679–686.
7. Ekins, R. P. (1975): Discussion. In *Steroid Immunoassay,* edited by E. H. D. Cameron, S. G. Hillier, and K. Griffiths, p. 83. Alpha Omega Publishing, Cardiff, Wales, U.K.
8. Ekins, R. P. (1975): Discussion. In *Steroid Immunoassay,* edited by E. H. D. Cameron, S. G. Hillier, and K. Griffiths, pp. 172–176. Alpha Omega Publishing, Cardiff, Wales, U.K.
9. Ekins, R. P. (1975): Discussion. In *Steroid Immunoassay,* edited by E. H. D. Cameron, S. G. Hillier, and K. Griffiths, pp. 311–313. Alpha Omega Publishing, Cardiff, Wales, U.K.
10. Ekins, R. P., Newman, G. B., and O'Riordan, J. L. H. (1968): Theoretical aspects of "saturation" and radioimmunoassay. In *Radioisotopes in Medicine: In Vitro Studies,* edited by R. L. Hayes, F. A. Gosewitz, and B. E. P. Murphy. U.S. Atomic Energy Commission Conference 67111, 59–100.
11. Erlanger, B. F. (1973): Principles and methods for the preparation of drug protein conjugates for immunological studies. *Pharmacol. Rev.* 25:271–280.
12. Ertinghausen, G., Shapiro, S. I., Green, G., and Zborowski, G. (1975): Adaptation of a T_3-uptake test and of radioimmunoassays for serum digoxin, thyroxine and triiodothyronine to an automated radioimmunoassay system—"Centria." *Clin. Chem.,* 21:1305–1313.
13. Fernandez, A. A., and Loeb, H. G. (1975): Practical applications of radioimmunoassay theory. A simple procedure yielding linear calibration curves. *Clin. Chem.,* 21:1113–1120.
14. Hunter, W. M., Nars, P. W., and Rutherford, F. J. (1975): Preparation and behavior of ^{125}I-labeled radioligands for phenolic and neutral steroids. In *Steroid Immunoassay,* edited by E. H. D. Cameron, S. G. Hillier, and K. Griffiths, pp. 141–152. Alpha Omega Publishing, Cardiff, Wales, U.K.
15. International Atomic Energy Agency (1974): *Radioimmunoassay and Related Procedures in Medicine,* Vols. I and II. Unipub, New York.
16. International Atomic Energy Agency Panel (1974): Standardization of radioimmunoassay procedures. *Int. J. Appl. Rad. Isotopes,* 25:145–160.
17. Jaffe, B. M., and Behrman, H. R., editors (1974): *Methods of Hormone Radioimmunoassay.* Academic Press, New York.

18. Jeffcoate, S. L., Edwards, R., Gilby, E. D., and White, N. (1975): The use of [^{3}H]-labelled ligands in steroid radioimmunoassays. In *Steroid Immunoassay,* edited by E. H. D. Cameron, S. G. Hillier, and K. Griffiths, pp. 133–140. Alpha Omega Publishing, Cardiff, Wales, U.K.
19. Lader, S., Hurn, B. A. L., and Court, G. (1974): A comparative assessment of immunization procedures for radioimmunoassay. In *Radioimmunoassay and Related Procedures in Medicine,* edited by International Atomic Energy Agency, Vol. I, pp. 31–44. Unipub, New York.
20. Landsteiner, K. (1962): *The Specificity of Serological Reactions.* Dover Press, New York.
21. Marschner, I., Erhardt, F., and Scriba, P. C. (1974): Calculation of the radioimmunoassay standard curve by "spline function." In *Radioimmunoassay and Related Procedures in Medicine,* edited by International Atomic Energy Agency. Unipub, New York.
22. Moss, Jr., A. J., Dalrymple, Glenn V., and Boyd, Charles M. (1976): *Practical Radioimmunoassay.* C. V. Mosby Co., St. Louis, Mo.
23. Odell, W., Skowsky, R., Abraham, G., Hescox, M., Fisher, D., and Grover, P. K. (1972): Production of antisera for polypeptide and steroid radioimmunoassays. *Biol. Reprod.,* 6:427–442.
24. Orme, M. L'E., Borgå, O., Cook, C. E., and Sjöqvist, F. (1976): Measurement of diphenylhydantoin in 0.1 ml plasma samples: Gas chromatography and radioimmunoassay compared. *Clin. Chem.,* 22:246–249.
25. Peron, F. G., and Caldwell, B. V. (1970): *Immunologic Methods in Steroid Determination.* Appleton-Century-Crofts, New York.
26. Ratcliffe, J. G. (1974): Separation techniques in saturation analysis. *Br. Med. Bull.,* 30:32–37.
27. Rodbard, D. (1974): Statistical quality control and routine data processing for radioimmunoassays and immunoradiometric assays. *Clin. Chem.,* 20:1255–1270.
28. Rodbard, D., and Faden, V. B. (1975): *Radioimmunoassay Data Processing, 3rd. ed.* National Technical Information Service, Springfield, Va.
29. Rodbard, D., Lenox, R. H., Wray, H. L., and Ramseth, D. (1976): Statistical characterization of the random errors in the radioimmunoassay dose-response variable. *Clin. Chem.,* 22:350–358.
30. Schiller, H. S., Hasselbrack, R., Riggs, R. S., and Brammall, M. A. (1976): A faster radioimmunoassay of progesterone in plasma, with use of polyethylene glycol as precipitant. *Clin. Chem.,* 22:1659–1663.
31. Skelley, D. S., Brown, L. P., and Besch, P. K. (1973): Radioimmunoassay. *Clin. Chem.,* 19:146–186.
32. Spector, S., Berkowitz, B., Flynn, E. J., and Peskar, B. (1973): Antibodies to morphine, barbiturates and serotonin. *Pharmacol. Rev.,* 25:281–291.
33. Spiehler, V., Sun, L., Miyada, D. S., Sarandis, S. G., Walwick, E. R., Klein, M. W., Jordan, D. B., and Jessen, B. (1976): Radioimmunoassay, enzyme immunoassay, spectrophotometry and gas-liquid chromatography compared for determination of phenobarbital and diphenylhydantoin. *Clin. Chem.,* 22:749–753.
34. Tyler, J. P. P., Hennam, J. F., Newton, J. R., and Collins, W. P. (1973): Radioimmunoassay of plasma testosterone without chromatography: A comparison of four antisera, and the evaluation of a novel approach to liquid scintillation counting. *Steroids,* 22:871–889.
35. Yalow, R. S., and Berson, S. A. (1959): Assay of plasma insulin in human subjects by immunological methods. *Nature,* 184:1648–1649.

Antiepileptic Drugs: Quantitative Analysis and Interpretation, edited by C. E. Pippenger, J. K. Penry, and H. Kutt, Raven Press, New York, © 1978.

Chapter 16

Ultraviolet Spectrophotometric Quantitation of Phenytoin and Phenobarbital

Horace E. Hamilton and Jack E. Wallace

Early methods developed for the analysis of phenytoin (Dilantin®, diphenylhydantoin) lacked sufficient sensitivity to be of clinical use (10). The first effective procedures for determining phenytoin in biologic specimens were reported in 1956 separately by two different groups (6,15); both methods were based on spectrophotometric measurements, one in the visible (6) and the other in the ultraviolet (15) region. Quantitation of phenytoin by the method of Dill et al. (6) was based on a lengthy and nonspecific colorimetric reaction, whereas detection and quantification by the method of Plaa and Hine (15) were dependent on the slope of the absorption spectra. The former procedure involves nitration of the extracted hydantoin, reduction of the subsequent nitro derivative to an aromatic amine, diazotization with nitrous acid, and coupling with the Bratton-Marshall reagent (2) to form a highly colored azo dye. The reaction is capable of reacting with any aromatic amine, thus affording no specificity for phenytoin. Even phenobarbital will give a product with an almost identical absorption maximum, and certain metabolites of phenytoin will also give the same colored azo-dye product. A relatively high degree of specificity (11) was achieved through the utilization of a three-plate countercurrent extraction procedure capable of separating phenytoin from phenobarbital, a drug often administered concommitantly. The procedure of Plaa and Hine (15) is less specific, the slope of the ultraviolet absorption spectra between 250 and 235 nm being the basis for the analytical measurement. Traces of many compounds, including any barbiturate, will contribute significantly to the slope of this curve. A partial, though incomplete, separation of phenobarbital from phenytoin was achieved by back-extracting the initial organic solvent into dilute hydrochloric acid to remove the barbiturate and then into an aqueous carbonate buffer solution to remove the phenytoin. The procedure allowed a 10% carryover of phenobarbital into the phenytoin fraction (18).

Several modifications of these early spectrophotometric procedures for phenytoin have been proposed. Svensmark et al. (22) combined the countercurrent extraction procedure of Dill et al. (6) with the spectrophotometric method of Plaa and Hine (15). Schiller and Buchthal (18) achieved a better separation of phenobarbital from phenytoin through a differential back-extraction into a pH 9 borate buffer and a pH 11 carbonate buffer. Svensmark and Kristensen (21) utilized the difference in absorbance at 235 and 260 nm following a partial separation of phenobarbital based on the back-extraction of chloroform into a phosphate buffer, of which the pH was critical (Fig. 1). Olesen (14) made some additional minor modifications to the method of Svensmark and Kristensen (21) to achieve routine clinical applications, but the problem of carryover in the final extract of barbiturates and other hydantoins remained a severe limitation to the accurate determination of phenytoin in biologic specimens containing other pharmacologic agents. Dill et al. (3) later developed an extraction procedure for separating phenytoin from its principal metabolite, 5-hydroxyphenyl-5-phenylhydantoin, prior to the application of the Bratton-Marshall colorimetric reaction. Of the aforementioned colorimetric (3,6) and ultraviolet spectrophotometric (11,14,15,18,21,22) procedures, the methods of Dill et al. (6) and Svensmark and Kristensen (21) appear to have received more widespread application in the clinical laboratory, and consequently have contributed most heavily to our early knowledge concerning clinical dose-plasma level relationships for phenytoin (7).

Wallace et al. (26) proposed a unique method of quantitating phenytoin in biologic specimens based on the conversion of the drug to benzophenone, a compound having a distinct absorption spectra and a high absorption coefficient. The procedure involved the alkaline hydrolysis of the hydantoin to an amine, and the subsequent reaction with bromine via the Hoffmann degradation to form benzophenone, which was removed from the reaction mixture by steam distillation. The Wallace method was eightfold more sensitive than the method of Svensmark and Kristensen and provided a low blank (21). The recovery of phenytoin from blood specimens by this method (90%) was comparable to that achieved by the tedious multistep countercurrent extraction procedure of Dill et al. (6), and superior to that of other spectrophotometric methods, 72 to 78% (11,14,15,18,21,22). Most impor-

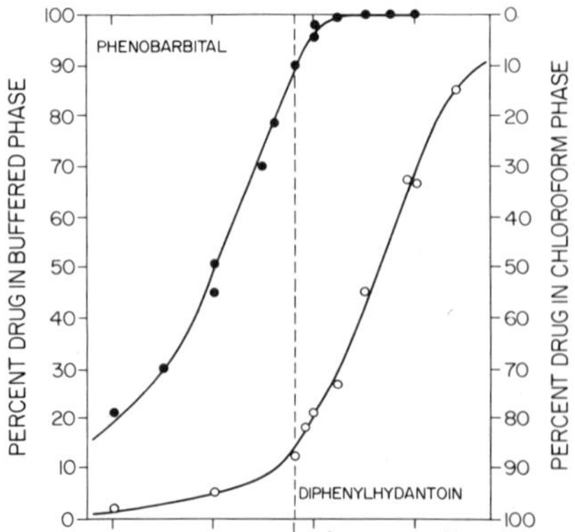

FIG. 1. Concentration of phenytoin and phenobarbital in 0.1 M borate buffers of different pH after equilibration with equal volumes of chloroform containing 20 μg/ml of phenytoin or phenobarbital. From Svensmark and Kristensen (21).

tant, however, was the specificity of this method; neither phenytoin metabolites, phenobarbital (and other barbiturates), nor other anticonvulsants commonly administered in conjunction with phenytoin adversely affect the quantitation of this important drug even at high concentrations in the biologic extract.

Although the production of benzophenone via alkaline hydrolysis and subsequent Hoffmann degradation provided the most sensitive method then available for the determination of phenytoin, the procedure did require 10 ml of blood per determination and still necessitated a postderivatization concentration step for the determination of therapeutic levels. Further, the procedure required the use of potentially hazardous molecular bromine and a steam distillation with a relatively critical distillation rate. These factors tended to limit the routine use of the method in clinical laboratories. Wallace and coworkers consequently published a series of modifications, making the method less tedious, more rapid, less critical of changes in reaction conditions, and markedly increasing the sensitivity of the method. The use of alkaline permanganate in lieu of bromine both removed a potential hazard and resulted in a 25% increase in sensitivity (23). The steam distillation was replaced by a less tedious and more reliable reflux for an additional 15% enhancement in sensitivity (24,25). Dichloroethane was substituted for chloroform to eliminate the necessity for evaporation of solvent to remove traces of alcohol normally present in chloroform prior to oxidation, and the aqueous alkali solution and solid potassium permanganate were added separately to eliminate problems of reagent stability (27). The incorporation of these separate modifications into a procedure utilizing a micro reflux condenser resulted in an extremely sensitive method that provided a 94% mean recovery of phenytoin from serum or plasma, and that provided a limit of sensitivity of 0.5 μg/ml for a 0.1-ml specimen (28).

Several other investigators have also proposed minor modifications of the Wallace procedure. Bock and Sherwin (1) and Lee and Bass (12) proposed the utilization of modified micro-Kjedahl flasks in lieu of the reflux flask-condenser combination. Saitoh et al. (17) and Dill et al. (4) proposed that the reactions be performed in test tubes rather than via reflux with continuous magnetic stirring; Wallace and Hamilton (28) demonstrated that the latter technique enhanced both sensitivity and precision over that achieved with sealed tubes. Morselli (13) used reflux with continuous stirring, but used a thermostirring bath with ice-packed condensers. Morselli used benzene as the extracting solvent to avoid the need to evaporate prior to oxidation; however, benzene appears to be a rather poor solvent for the extraction of phenytoin (7). An interesting and unique modification of the Wallace method is the method of Dill and Glazko (5), in which the benzophenone is extracted from *n*-heptane into sulfuric acid and the resulting fluorescent product measured spectrofluorometrically (360 nm activation, 490 nm emission). The method provides sufficient sensitivity for determination of therapeutic levels of phenytoin in fingerstick specimens, and also provides an exceptionally low blank reading for serum specimens containing no phenytoin.

A unique specificity, that is, lack of interference from barbiturates and other anticonvulsant drugs, characterizes the procedures that determine phenytoin as benzophenone which is a marked contrast with other spectrophotometric methods for determining this anticonvulsant. Richens (16) stated that "The inaccuracy of the spectrophotometric techniques, excluding the Wallace technique, is striking." In an interlaboratory quality control program, Richens observed that the percentage of phenytoin estimations that were outside the 95% confidence limits were approximately quadrupled for other spectrophotometric methods as opposed to the benzophenone method. Consequently, procedures for determining phenytoin by the ultraviolet spectrophotometric measurement of benzophenone have been listed as "state-of-the-art" methodologies in several recent monographs (9,29).

Phenytoin does not pose a similar interference with the spectrophotometric analysis of phenobarbital as determined by the method of Goldbaum (8). The barbiturates as undissociated molecules do not exhibit ultraviolet absorption in acidic solution; when ionized in alkaline solution, their ultraviolet absorption (i.e., wavelength, intensity, and stability) is very much dependent on pH. Barbiturates by this method are determined by a differential ultraviolet spectra with measurements at pH 10.5 and 13; although hydantoins and certain other drugs may interfere with the spectra at a given pH, they do not alter the spectra of pH 10.5 relative to that at pH 13. This method gives a quantitative estimate for all barbiturates. A limited differentiation between individual barbiturates may be achieved on the basis of relative pH-induced differences in absorbance at various wavelengths (8), differences in the partitioning of the barbiturate between organic solvent and specific buffer or alkali solutions (20), or the stability of the absorption in the presence of strong alkali (19); the latter method has had the greater utilization in clinical and forensic laboratories. Certain other compounds, notably the salicylates, also have characteristic absorption spectra at different pH values, and consequently their presence may influence the spectrophotometric determination of phenobarbital. However, ionization of the barbiturates begins at pH levels above 9.5, with essentially all of the compound in the undissociated form at pH 8.6; thus a sodium bicarbonate solution may be used to remove salicylates from the organic extracting solvent prior to back-extraction of the barbiturate into alkali.

This chapter describes two modifications of the ultraviolet spectrophotometric technique utilizing benzophenone as the product for final estimation (28). Only the modified nonreflux techniques (4,17) or the spectrophotofluorometric techniques of Dill and Glazko (5) are recommended as alternative ways to determine phenytoin spectrophotometrically. Each of these procedures depends on the oxidation of the drug to benzophenone.

EXPERIMENTAL

Apparatus

Reflux condensers are mounted on a Flexaframe support. The semimicro determination utilizes a conventional Allihn condenser, whereas the micro determination employs an "external cold finger" reflux condenser (28). Glas-Col heating mantles (Terre Haute, Ind.) in each procedure are positioned on magnetic stirrers beneath the respective condensers. Six to twelve reflux units can be attached through a single variable Staco transformer, which applies voltage to each heating mantle through the use of a multiple electric outlet. With this type of setup as many as 12 phenytoin analyses can be run simultaneously within 4 to 5 ft of linear bench space. The use of small shot pellets (BB's) as a heat-transfer medium permits one size heating mantle to be used with varying flask sizes.

Spectrophotometric measurements are best performed on a ratio-recording spectrophotometer equipped with a microcell holder. A Beckman Acta III is used in the laboratory of the authors.

Microdetermination of Phenytoin

Five milliliters of dichloroethane, 0.1 to 0.2 ml of plasma, serum, or whole blood, and 0.1 ml of 1 N HCl are pipetted into a 15-ml glass-stoppered tube. The tube is stoppered, shaken vigorously for 1 min, and following removal of the stopper, centrifuged for 2 min at 2,000 rpm. Then 4.5 ml of the dichloroethane layer is transferred to a second tube and similarly extracted into 2.5 ml of 5 N NaOH. Two milliliters of the sodium hydroxide extract, approximately 0.2 g of potassium permanganate, 1.0 ml of spectrograde *n*-heptane, and a 1.3-cm (0.5-in.) Teflon-coated magnetic stirring bar are placed in a 50-ml round-bottom flask fitted with a 24/40 ground-glass joint.

Semimicrodetermination of Phenytoin

With 25 ml of dichloroethane, 1 ml of plasma or serum, and 0.5 ml of 1 N HCl, extraction and centrifugation are performed in a 50-ml round-bottom centrifuge tube. The aqueous layer may be aspirated and the solvent filtered into a stoppered 50-ml graduated cylinder. At this point the recovered solvent in each cylinder should be adjusted to identical volumes (20 to 24 ml) before back-extraction with 5 N NaOH is initiated. The equalization of solvent volumes at this point simplifies the calculation of results. Ten milliliters of 5 N NaOH is added and the cylinders are stoppered, shaken vigorously for 1 to 2 min, and subsequently centrifuged for 2 min at 2,000 rpm. Nine milliliters of the aqueous layer is transferred to a 50-ml round-bottom flask, to which are added a magnetic stirring bar, 3 ml of *n*-heptane, and approximately 0.2 g (0.1 to 0.4 g) of potassium permanganate.

The boiling flask is attached to the reflux condenser and secured into a heating mantle, which is supported by the top surface of a magnetic stirrer. After the mixture has refluxed with vigorous stirring for 25 min, optimally achieved with 40 V AC applied to the heating mantles, the heating mantles are removed and the flasks are allowed to cool for 5 to 10 min. Then 10 to 25 ml of water is poured into the flasks through the open end of the reflux columns. The flasks are removed, sufficient water is added to float the heptane layer just into the neck of the flask, and the heptane layer is transferred to the quartz cells. The heptane layer is scanned spectrophotometrically over the 310- to 230-nm range, or the absorbance is measured at 247 nm. Since all standards and unknowns are treated identically, calculations are accomplished by application of a simple ratio:

$$\frac{\text{absorbance of unknown}}{\text{absorbance of standard}} \times \text{concentration of standard} = \begin{array}{l}\text{concentration}\\ \text{of specimen}\end{array}$$

If different volumes of specimen and standard are used, or if different volumes of solvent are recovered, appropriate corrections must be made in the final calculation.

Analysis of Phenobarbital by Ultraviolet Spectrophotometry

The solvents used to extract phenytoin from biologic specimens can be utilized for extraction of the barbiturates, particularly phenobarbital. A minimum of about 10 μg is required. A 1.0- to 2.0-ml sample of whole blood or serum (no pH adjustment) is extracted with 25 ml of dichloroethane. This mixture is shaken vigorously for 1 to 2 min and the organic layer is removed and filtered through Whatman no. 1 filter paper into a graduated cylinder and the volume of dichloroethane adjusted to a specific volume as outlined in the extraction procedure for phenytoin. This is an excellent stopping point in the analysis. The dichloroethane is subsequently extracted with 5 ml of 0.45 N NaOH. At this point the analysis should be taken to rapid completion. After 1 to 2 min of vigorous shaking the NaOH layer is removed. Into each of two semimicrocuvettes (2.4-ml capacity), place 1.0 ml each of the aqueous layer. To one cuvette add 0.17 ml of 0.45 N NaOH and to the other add 0.17 ml of 16% ammonium chloride solution. The cuvette containing only NaOH solution is placed in the sample compartment of a double-beam ratio-recording ultraviolet spectrophotometer capable of scanning from 210 to 340 nm. The cuvette containing the NaOH solution diluted with the NH_4Cl solution is placed in the reference compartment. The difference in absorbance between the two solutions at 260 nm is used to calculate the phenobarbital concentration. The remaining volume of 0.45 N

NaOH solution can be quantitatively transferred to a 50-ml round-bottom flask for analysis of phenytoin as described above.

GENERAL DISCUSSION—COMMENTS

Both the semimicro- and microprocedures provide quantitative recovery of phenytoin at subtherapeutic through toxic levels from small volumes of plasma (Tables 1 and 2, respectively). The method provides a mean recovery of 94% and a sensitivity limit of approximately 0.5 μg/ml for a 0.2-ml specimen. Coefficients of variation for replicate determinations are typically less than 4%.

Earlier spectrophotometric determinations for phenytoin based on the conversion to benzophenone utilized large solvent volumes for steam distillation or reflux, resulting in an extensive dilution of the benzophenone product. Use of 50-ml boiling flasks with the standard Allihn condenser requires only 3 ml of heptane, which results in a significant increase in sensitivity. However, a further decrease in the solvent volume to 2 ml, when using the standard condenser, more than doubles the coefficient of variation that is achieved with 3 ml of solvent, apparently because of an insufficient amount of liquid solvent available for the continuous extraction of benzophenone. Utilization of an "external cold finger" reflux condenser induces a more rapid condensation of solvent vapors, which permits the effective utilization of smaller volumes of solvent (that is, 0.5 to 1.0 ml) and results in a consequent enhanced sensitivity.

Studies have indicated that decreased sensitivity (approximately 70% of that achieved via reflux with continuous magnetic stirring) is obtained in

TABLE 1. *Phenytoin determination by semimicroprocedure*

Concentration[a] (μg/ml)	Absorbance[b,c]	Absorbance/ concentration	Recovery[c] (%)
2.5	0.057 ± 0.009	0.0764	103.5 ± 15.8
5	0.105 ± 0.003	0.0700	94.9 ± 3.1
10	0.211 ± 0.003	0.0702	95.2 ± 1.0
20	0.421 ± 0.005	0.0701	95.0 ± 1.1
30	0.620 ± 0.018	0.0689	93.3 ± 2.7
40	0.810 ± 0.020	0.0675	91.4 ± 2.3
60	1.267 ± 0.036	0.0703	95.3 ± 2.7
80	1.655 ± 0.016	0.0691	93.6 ± 1.3
Mean		0.0703 ± 0.0044 (6.3%)	95.3 ± 6.0 (94.1 ± 2.0 over the range 5–80 μg/ml)

[a] Determinations performed on 1.0 ml of plasma.
[b] Absorbance at 247 nm, adjusted for mean plasma blank of 0.012.
[c] Mean of triplicate determinations ± standard deviation.

TABLE 2. *Phenytoin determination by microprocedure*

Concentration[a] (μg/ml)	Absorbance[b]	Absorbance/ concentration	Recovery (%)
5	0.050 ± 0.008	0.0694	94.4
10	0.099 ± 0.002	0.0688	93.5
20	0.196 ± 0.002	0.0680	92.6
30	0.302 ± 0.012	0.0699	95.1
40	0.392 ± 0.003	0.0680	92.6
60	0.598 ± 0.007	0.0692	94.1
80	0.793 ± 0.017	0.0688	93.7
Mean		0.0689 ± 0.0027	93.7 ± 3.6

[a] Triplicate plasma determinations performed on 0.2-ml specimens.
[b] Absorbance at 247 nm ± standard deviation, adjusted for mean plasma blank of 0.002.

the nonreflux technique and is a consequence of benzophenone overoxidation (product degradation), rather than its volatility (28). A decreased yield of benzophenone is also obtained if the magnetic stirrers are temporarily stopped during reflux. Although the nonreflux technique does not provide the sensitivity obtained through reflux, it does offer the advantage of not requiring the more expensive reflux apparatus. For laboratories having a limited budget and not possessing reflux apparatus, the nonreflux technique may be the most appropriate method. But for those laboratories possessing the necessary apparatus, the enhanced sensitivity and reproducibility achieved by the reflux method may more than offset the modest additional analysis time. The utilization of the cold finger condenser provides a micromethod that is unequaled in sensitivity by the sealed oxidation techniques.

ACKNOWLEDGMENT

This research was supported in part by Grant RO1 MH 2643–0111 from the National Institute of Health, Bethesda, Maryland.

REFERENCES

1. Bock, G. W., and Sherwin, A. L. (1971): The rapid quantitative determination of diphenylhydantoin in plasma, serum, and whole blood of patients with epilepsy. *Clin. Chim. Acta,* 34:97–103.
2. Bratton, A. C., and Marshall, E. K., Jr. (1939): A new coupling component for sulfanilamide determination. *J. Biol. Chem.,* 128:537–550.
3. Dill, W. A., Baukema, J., Chang, T., and Glazko, A. J. (1971): Colorimetric assay of 5,5-diphenylhydantoin (Dilantin®) and 5-(*p*-hydroxyphenyl)-5-phenylhydantoin. *Proc. Soc. Exp. Biol. Med.,* 137:674–679.
4. Dill, W. A., Chucot, L., Chang, T., and Glazko, A. J. (1971): A simplified benzophenone procedure for diphenylhydantoin assays in plasma. *Clin. Chem.,* 17:1200–1201.
5. Dill, W. A., and Glazko, A. J. (1972): Fluorometric assay of diphenylhydantoin in plasma or whole blood. *Clin. Chem.,* 18:675–676.

6. Dill, W. A., Kazenko, A., Wolf, L., and Glazko, A. (1956): Studies on 5,5-diphenylhydantoin (Dilantin®) in animals and man. *J. Pharmacol. Exp. Ther.*, 118:270–279.
7. Glazko, A. J. (1972): Diphenylhydantoin: Chemistry and methods for determination. In *Antiepileptic Drugs,* edited by D. M. Woodbury, J. K. Penry, and R. P. Schmidt. Raven Press, New York.
8. Goldbaum, L. R. (1952): Determination of barbiturates. *Anal. Chem.,* 24:1604.
9. Hepler, B. R., and Wallace, J. E. (1975): Diphenylhydantoin. In *Methodology for Analytical Toxicology,* edited by I. Sunshine, p. 132. Chemical Rubber Co., Cleveland, Ohio.
10. Kozelka, F. L., and Hine, C. H. (1941): A method for determination of 5,5-diphenylhydantoin in biological material. *J. Biol. Chem.,* 72:276–279.
11. Kristensen, M., Hansen, J. M., Hansen, O. E., and Lund, V. (1967): Sources of error in the determination of phenytoin (Dilantin®) by Svensmark and Kristensen's method. *Acta Neurol. Scand.,* 48:447–450.
12. Lee, S. E., and Bass, N. H. (1970): Microassay of diphenylhydantoin. *Neurology* (Minneap.), 20:115–124.
13. Morselli, P. L. (1970): An improved technic for routine determinations of diphenylhydantoin in plasma and tissues. *Clin. Chim. Acta,* 28:37–40.
14. Olesen, O. V. (1967): Determination of phenobarbital and phenytoin in serum by ultraviolet spectrophotometry. *Scand. J. Clin. Lab. Invest.,* 20:63.
15. Plaa, G. L., and Hine, C. H. (1956): A method for the simultaneous determination of phenobarbital and diphenylhydantoin in blood. *J. Lab. Clin. Med.,* 47:649–657.
16. Richens, A. (1975): Quality control of drug estimations. *Acta Neurol. Scand., Suppl.* 60:81–84.
17. Saitoh, Y., Nishibara, K., Nakagawa, F., and Suzuki, T. (1973): Improved microdetermination for diphenylhydantoin in blood by UV spectrophotometry. *J. Pharm. Sci.,* 62:206–210.
18. Schiller, P. J., and Buchthal, F. (1958): Diphenylhydantoin and phenobarbital in serum in patients with epilepsy. *Dan. Med. Bull.,* 5:161–163.
19. Stainier, C., Bosly, J., Dutrieux, F., and Stainier, R. (1963): Influence des substituants sur la stabilité des barbituriques en milieu alcalin. *Pharm. Acta Helv.,* 38:587.
20. Stevenson, G. W. (1961): Spectrophotometric determination of blood barbiturates. *Anal. Chem.,* 33:1374.
21. Svensmark, O., and Kristensen, P. (1963): Determination of diphenylhydantoin and phenobarbital in small amounts of serum. *J. Lab. Clin. Med.,* 61:501–507.
22. Svensmark, O., Schiller, P. J., and Buchthal, F. (1960): 5,5-Diphenylhydantoin (Dilantin®) blood levels after oral or intravenous dosage in man. *Acta Pharmacol. Toxicol.* (Kbh.), 16:331–346.
23. Wallace, J. E. (1966): Spectrophotometric determination of diphenylhydantoin. *J. Forensic Sci.,* 11:552–559.
24. Wallace, J. E. (1968): Microdetermination of diphenylhydantoin in biological specimens by ultraviolet spectrophotometry. *Anal. Chem.,* 40:978–980.
25. Wallace, J. E. (1969): Simultaneous spectrophotometric determination of diphenylhydantoin and phenobarbital in biologic specimens. *Clin. Chem.,* 15:323–330.
26. Wallace, J. E., Biggs, J. D., and Dahl, E. V. (1965): Determination of diphenylhydantoin by ultraviolet spectrophotometry. *Anal. Chem.,* 37:10–13.
27. Wallace, J. E., Farquhar, J. K., Hamilton, H. E., and Everhart, B. A. (1974): Comments on the determination of diphenylhydantoin. *Clin. Chem.,* 20:515–516.
28. Wallace, J. E., and Hamilton, H. E. (1974): Diphenylhydantoin microdetermination in serum and plasma by UV spectrophotometry. *J. Pharm. Sci.,* 63:1795–1798.
29. Williams, L. A. (1971): Diphenylhydantoin. In *Manual of Analytical Toxicology,* edited by I. Sunshine, p. 128. Chemical Rubber Co., Cleveland, Ohio.

ANTIEPILEPTIC DRUG QUALITY CONTROL

Antiepileptic Drugs: Quantitative Analysis and Interpretation, edited by C. E. Pippenger, J. K. Penry, and H. Kutt, Raven Press, New York, © 1978.

Chapter 17

Antiepileptic Drug Levels Quality Control Program: Interlaboratory Variability

C. E. Pippenger, H. Paris-Kutt, J. Kiffin Penry, and David D. Daly

Over the past several years, the value of monitoring serum antiepileptic drug concentrations as an adjunct to the provision of better care for epileptic patients has been clearly demonstrated (3,6,14). As a consequence, physicians, particularly neurologists, have demanded the availability of services for monitoring serum antiepileptic drug concentrations. This demand has stimulated a large number of laboratories to establish testing procedures for the various antiepileptic drugs.

In 1972, participants at a workshop on the determination of antiepileptic drugs in serum expressed concern about the reliability of laboratories that routinely perform antiepileptic drug assays (7). Subsequently, a European survey of proficiency in antiepileptic drug assays demonstrated wide interlaboratory variability. A European quality control program for antiepileptic drugs was instituted under the supervision of Dr. A. Richens, St. Bartholomew's Hospital, London. The results have been described (10,11).

Much of the interlaboratory variability in therapeutic drug monitoring is attributable directly to the lack of appropriate proficiency regulations and cooperation between laboratories to assure uniform performance regardless of the laboratories' geographical locations. Because laboratory licensure regulations are rather broad and differ widely among states or cities, the establishment of a new laboratory is not difficult. To open a therapeutic drug monitoring laboratory, basically all the operator has to do is find a pathologist who will nominally "supervise" the laboratory and allow utilization of his licenses, buy the appropriate analytical equipment, and hang a sign outside the door that says "drug levels." The opening of a hot dog stand in any city is more stringently regulated. The vendor needs numerous licenses from the city and state that certify the operator's health, the sanitation of the physical facilities, and numerous other requirements before the establishment is allowed to conduct business. The requirements for certification of an established laboratory also vary from state to state, depending on the interest and concern of the regulating agencies involved.

In order to assess the accuracy of laboratories performing antiepileptic drug assays, in 1974, a series of three "patient" specimens were blindly evaluated by a number of laboratories that routinely analyzed antiepileptic drug levels. All samples were submitted under a physician's letterhead, and all laboratory fees were paid. The results of this survey are summarized in Table 1. A detailed description of this survey has been reported (9).

Table 1 shows that the number of laboratories performing assays of phenytoin, phenobarbital, primidone, carbamazepine, and ethosuximide decrease in order of the drugs named. The coefficient of variation for a given assay tends to increase when fewer laboratories are performing the assay. This decreasing performance appears to be related to the frequency of requests for a given assay, and primidone, carbamazepine, and ethosuximide assays are performed less frequently by most laboratories. Consequently, many of the laboratories performing these assays did not appear to have well-established or well-controlled methodologies or were not really aware of potential problems associated with the assays. An unacceptable range of values was reported for each drug (Table 1). It is not difficult to imagine what such values would mean in the treatment of patients if they were accepted as correct by the attending physician.

This survey also demonstrated that some laboratories had no concept of the optimal therapeutic ranges of the drug they were assaying. Less than 10% of the reporting laboratories commented on durg concentrations that were significantly above the therapeutic range. One laboratory wrote a note on the physician's report with regard to an ethosuximide concentration of 836 μg/ml which said: "my standards were a little off today, but this level is high." The survey clearly established, however, that there are both good laboratories (within ±1 SD of the reference value) and bad laboratories (over ±1 SD of the reference value). Unfortunately, both types are reporting serum drug levels that are utilized by the attending physician to adjust the patient's medication regimen.

TABLE 1. ***Results from blind survey of antiepileptic drug-level determinations in three pooled plasma samples***

	Drug	Number of laboratories reporting	Mean (μg/ml)	Standard deviation	Range (μg/ml)	Coefficient of variation (%)
Sample 1	Phenytoin	109	13.1	7.5	0.0– 70.0	57.3
	Phenobarbital	108	49.0	24.9	0.0–264.0	50.8
	Primidone	93	12.3	9.5	0.0– 83.0	77.2
	Ethosuximide	71	14.9	75.2	0.0–633.0	504.7
Sample 2	Phenytoin	107	24.8	10.1	0.0– 76.8	40.7
	Phenobarbital	107	21.7	23.0	0.0–246.4	106.0
	Primidone	93	5.1	10.1	0.0– 73.0	198.0
	Ethosuximide	74	49.9	97.3	0.0–836.0	195.0
Sample 3	Phenytoin	108	12.5	5.1	0.0– 29.0	49.8
	Phenobarbital	109	26.0	9.8	0.4– 64.8	37.7
	Primidone	93	3.7	9.2	0.0– 65.0	248.6
	Ethosuximide	71	52.4	56.7	0.0–439.2	108.2

Modified from [9].

As a consequence of the results obtained in the blind survey, a voluntary Antiepileptic Drug Levels Quality Control Program (AEDL-QC) was established in April 1975 under the auspices of the Epilepsy Foundation of America, with an initial enrollment of 125 laboratories. By July 1976, there were 187 participating laboratories. The program was then expanded by active recruitment, and 550 laboratories are currently participating in the AEDL-QC program.

Each month, we mail three spiked serum samples to all participating laboratories. Each laboratory analyzes the sample and immediately reports the results to us. We report the actual spiked values by return mail, so that the laboratories know immediately whether their values are consistent with the control values.

One of the requirements for participation in the quality control program is completion of a questionnaire that describes various aspects of each laboratory's operations, including the methodology. As of November 1, 1976, laboratories performing antiepileptic drug levels were utilizing the following methods: gas liquid chromatography, 213; homogeneous enzyme immunoassay (EMIT), 145; ultraviolet spectrophotometry, 50 (primarily for phenobarbital, although some were using UV for both phenytoin and phenobarbital); radioimmunoassay, 26 (phenytoin only); high-pressure liquid chromatography, 4; thin-layer chromatography, 3. Each of these methodologies has been extensively reviewed in this volume. The following general conceptions are based on our observations of the methodologies in the quality control program:

The thin-layer chromatographic (TLC) assays are readily susceptible to error. Because many classes of drugs have migration patterns similar to those of antiepileptic drugs, in the commonly employed solvent systems, it is difficult to quantitate serum antiepileptic drug levels with TLC. To quantitate antiepileptic drugs successfully by this method, the laboratory must know specifically what drugs the patient is taking, and establish whether or not these agents interfere in the assay.

The radioimmunoassay (RIA) is a highly sensitive and specific procedure, but it is limited in three respects:

1. Phenytoin is the only commercially available RIA assay. Other antiepileptic drugs found in patients on multiple-drug therapy must be analyzed by another method.
2. Some RIA kits for phenytoin cross-react with the major metabolite of phenytoin (parahydroxyphenytoin, HPPH), which is present in small quantities in serum, whereas other kits do not (see Chapter 15).
3. RIA assays require special equipment, special precautions, and highly skilled technicians.

The clinical applicability of high-pressure liquid chromatography (HPLC) to the analysis of antiepileptic drug concentrations currently cannot be determined because of insufficient data. Preliminary reports suggest that HPLC is applicable not only to quantitation of antiepileptic drugs but also to analysis of their major metabolites (see Chapter 14).

The most common spectrophotometric methods for antiepileptic drug analysis are the colorimetric method of Dill et al. (1) and the ultraviolet spectrophotometric technique of Svensmark and Kristensen (13). These methods are restricted primarily to the analysis of phenytoin and phenobarbital. If careful procedures are followed and the limitations of these assays are recognized, both phenytoin and phenobarbital may be quantitated accurately by the colorimetric or UV method. However, the laboratory must know what other drugs the patient is receiving. For example, primidone is not completely separated by countercurrent extraction methods employing the commonly used partition solvents, which results in an apparent elevation of both phenytoin and phenobarbital concentrations. Unless the UV assay is in the hands of an extremely good analyst, we would not encourage its use. The fluorometric assay of Dill et al. (2) is simple and specific for phenytoin but it is not applicable to other drugs the patient may be receiving.

The homogeneous enzyme immunoassay (EMIT) is rapid and specific, and allows the five major antiepileptic drugs to be determined in one 50-μl serum specimen (8) (see Chapter 10). If the drugs that the patient is receiving are known, it is possible to assay for only those drugs. The EMIT system is simple to use and therefore readily adaptable to the small hospital laboratory. It should be noted that quality control is essential to the successful employment of the EMIT system (see Chapter 18).

Gas-liquid chromatographic (GLC) assays are rapid and specific when properly performed. With the recent and rapid technological advances in antiepileptic drug analysis, it is difficult to realize the role that the GLC methods, developed between 1969 and 1971, have had in allowing the widespread routine therapeutic monitoring of antiepileptic drugs to become a reality. Although initially many of the potential errors related to GLC analysis of antiepileptic drugs were not recognized, improved extraction techniques and the development of appropriate internal standards have substantially refined the GLC methodology. GLC remains a valuable and reliable technique for the determination of antiepileptic drugs and their metabolites.

One of the major factors contributing to interlaboratory variability is the type of GLC methodology used. Basically, there are three types of GLC methods for analyzing antiepileptic drugs: (a) derivatization with trimethylphenylammonium hydroxide (TMPAH) (5), (b) derivatization with tetramethylammonium hydroxide (TMAH) (12), or (c) underivatized (4). The application of each of these methods to antiepileptic drug analysis has been well described. With appropriate care all three methods are quite satisfactory.

It appears that almost every laboratory has modified the basic methods described in the literature. The initial methods were originally designed to eliminate problems in GLC analysis of antiepileptic drugs, but most of the modifications have succeeded in reintroducing the problems. Generally, the changes have been made to achieve shorter extraction or analysis times. The modifications are generally at the expense of procedures that were designed to remove interfering components from the serum. Some laboratories use procedures that remove only part of the naturally interfering compounds. Others operate the chromatographic equipment at elevated temperatures to decrease analysis time, without realizing that interfering peaks may be driven under the drug peaks.

In order to assess the continuing performance of the laboratories participating in the quality control program, we developed the concept of a performance index. The performance index (PI) is defined as the sum of the absolute differences between reported concentrations and spiked values for a given month divided by the sum of the spiked values for that month:

$$\mathrm{PI} = \frac{\sum_{i}^{n} = 1\ |R_i - S_i|}{\sum_{i}^{n} = 1\quad S_i}$$

where R_i = the recorded laboratory value and S_i = the spiked value.

Based on our experience with performance index patterns, we believe that a PI of less than 10 is exceptionally good, 10 to 20 is satisfactory, and above 20 is unacceptable when the results are applied to patient management.

Figure 1 shows the performance index patterns for five antiepileptic drugs analyzed in both an "excellent" laboratory and an "unsatisfactory" laboratory. The "excellent" laboratory routinely conducts a good internal quality control program and takes care in the extraction and analysis of the drugs. The "unsatisfactory" laboratory modified the simplest method it could find and had no internal quality control program. The laboratory's performance improved following technician training, but relapsed when the trained technician quit. The patterns presented in Fig. 1 are characteristic of laboratories with satisfactory and unsatisfactory PI patterns regardless of the analytical methodology employed in antiepileptic drug analysis.

One of the most gratifying experiences of the quality control program has been the improvement in performance exhibited by many laboratories that corrected or improved their methodologies upon receiving their performance results. Unfortunately, others have maintained poor performance indexes throughout the program and have made no attempt to correct their errors.

The PI patterns of the laboratories participating in the quality control program clearly demonstrate that intralaboratory variability in many laboratories is excessive. Intralaboratory variability is correctable, and it is the responsibility of each laboratory to institute the appropriate quality control

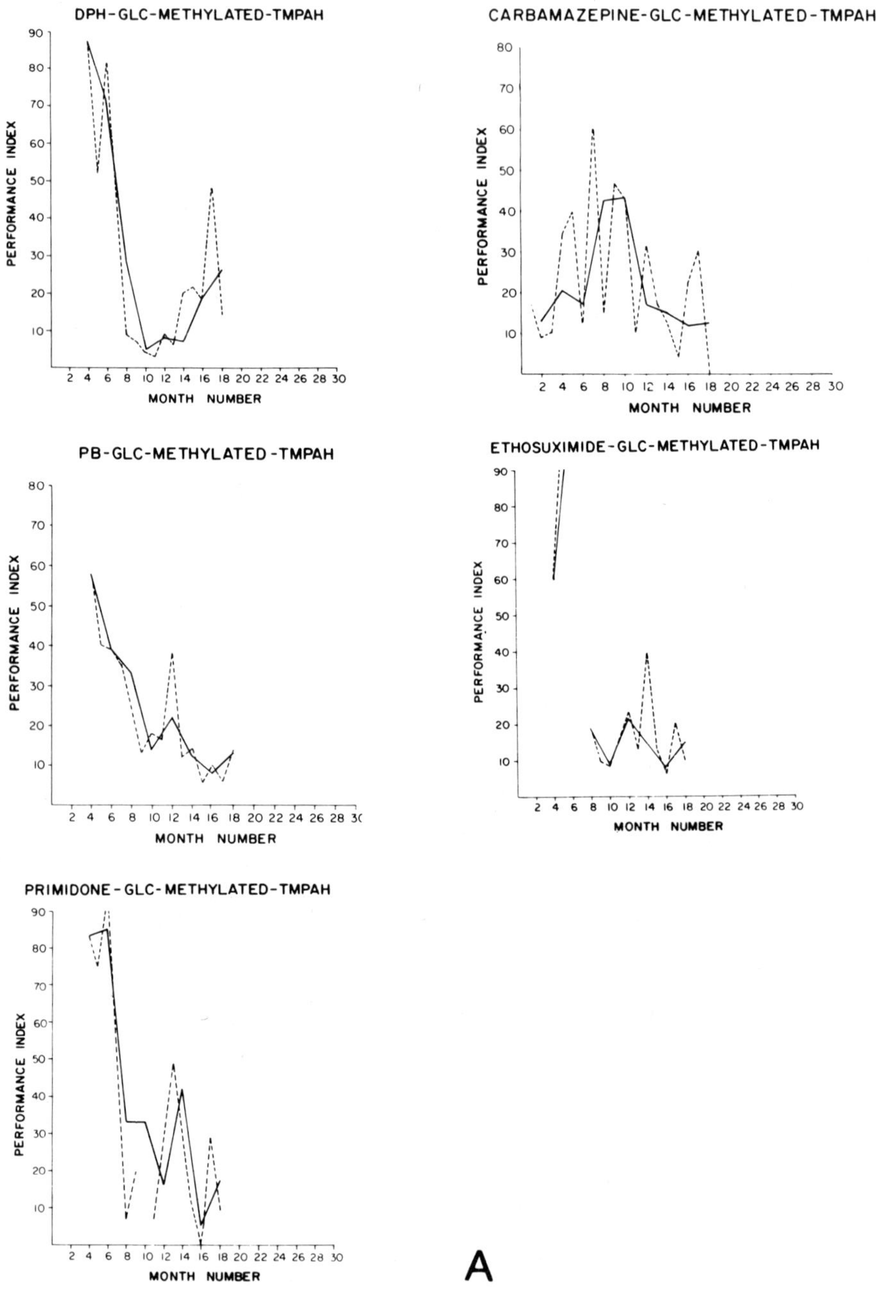

FIG. 1A. See legend to 1B (facing).

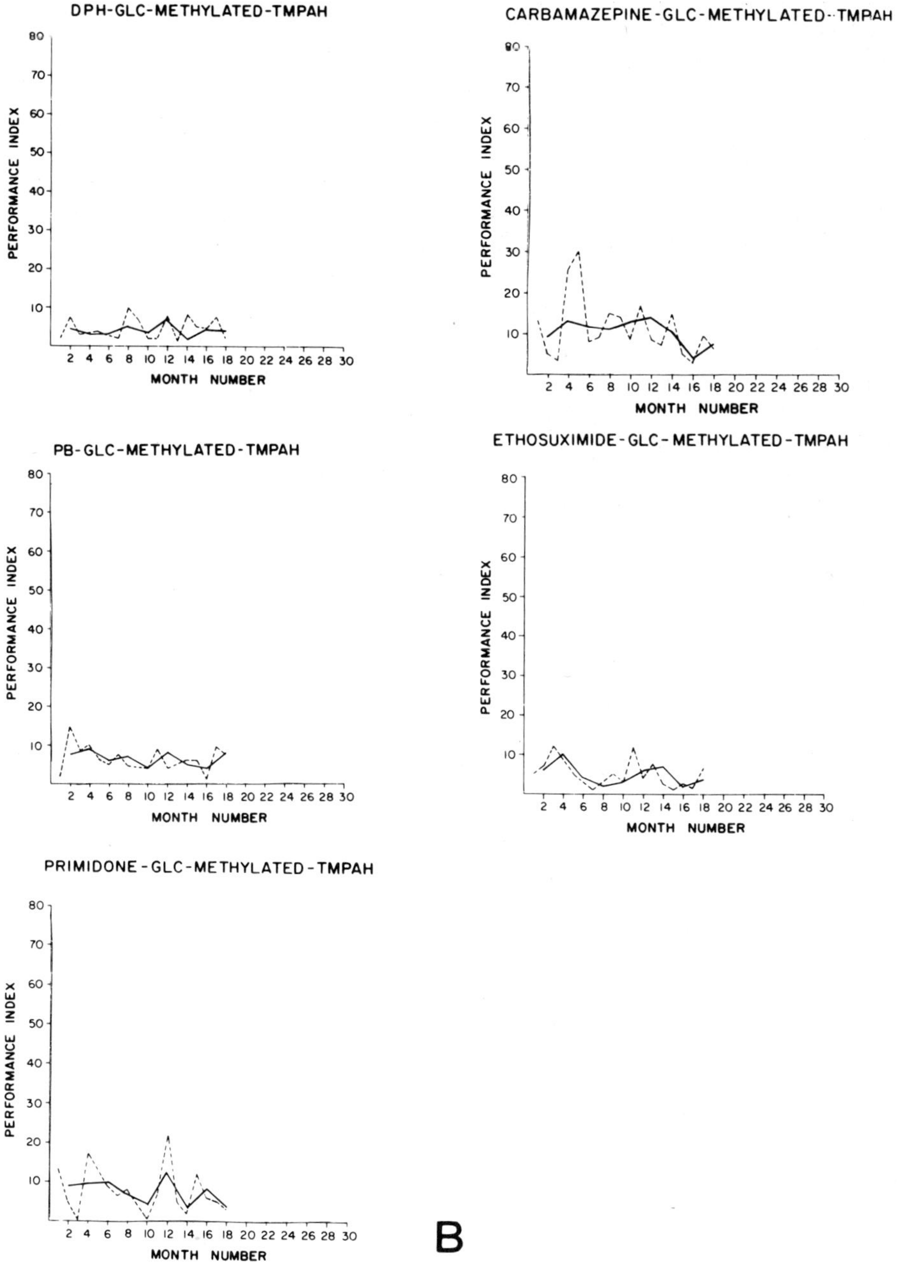

FIG. 1B. Performance index patterns for an "excellent" (A) and an "unsatisfactory" (B) laboratory, both utilizing identical GLC derivatization techniques with trimethylphenylammonium hydroxide (TMPAH).

schemes to curtail the month-to-month performance index variations that we have observed.

Intralaboratory quality control is such a simple procedure that we cannot understand why some laboratories fail to practice it. The internal quality control program in our laboratory serves as an example. Every day, whether drugs are assayed by gas chromatography or EMIT, a standard curve is obtained from a biological matrix (EMIT calibrators) prior to analysis of patient samples. With each day's run, three quality control specimens containing subtherapeutic, therapeutic, and toxic drug concentrations are carried through the analytical procedure. Quality control specimens are prepared by pooling specimens or spiking plasma with the appropriate drug concentrations (see Dudley and Bius, Appendix II). The run is repeated if the reported concentration of the controls exceeds 10% of the expected control values. Control values are plotted each day to identify possible trends indicative of potential analytical problems. Any laboratory encounters problems with day-to-day internal quality control. When the quality control values are incorrect, patient specimens should not be assayed until the problem is resolved and control is reestablished. Although laboratories are under pressure to report results to the physician, they must take time to correct the assay rather than report an erroneous level. One quality control specimen is not sufficient. For example, it is possible to be in control at therapeutic concentrations and out of control at lower or toxic concentrations. The same quality control criteria are applicable to any analytical method for antiepileptic drugs.

Another problem related to quality control is that not everyone uses an analytical balance properly in weighing drugs for use as standards. Currently, the only good antiepileptic drug calibrators in a biological matrix are those available from Syva Co. (Palo Alto, Ca.). Commercially marketed toxicology controls are of limited value and should not be utilized as controls for antiepileptic drug assays, even though they may contain these agents, unless they have been thoroughly evaluated. For example, the Lederle and Ortho toxicology controls contain both phenobarbital and glutethimide (Doriden). Methylation of a serum extract methylates all components that will react with the derivatizing agent, including other drugs and fatty acids. Both gluthethimide and phenobarbital are extracted and methylated in many GLC procedures. Because the difference in retention time between the methylated derivatives of glutethimide and phenobarbital is 0.03 min, these compounds are not separated under routine GLC operating conditions. Consequently, the erroneously high calibration for phenobarbital, if either the Lederle or Ortho toxicology controls are used, would result in an inaccurate report of a low phenobarbital level in the patient. The physician might then make inappropriate adjustments in the patient's phenobarbital regimen.

A substantial improvement in the performance of many laboratories participating in the AEDL-QC program is clearly evident. When the pilot program was initiated in 1975, more than half of the laboratories surveyed were producing unreliable antiepileptic drug levels. Blood-level monitoring reports produced by an unreliable laboratory could lead the physician to inaccurate adjustments of antiepileptic drug dosages, perhaps resulting in increased seizure frequency or drug toxicity for the patient.

An analysis of the performance of laboratories based on the monthly PI pattern shows a significant improvement in laboratory performance (Table 2). Laboratories in the "excellent" and "satisfactory" categories are routinely producing reliable results. This improved performance is especially significant for laboratories determining levels of phenytoin and phenobarbital, the two most widely prescribed antiepileptic drugs. Improvement in performance of laboratories assaying carbamazepine levels is less dramatic, but understandably so because the methodology for assaying this drug presents the greatest number of analytical problems and is prone to error if not carefully performed (see Chapter 18).

An important consideration of antiepileptic drug levels in patient management is the cost of the determination. Based on information from the quality control program, patients taking only one antiepileptic drug would be charged from $3 to $38 for determination of the drug level. If the patient is receiving two drugs, however, the cost ranges from $9 to $80, and for three drugs, the range is $13 to $150. If a patient is taking phenytoin and primidone and the physician requests determination of three drug levels (phenytoin, primidone, and phenobarbital), the cost to the patient is $50 to $150. Unfortunately, this pricing structure denies the patient proper medical care. Many patients need a series of antiepileptic drug-level determinations over a period of a few weeks or months for proper regulation of their drug dosages. How can epileptic patients manage to achieve seizure control through adjustment of medication dosages when they cannot afford to pay for the analysis of antiepileptic drug levels?

Two years ago one hospital was charging a fee of $20 for each specimen, regardless of the number of drugs in the sample. The hospital administration elected to raise the price to $42 without consulting anyone. Fee raises are always justified by referring to the inflation rate; it costs more to run the

TABLE 2. *Typical monthly performance of laboratories participating in the AEDL-QC program*

Drug	Number of laboratories (N)	Excellent (%N)	Satisfactory (%N)	Unsatisfactory (%N)	Extremely poor (%N)
Phenytoin	367	49.0 (180)	39.2 (144)	10.2 (38)	1.4 (5)
Phenobarbital	374	40.4 (151)	34.0 (127)	24.9 (93)	0.8 (3)
Carbamazepine	194	20.1 (39)	42.8 (83)	29.4 (57)	7.7 (15)
Primidone	286	33.2 (98)	28.0 (80)	33.9 (97)	3.8 (11)
Ethosuximide	179	42.4 (76)	27.4 (49)	30.2 (54)	0.0 (0)

Number of laboratories shown in parentheses.

tests. As a result of these fee increases, there was essentially no growth in the number of patient specimens processed over a 1-year period. The analysis of inpatient specimens increased, but physicians stopped submitting outpatient samples, except in extreme situations, because the patients could not afford to have the drug levels analyzed. There is no justifiable reason why the determination of an antiepileptic drug level should cost significantly more than an SMA 12–60 profile. As long as antiepileptic drug assays are exhorbitantly priced, patients are denied the care to which they are entitled.

Many laboratories defend their pricing systems by stating that "we have to make a profit, we have to support our laboratory, we have to cover our costs." The cost of reagents for GLC analysis of anticonvulsant is 14¢; the cost of the EMIT reagents for three drugs run in duplicate is $9. What is a fair price? That may be difficult to say, but we do not believe that patients should be charged more for assay of multiple drugs than for single drugs, or certainly not much more. Nor do we believe that assays should be denied to patients who cannot afford them, because they are necessary for good patient care. Should analysis of antiepileptic drug levels be denied the child with uncontrolled grand mal seizures whose parent is making $5,328 a year, does not qualify for Medicaid, and has no hospitalization insurance? Should we charge the parent $210 for five determinations over a 6-week period? There needs to be some judiciousness and fairness in laboratory fees for analysis of antiepileptic drugs. Fair laboratory fees will not come from the physician but from the laboratories who admit "this is an excessive fee for the patient to pay, surely we can do it for less."

The improvement of inter- and intralaboratory performance in the analysis of antiepileptic drugs depends on all laboratories working together. We urge laboratories engaged in antiepileptic drug monitoring to adopt the following policies: Institute an internal quality control program. Do not hesitate to ask questions if you need help. Never be afraid to disagree with established methods. Learn as much as possible, which will improve your laboratory's performance. Keep in contact with the people in your region who are assaying antiepileptic drugs. Encourage laboratories to cooperate, and help other laboratories if they need help. Ensure fair pricing practices in your laboratory.

Only through the cooperative efforts of concerned laboratories will antiepileptic drug levels become reliable and reproducible. Then, failure to use antiepileptic drug-level determinations could no longer be attributed to lack of trust in laboratory results. Improved laboratory performance assures the patient of the best possible care. It requires accurate and reliable quantitation of antiepileptic drugs, and this is our responsibility.

REFERENCES

1. Dill, W. A., Baukema, J., Chang, T., and Glazko, A. J. (1971): Colorimetric assay of 5,5-diphenylhydantoin (Dilantin) and 5-(*p*-hydroxyphenyl)-5-phenylhydantoin. *Proc. Soc. Exp. Biol. Med.,* 137:674–679.

2. Dill, W. A., Leung, A., Kinkel, A. W., and Glazko, A. J. (1976): A simplified fluorometric assay for diphenylhydantoin in plasma. *Clin. Chem.*, 22:908–911.
3. Eadie, M. J., and Tyrer, J. H. (1974): *Anticonvulsant Therapy—Pharmacological Basis and Practice.* Churchill Livingstone, London.
4. Evenson, M. A., Jones, P., and Darcey, B. (1970): Simultaneous measurement of diphenylhydantoin and primidone in serum by gas-liquid chromatography. *Clin. Chem.*, 16:107.
5. Kupferberg, H. J. (1970): Quantitative estimation of diphenylhydantoin, primidone and phenobarbital in plasma by gas-liquid chromatography. *Clin. Chem. Acta,* 29: 283–288.
6. Kutt, H., and Penry, J. K. (1974): Usefulness of blood levels of antiepileptic drugs. *Arch. Neurol.,* 31:283–288.
7. Penry, J. K. (1973): Workshop on laboratories for determination of antiepileptic drugs in serum. *Epilepsia,* 14:118–121.
8. Pippenger, C. E. (1976): Homogenous enzyme immunoassays for the quantitation of diphenylhydantoin, phenobarbital, and primidone in serum or plasma: An overview. In *Quantitative Analytic Studies in Epilepsy,* edited by P. Kellaway and I. Petersen. Raven Press, New York.
9. Pippenger, C. E., Penry, J. K., White, B. G., Daly, D. D., and Buddington, R. (1976): Interlaboratory variability in determination of plasma antiepileptic drug concentrations. *Arch. Neurol.,* 33:351–355.
10. Richens, A. (1975): Results of a phenytoin quality control scheme. In *Clinical Pharmacology of Anti-Epileptic Drugs,* edited by H. Schneider, D. Janz, C. Gardner-Thorpe, H. Meinardi, and A. L. Sherwin. Springer-Verlag, Berlin, Heidelberg, New York.
11. Richens, A. (1975): Quality control of drug estimations. *Acta Neurol. Scand.,* Suppl. 75:81–84.
12. Solow, E. B., and Green, J. B. (1972): The simultaneous determination of multiple anticonvulsant drug levels by gas-liquid chromatography: Method and clinical application. *Neurology* (Minneap.), 22:540–550.
13. Svensmark, O., and Kristensen, P. (1963): Determination of diphenylhydantoin and phenobarbital in small amounts of serum. *J. Lab. Clin. Med.,* 61:501–507.
14. Woodbury, D. M., Penry, J. K., and Schmidt, R. P., editors (1972): *Antiepileptic Drugs.* Raven Press, New York.

Antiepileptic Drugs: Quantitative Analysis and Interpretation, edited by C. E. Pippenger, J. K. Penry, and H. Kutt, Raven Press, New York, © 1978.

Chapter 18
Common Errors in the Analysis of Antiepileptic Drugs

C. E. Pippenger and H. Kutt

Any analytical procedure used for therapeutic drug monitoring is prone to error. Laboratory errors can arise, for example, from instrument failure, inappropriate analytical procedures, a technician's mistake, or a mistranscription of results. Many errors can be traced to a relatively minor event such as inappropriate preparation of standard curves. One of the major goals of every laboratory should be to minimize the occurrence of laboratory errors. With the rapid increase in the number of routine clinical chemistry services engaged in therapeutic drug monitoring, many laboratories have entered into drug analysis without the training or expertise commonly associated with these assays in research laboratories. Because of the increased demand from physicians for antiepileptic drug monitoring as an aid in the management of their epileptic patients, the volume of assay specimens has exceeded the capacity of basic research laboratories, and service laboratories have had to assume the responsibility for routine drug monitoring.

Prevention of the intra- and interlaboratory variability commonly associated with antiepileptic drug monitoring (8) requires that every laboratory be aware of potential sources of error that may occur during routine antiepileptic drug analysis. This chapter describes some common errors than can occur at any point within the analytical procedure, from the time the specimen arrives in the laboratory until the final report is issued.

REQUISITION FORMS

One of the major problems associated with antiepileptic drug analysis is the failure of the analytical laboratory to be cognizant of all medications that the patient might be receiving. Many drugs have common ultraviolet spectra which can interfere with UV procedures. For instance, primidone in most extraction procedures is not separated from phenytoin or phenobarbital, and the results for these drugs may be erroneously elevated as a consequence of the UV absorption of primidone. Under common gas chromatographic conditions, mephenytoin and its major metabolite 5-ethyl-5-phenylhydantoin (Nirvanol) are both methylated to the same end product with alkylating reagents. Mephenytoin will elute as a leading shoulder or directly under the phenobarbital peak, thus leading to an erroneous report of an elevated phenobarbital level. Laboratories should evaluate in their analytical systems all currently marketed antiepileptic drugs and their metabolites to assess possible interferences in the assay.

We recommend that laboratories engaged in therapeutic monitoring of antiepileptic drugs use a general requisition form that requires the patient's age, weight, and sex, and a listing of all drugs (including adjunctive agents)

THE PRESBYTERIAN HOSPITAL - CLINICAL CHEMISTRY SERVICE

ANTICONVULSANT DRUG LEVEL REQUEST

Name ______________________ Levels Requested: Diphenylhydantoin ( )

Unit No. ______________________ Phenobarbital ( )

Sex M ____ F ____ Primidone ( )

Age ____________ Ethosuximide ( )

Body Weight ________ Carbamazepine ( )

List ALL medications including non-anticonvulsants and dosages the patient is receiving or has received in the past 14 days.

Medication:	Total Daily Dosage	Time of Last Dose	Other Drugs	Total Daily Dosage	Time of Last Dose
Diphenylhydantoin	______	______	______	______	______
Phenobarbital	______	______	______	______	______
Primidone (Mysoline)	______	______	______	______	______
Ethosuximide (Zarontin)	______	______	______	______	______
Carbamazepine (Tegretol)	______	______	______	______	______
Diazepam (Valium)	______	______	______	______	______

Types of Clinical Seizures: (Check as many as are applicable)

1. Generalized Major Motor ( )
2. Short Absence ( )
3. Focal motor ( )
4. Focal sensory ( )
5. Special sensory or psychical ( )
6. Automatisms ( )
7. Myoclonic ( )
8. Infantile spasms ( )
9. Other (specify) ______________

Etiology: Unknown ( ) Known ( ) (What?) __________

Seizure Control: Complete ( ) Incomplete:
Good ( ) Fair ( ) Poor ( )
How frequent ? __________

Signs of toxicity: No ( )
Yes (What?)
Nystagmus ( ) Ataxia ( ) Lethargy ( ) Headaches ( )
Nausea ( ) Vomiting ( ) Others: __________

Time sample drawn: ________ A.M. P.M.

Comments:

Physician requesting test: ______________ (please print) ________ (date of sample) ________ (Tel. Ex.)

Local Address: N. I. ________ Other ______________

NOTE: ACD LEVELS WILL NOT BE ASSAYED UNLESS ACCOMPANIED BY THIS COMPLETED FORM

FIG. 1. An example of an antiepileptic drug-level request form that provides sufficient information to evaluate the pharmacological status of a patient in relation to serum drug concentration.

and their daily dosages that the patient is receiving. The requisition form used at Columbia University's laboratory is illustrated in Fig. 1. The list of antiepileptic drugs on the request form alerts the laboratory to specimens that contain potentially interfering drugs. Such request forms are also helpful in identifying patients who may have abnormal drug levels as a result of drug interactions, iatrogenic overdosage or underdosage, patient noncompliance, and disease. The interpretation of serum antiepileptic drug concentrations with respect to these factors has been extensively reviewed (3,5,13).

SAMPLE CONDITION

When the specimen arrives in the laboratory, it should be inspected for the appearance of hemolysis and lipemia. A badly hemolyzed sample greatly enhances the possibility of erroneously low phenytoin levels, because phenytoin is unequally distributed between erythrocytes and plasma (9). Hemolysis dilutes the plasma with the erythrocytes' intracellular fluid. Phenytoin levels from whole blood specimens are not comparable to plasma or serum phenytoin concentrations, unless the assayed concentration is corrected based on the hematocrit.

Lipemic samples contain a large quantity of fatty acids that will not be removed during extraction procedures prior to gas-chromatographic analysis. Because the column packings routinely used for drug analysis are also used for fatty acid analysis, the fatty acids can elute near or under any of the antiepileptic drug peaks, most commonly phenobarbital, and thus alter the chromatographic response. Lipemic samples should be thoroughly washed with hexane, or other appropriate materials, prior to GLC analysis to avoid the possibility of interfering lipids. Lipemic specimens may also interfere with EMIT assays because of light scattering in the cuvette.

PREPARATION OF STANDARDS

A cardinal rule of analytical chemistry is that standard curves must be prepared in the same biological matrix as will be used to assay specimens. Some laboratories prepare standard curves that have been extracted from buffered drug solutions and then use these curves to calculate concentrations from serum specimens. As emphasized by Dudley (Chapter 3) and Dudley and Bius (Appendix II), the nature of any biological matrix is such that it can alter drug extraction efficiencies and thereby lead to erroneous results. A detailed description of the preparation of antiepileptic drug standards in a biological matrix is given by Dudley and Bius in Appendix II. We urge everyone to prepare their standards in a similar manner. GLC calibrators and controls in a biological matrix are available from various manufacturers (see Appendix II).

QUALITY CONTROL

The importance of an active intralaboratory quality control program cannot be overemphasized. We recommend that controls be run daily on whatever system is used. Certainly, one cannot run a standard curve once a month and expect the performance of a gas chromatographic column, for example, to be the same on the last day of the month as it was on the first day of the month, when a large number of samples have been processed through the system. Controls and preferably one or two standards should be run daily in order to assure that the calibration curves are correct. If the controls do not meet performance specifications, appropriate steps should be taken immediately to correct the problem.

Before a commercial control is used in a quality control program, the components of the control must be evaluated. For example, the Lederle Toxicology Control currently marketed contains phenytoin, phenobarbital, and glutethimide, each at a concentration of 20 μg/ml. Laboratories using methylation techniques in the analysis of antiepileptic drugs may find elevated phenobarbital levels with the Lederle control, because both chemical structure and extraction characteristics of glutethimide and phenobarbital are almost identical. On most columns used in the methylation techniques, the difference in retention time between phenobarbital and glutethimide is 0.03 min. It is quite possible, then, that glutethimide and phenobarbital will elute together, giving an erroneously high value. If the Lederle control is used as a calibrator for phenobarbital, the reported phenobarbital levels could be approximately half their true values. We emphasize that every laboratory, before using any commercial control, should carefully assess the other drugs in that control to establish whether or not these compounds interfere in the laboratory's routine drug monitoring procedures.

THE EXTRACTION

Most analytical procedures, including gas chromatographic analysis, require extraction of the biological matrix to isolate the monitored drugs from interfering materials. The analytical methods for routine drug analysis have been extensively reviewed in Chapter 2. Most of these methods were developed in basic research laboratories and were designed to eliminate possible interferences in the assay from extraneous materials. Many of the procedures are time consuming and require thorough knowledge of the chemical characteristics of the compounds under analysis.

One of the most common errors associated with routine drug analysis is the modification of established methods in order to achieve shorter analysis times. The results of such modifications can be disastrous, because failure to remove lipids or other substances that chromatograph on most GLC columns or alter UV spectra can alter the analytical response. Excellent methods for the analysis of antiepileptic drugs have been well established, including those of Kupferberg (4), Dudley et al. (Chapter 4), Solow and Green (11), Booker and Darcey (Appendix II), and Dill et al. (1,2). These methodologies have all proved to yield good quantitative results, provided that the instructions are followed carefully. When an established method is altered or a new analytical technique is developed by a laboratory, it should be carefully assessed for reproducibility, the possibility of interfering substances in the biological matrix, and potential interference from adjunctive medication. Failure to evaluate these factors will only lead to an erroneous analytical technique, which may endanger the patient's proper medical management.

Many GLC procedures utilize on-column methylation or other derivatization techniques to enhance the gas chromatographic analysis of drugs. The most common error associated with derivatization procedures is the failure to use appropriate internal standards. Many investigators have described the decomposition of phenobarbital in an alkaline medium (6,12,14). Phenobarbital decomposes quite erratically in the presence of water and alkaline methylating agents during on-column methylation. The only successful solution to this problem is the use of *p*-tolylphenobarbital as the internal standard for the gas chromatographic quantitation of phenobarbital. Table 1 shows a comparison of serum phenobarbital levels obtained in our laboratory, utilizing on-column methylation with 0.2 M trimethylphenylammonium hydroxide as the derivatizing agent. Phenobarbital concentrations were calculated with either *p*-tolylphenobarbital or *p*-tolylphenytoin (methylphenylphenylhydantoin) as the internal standard. The same samples were analyzed by EMIT methodology for phenobarbital. The results clearly show that the levels were erratic and inconsistent when *p*-tolylphenytoin was used as the internal standard for phenobarbital calculations, compared with the levels obtained when *p*-tolylphenobarbital was used as the internal standard. In contrast, the use of *p*-tolylphenobarbital as the internal standard yielded results that were consistent and comparable with the EMIT system. Obviously, the *p*-tolylphenytoin does not undergo the same decomposition reactions in an alkaline medium as does phenobarbital. The decomposition of phenobarbital and *p*-tolylphenobarbital is consistent and reproducible, because the chemical characteristics of both compounds are comparable. Failure to use *p*-tolylphenobarbital as the internal standard for phenobarbital in derivatization procedures precludes accurate phenobarbital quantitation. Dudley (Chapter 3) has extensively reviewed the use of internal standards in antiepileptic drug monitoring. We urge that every laboratory utilize the appropriate internal standards for therapeutic drug monitoring.

Carbamazepine assays are particularly prone to error in the derivatization procedures because in the presence of alkaline methylating agents carbamazepine is converted to iminostilbene and methylated iminostilbene (10). The proportion of iminostilbene to methyliminostilbene seems to depend on the injection technique and the geometry of the injection port of the gas chromatograph. It has been our experience that laboratories with automatic in-

TABLE 1. *Comparison of phenobarbital concentrations obtained from the same plasma specimens by gas-liquid chromatography with different internal standards and EMIT*

Specimen no.	MPPH-PB[a] (μg/ml)	PTPB-PB[b] (μg/ml)	EMIT-PB[c] (μg/ml)
1	22.9	47.1	45.6
2	2.4	13.0	13.6
3	13.0	14.0	17.1
4	12.4	20.9	19.8
5	4.9	12.6	14.7
6	3.4	8.4	9.9
7	10.3	12.4	12.6
8	40.1	43.0	43.6
9	13.4	17.1	19.1
10	7.1	11.6	12.0
11	34.7	51.2	54.1
12	6.3	10.6	9.7
13	15.2	21.6	25.7
14	10.7	12.3	13.4
15	7.9	11.6	9.2
16	32.0	31.1	27.9
17	53.0	70.1	75.8
18	5.1	16.8	17.7
19	34.4	43.1	34.8
20	11.6	16.8	16.3
Mean	17.0	24.3	25.0
Standard deviation	14.2	17.3	17.5

[a] GLC analysis of phenobarbital (PB) with methylphenylphenylhydantoin (MPPH) as the internal standard.

[b] GLC analysis of phenobarbital (PB) with p-tolylphenobarbital (PTPB) as the internal standard.

[c] EMIT analysis of phenobarbital.

jectors, which give consistently smooth injections, determine carbamazepine levels satisfactorily by gas chromatography in the presence of methylating agents. However, laboratories that manually inject carbamazepine in methylating agents may encounter substantial errors, because the length of time carbamazepine is in the injection port alters its decomposition profile. Other, unknown factors may be directly or indirectly involved in the problems encountered in this assay. Because no compound with properties similar to carbamazepine is currently available as an internal standard, laboratories using gas chromatography for carbamazepine analysis should proceed with caution. The silylation technique described by Dudley and Bius (Appendix II) is satisfactory, but requires a separate extraction and derivatization procedure for carbamazepine analysis.

UNDERIVATIZED GLC ANALYSIS

Laboratories that perform underivatized assays do not encounter the problems associated with derivatization. They do face other problems, however, which may include interfering peaks if the samples are not highly purified prior to GLC analysis and small tailing peaks that are difficult to quantitate. If interfering substances are not removed from specimens by the appropriate extraction techniques, and specimens are injected every 15 min, it is possible that 40 min later a series of peaks representing impurities in the first specimen injected will be eluted and interfere with the quantitation of a specimen that has just been injected. There are also problems associated with ghosting in certain gas chromatographs because of the configuration of the injection ports. Many of the problems commonly associated with underivatized analysis can be eliminated by carefully selecting the appropriate conditions and column packings, as described by Darcey and co-authors (Chapter 7).

QUANTITATION

There are a number of ways in which raw analytical data can be reduced to yield serum concentrations. Gas chromatographic peaks can be measured by peak height or peak area and the appropriate standard curves constructed. An error in measurement of peak height or peak area is always possible. Manual peak height measurements made from an artificial baseline may be erroneous if interfering substances induce a baseline shift. Peak height measurements should always be made with respect to the actual baseline and not to an arbitrary "zero" baseline.

The introduction of automated data reduction systems for integration of peak areas (such as the Hewlett Packard integrator series) does not eliminate quantitation errors. Such errors usually result from the failure of an automatic integrator to start or stop integrating at the appropriate point in relation to the symmetry of the peak. Any laboratory employing automatic data reduction systems should always examine the actual recorder tracings with respect to the printed integrator concentrations to assure that proper data reduction has occurred. In our experience, visual examination of the recorder tracing has identified potential errors and indicated malfunctioning of the data reduction system.

In addition, automatic data reduction systems should be run through their own test procedures periodically to assure proper functioning. These systems often show intermittent malfunctions late in the afternoon, after having operated for several hours. Intermittent problems can often be identified by running the same control at different points in the analytical run.

REPORTING ERRORS

Once the serum concentrations have been generated by an analytical technique, the possibility of transcriptional errors remains. The laboratory must constantly be on guard, double checking to be sure that calculations are correct and have not been erroneously transcribed. Daily log sheet results should always be checked against the physician's report form before the reports are released from the laboratory.

THE EMIT SYSTEM

Recent development of the homogenous enzyme assays (EMIT) has been a major advance in the rapid and accurate analysis of microsamples. The theory and application of EMIT assays to antiepileptic drug analysis have been described by Schottelius (Chapter 10) and by Pippenger et al. (7). It must be emphasized, however, that the EMIT system was not designed as an absolute quantitative system. It is only accurate within the range of the calibrators supplied with the system. As pointed out in the package insert, the laboratory cannot accurately quantitate below the lowest calibrator or above the highest calibrator. Automatic data reduction systems used with EMIT assays will give concentrations both below and above the range of the calibrators. Such results should be verified by appropriate dilutions or recalibration before reporting.

Those laboratories utilizing the EMIT system are well aware that as concentrations associated with the higher calibrators are approached (particularly in the phenobarbital and ethosuximide assays), small changes in enzyme activity as reflected by the R-Ro values can yield significant changes in apparent drug concentrations read from the graph paper or data reduction system.

EMIT graph paper is derived from a logit transform and is individualized for each of the antiepileptic drug assays. Typically, the plot of response versus concentration in immunochemical reactions is sigmoidal. The logit graph paper of the EMIT system transforms the characteristic S-shaped curve into a straight line. However, maximum response per concentration unit is achieved in the middle of the curve and may decrease at the extremes, a phenomenon independent of the graph paper used. The EMIT antiepileptic drug assays are designed so that optimal quantitation is achieved within the therapeutic range. Therefore, for more accurate quantitation of specimens with high drug concentrations, the specimen should be diluted 1:1 with blank serum or with the appropriate dilution factor necessary to reduce the concentration of the specimen to the optimum therapeutic range. Application of the appropriate dilution factors yields an accurate assessment of the actual drug concentration.

The condition of the sample can affect the performance of the EMIT system. Both lipemic and severely hemolyzed specimens may give erroneous results because of light scattering by particulate matter in the cuvette light path and very high initial absorbances, resulting in nonlinear spectrophotometric response. Rarely, for unknown reasons, samples that appear normal may not yield acceptable values. Certainly, if the laboratory results do not agree with the clinical status of the patient, the specimen should be reevaluated or another specimen analyzed.

We have recently observed that the EMIT ethosuximide assay cross-reacts equivalently with desmethylmethsuximide, the active metabolite of methsuximide (Celontin). The response is linear, and ethosuximide reagents can be used to quantitate desmethylmethsuximide. This cross-reactivity emphasizes the importance of using a general requisition form to assess the patient's medication regimen. Generally, methsuximide and ethosuximide are not administered in combination, but every laboratory should be alert to such a possibility. With preparation of the appropriate serum standards containing desmethylmethsuximide, serum concentrations of this compound can be accurately and routinely assayed with the EMIT ethosuximide assay.

Quality control is as essential with the EMIT system as it is with any other analytical technique. The ease of operation of the system tends to encourage carelessness in quality control. Controls should be run every day, and the calibration curve should be checked daily before analytical results are reported. The instrumentation should be checked carefully, particularly the dilutors, because it is possible that erratic results can be obtained as a consequence of a leaking dilutor. Dilutor malfunction may be readily indentified by erratic results between duplicate specimens. Accumulation of a crystalline deposit at the base of the sampling syringe plunger is also indicative of dilutor problems. Laboratories using the EMIT system are strongly urged to become thoroughly familiar with the troubleshooting sections of the EMIT package inserts, which clearly define problems that may arise. The manufacturer provides a daily checklist for the EMIT antiepileptic drugs system, which aids the operator in organizing daily quality control and calibration. Use of this checklist will help minimize operator error during daily standardization.

It is possible to measure concentrations lower than the lowest calibrator by adding the antibody and enzyme to the initial (first cup) dilution of the specimen. However, if this is done, a new calibration curve must be constructed with the appropriate drug concentrations to cover the desired range. We use a 1:10 dilution of EMIT calibrators for the range 0.25 to 3 μg/ml.

SUMMARY

This description of potential laboratory errors provides an overview of some of the more common errors encountered in the routine analysis of antiepileptic drugs. Although we have highlighted only a few of the possible errors that can occur, we emphasize that every laboratory must engage in an intensive internal quality control program on a daily basis to assure that variability is kept to a minimum and high standards of accuracy are maintained.

Without constant vigilance, laboratories can become so error prone that the welfare of the patient may be endangered. For example, a 30% error in a serum phenytoin level could result in a radical alteration of the patient's medication regimen, whereas a 30% error in an ethosuximide or phenobarbital level would not necessarily cause a major change in the physician's management of the patient.

Every laboratory should strive to reduce error to less than 10% to assure minimum intralaboratory variability. No laboratory is perfect, and an occasional mistake can always occur, but most laboratory errors are preventable. The object of quality control is to keep errors to an absolute minimum and to allow the laboratory to recognize and correct any loss of control as early as possible.

REFERENCES

1. Dill, W. A., Baukema, J., Chang, T., and Glazko, A. J. (1971): Colorimetric assay of 5,5-diphenylhydantoin (Dilantin) and 5-(*p*-hydroxyphenyl)-5-phenylhydantoin. *Proc. Soc. Exp. Biol. Med.*, 137:674–679.
2. Dill, W. A., Chucot, L., Chang, T., and Glazko, A. J. (1971): Simplified benzophenone procedure for determination of diphenylhydantoin in plasma. *Clin. Chem.*, 17:1200–1201.
3. Eadie, M. J., and Tyrer, J. H. (1974): *Anticonvulsant Therapy—Pharmacological Basis and Practice.* Churchill Livingstone, London.
4. Kupferberg, H. J. (1970): Quantitative estimation of diphenylhydantoin, primidone and phenobarbital in plasma by gas-liquid chromatography. *Clin. Chem. Acta,* 29: 283–288.
5. Kutt, H., and Penry, J. K. (1974): Usefulness of blood levels of antiepileptic drugs. *Arch. Neurol.,* 31:283–288.
6. Perchalski, R. J., Scott, K. N., Wilder, B. J., and Hammer, A. H. (1973): Rapid, simultaneous GLC determination of phenobarbital, primidone and diphenylhydantoin. *J. Pharm. Sci.,* 62:1735–1736.
7. Pippenger, C. E., Bastiani, R. J., and Schneider, R. S. (1975): Evaluation of an experimental homogeneous enzyme immunoassay for the quantitation of phenytoin and phenbarbitone in serum or plasma. In *Clinical Pharmacology of Anti-Epileptic Drugs,* edited by H. Schneider, D. Janz, C. Gardner-Thorpe, H. Meinardi, and A. L. Sherwin. pp. 331–335. Springer-Verlag, New York, Heidelberg, Berlin.
8. Pippenger, C. E., Penry, J. K., White, B. G., Daly, D. D., and Buddington, R. (1976): Interlaboratory variability in determination of plasma antiepileptic drug concentrations. *Arch. Neurol.,* 33:351–355.
9. Pippenger, C. E., and Sichler, D. L. (1973): A comparison of the detection of anticonvulsant drugs in whole blood, hemolyzed blood and plasma by gas-liquid chromatography. *Clin. Chem.,* 19:660.
10. Roger, J. C., Rodgers, G., Jr., and Soo, A. (1973): Simultaneous determination of carbamazepine ("Tegretol") and other anticonvulsants in human plasma by gas liquid chromatography. *Clin. Chem.,* 19:590–592.
11. Solow, E. G., and Green, J. B. (1972): The simultaneous determination of multiple anticonvulsant drug levels by gas-liquid chromatography: Method and clinical application. *Neurology* (Minneap.), 22:540–550.
12. Van Meter, J. C., and Gillen, H. W. (1973): A source of variation in the gas chromatographic assay of phenobarbital treated with trimethylanilinium hydroxide. *Clin. Chem.,* 19:359–360.
13. Woodbury, D. M., Penry, J. K., and Schmidt, R. P., editors (1972): *Antiepileptic Drugs.* Raven Press, New York.
14. Wu, A. (1974): Concerning on column methylation of phenobarbital. *Clin. Chem.,* 20:630.

Antiepileptic Drugs: Quantitative Analysis and Interpretation, edited by C. E. Pippenger, J. K. Penry, and H. Kutt, Raven Press, New York, © 1978.

Chapter 19
Application of Statistical Methods to Antiepileptic Drug Analysis

Edward Fingl

Statistical analysis is sometimes equated merely with decisions about whether or not differences between experimental means are "statistically significant." This is unfortunate; "significance testing," as useful as it is, is only one important function of statistical analysis. Particularly, its role as the basis for experimental design is of equal or greater practical value. This chapter considers applications of statistical analysis that assist in the calculation of assay results, assessment of the reliability of these results, and design of assay procedures. Discussion focuses not on the calculations but on the "statistical thinking" that should accompany the calculations and their interpretation. Details of the calculations are available in many standard textbooks; Snedecor and Cochran (6) and Armitage (1) are excellent general references. Barnett (2) is especially recommended for its discussion of applications of statistics to the clinical laboratory.

DESCRIPTIONS OF VARIABILITY

The results of drug assays can be applied clinically only with regard for the reliability of the assays. For this reason, reports of drug assays should also include a description of the reliability of an individual assay result. Standard deviation, coefficient of variation, or, preferably, confidence limits are convenient and generally useful descriptions of the reliability of assay results but must be employed with recognition of their limitations. Nonstatistical and graphical descriptions of variability should not be neglected because of preoccupation with statistical procedures.

Parametric Methods

Statistical descriptions of variability and related significance tests based on standard deviations are termed *parametric* methods because they require the assumption that the measurements are normally distributed. Standard deviation and standard deviation of the mean (standard error) are attractive as measures of variability because they are readily converted to *confidence limits* for the mean,

$$\bar{Y} \pm ts_{\bar{Y}}$$

or *limits of dispersion* or *tolerance limits* for individual measurements,

$$\bar{Y} \pm ts$$

where $\bar{Y}$ is the mean of a series of measurements, s is the standard deviation, $s_{\bar{Y}}$ is the standard deviation of the mean, and t is a factor from the t-distribution corresponding to the degrees of freedom and the selected level of confidence (usually 95% or 99%).

Confidence limits for a mean represent the range expected to include the population mean, with the selected probability; and tolerance limits represent the range expected, on the average, to include any specified percentage of individual observations. For drug assays, an assay result and its standard deviation can also be converted to confidence limits that represent the range expected to include the "true" result, with the specified confidence.

Two points deserve emphasis. First, these limits are properly based on the t-distribution. They are underestimated if the familiar factors from the normal distribution (2 for 95% or 2.6 for 99%) are substituted. Second, limits based on standard deviations provide the desired interpretations only if the observations are, in fact, normally distributed. The practical consequences of incorrectly assuming that observations are normally distributed depend on the extent of departure from the assumption and the purpose of the analysis. The "normal range" and similar limits for individual measurements are more vulnerable to assumptions about distribution than are confidence limits for means.

Coefficient of variation is defined as the standard deviation divided by the mean ($s/\bar{Y}$); it is appropriately termed the *relative standard deviation.* Coefficient of variation is variously symbolized as C or CV and variously expressed as a fraction or percentage. These inconsistencies should not detract from its general usefulness as a shorthand description of standard deviation. Coefficient of variation is particularly convenient if standard deviation increases in proportion to the mean and coefficient of variation is constant over a range of values. If coefficient of variation is constant, limits for assay results are also conveniently expressed as a fraction or percentage of the mean.

Nonparametric Methods

Because experimental observations need not be normally distributed, many statisticians argue that preference should be given to *nonparametric* or *distribution-free* statistical methods that avoid stringent assumptions about the distribution of the observations. For descriptive summaries, they favor the median over the mean, and limits based on percentiles over those based on standard deviations; for significance tests, they favor nonparametric procedures over classical t-tests and analysis of variance. If the observations are not normally distributed, nonparametric procedures provide more reliable interpretation; if the observations are normally distributed, both are reliable, and the better nonparametric procedures are only slightly less efficient than the parametric methods.

Nonparametric significance tests are now widely employed in many disciplines. Other nonparametric procedures are utilized less frequently but can be expected to gain greater acceptance in the future.

Other Descriptions of Variability

Statistical descriptions of variability must not be overemphasized at the expense of nonstatistical and graphical procedures. The pattern of variability of experimental observations is sometimes such that the relationships cannot be simply and adequately expressed by a single statistical index, or even several together. In those cases, nothing may be as effective and as convenient as a *scatter diagram* or other graphical summary. Similarly, particularly when the observations are limited, the *range* of values actually encountered experimentally may be more meaningful than any statistical description.

EVALUATION OF DRUG ASSAYS

Drug assays are characterized and compared primarily in terms of precision and accuracy. Quality control procedures are employed for evaluation of precision and accuracy of an assay as for other analytical procedures.

Precision

Precision refers to the reproducibility of repeated *independent* measurements. Precision of an assay is reliably and most directly assessed by repeated analysis of one or more internal quality control samples with each series of test samples. As for other analytical procedures (3), replicate determinations of test samples can also provide an estimate of assay precision and may be more convenient. For laboratory purposes, variability of an assay can be expressed as the standard deviation or coefficient of variation for these assay results. For reports to the clinician, confidence limits for the individual assay result are likely to be less confusing and are probably preferred.

Precision of an assay can also be assessed indirectly from the calibration curve. This indirect estimate of precision cannot replace the direct estimate provided by repeated analysis of quality control samples or replicates of test samples, but the indirect estimate can be very useful during development of an assay procedure and whenever assay conditions are changed. If the various estimates of assay precision differ significantly, flaws in the experimental procedure should be suspected.

Accuracy

Accuracy refers to the agreement between experimental measurements and "true values" for the variable on an absolute scale. An assay may be precise yet not accurate if standards for the calibration curve are prepared incorrectly, or if a similar systematic error is introduced into the execution of the assay or the calculation of assay results.

Accuracy of an assay can be established only by analysis of samples also analyzed by other laboratories. External quality control samples provided by national or regional quality control programs serve this important function (4,5). Exchange of samples between laboratories can also provide evidence of assay accuracy and may be even more effective, since it permits comparison of a greater number and variety of samples.

Assessment of accuracy is mandatory when an assay procedure is first established, and external quality control should be continued routinely at regular intervals. Assay results for external quality control samples should agree with values reported by the reference laboratories within the limits of assay precision.

External quality control procedures cannot assure accuracy of individual test results. Inaccuracy of individual assays, because of misidentification of samples, errors of transcription, or similar blunders, can be minimized only by rigid adherence to laboratory protocol and an adequate system of laboratory checks.

Control Charts

Control charts should be constructed for all routine drug assays. Charts should be kept for the individual values for the internal quality control samples and for the differences between replicates for the test samples. Control charts should also be maintained for standard deviation, slope, and possibly intercept for the calibration curve. A plot of standard deviation/slope ratio (s/b) should also be informative.

When sufficient assays have been performed, lines can be added to the charts to represent the range within which the values are expected to vary by chance. Subsequent results beyond these limits become suspect, and possible explanations for the deviations should be explored. Less extreme, persisting trends in deviation should also be investigated.

Application of quality control procedures and control charts to drug assays is similar to that for other analytical procedures. Helpful discussions have been provided by Barnett (2) and by Toro and Ackermann (7).

Other Assay Characteristics

Sensitivity, specificity, time, cost, and other characteristics are also important for total evaluation and comparison of drug assays but are not germane for the present discussion. However, it should be noted that precision of an assay can be increased by replicate determinations. Replicate determinations by an inherently imprecise but simple and inexpensive assay may be less time consuming and less expensive than a single determination by a more precise but complicated and expensive procedure.

REGRESSION ANALYSIS

Simple graphical methods are commonly utilized for assay calculations. Assay results for the standards are plotted against drug concentration, the best-fitting line is drawn by eye, and results for the test samples are read from the graph. Although it is the most elementary form of regression analysis, graphical analysis is usually satisfactory and is favored because of its simplicity and convenience. Nevertheless, regression calculations need not be excessively complex and offer several advantages over graphical procedures. The textbook by Snedecor and Cochran (6) is recommended for general discussion of regression analysis.

Regression Calculations Versus Graphical Analysis

Regression calculations *facilitate automation* of assay calculations, and the convenience and saving of time can be significant even when the number of samples is small. It can also be argued that regression calculations are *more objective* than graphical procedures for determining the "best-fitting" calibration curve. However, calibration curves for most assays exhibit only moderate variation, and graphical procedures are usually as reliable as calculations.

Other advantages of regression calculations over graphical analysis are less apparent but nonetheless useful. If the observations are adequate in number, regression analysis can be employed as a *test for validity* of the calculations, by testing for significant deviation from linearity and/or for significant departure of the regression line from the origin. Moreover, regression analysis can provide an *estimate of assay precision* and can aid in *assay design.*

Conventional Linear Regression

Since the fundamentals of linear regression are familiar to most investigators, discussion in this section is limited to aspects of importance when applied to drug assays. Several basic characteristics of conventional linear regression are summarized in Fig. 1. The linear regression equation is

$$Y = a + bX$$

where Y is the dependent variable (assay endpoint), X is the independent variable (drug concentration), b is the regression coefficient (slope), and a is the intercept (value of Y when $X = 0$). When regression analysis is ap-

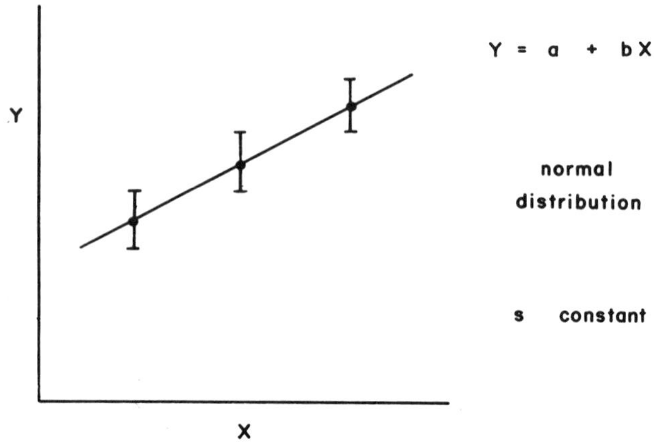

FIG. 1. Some basic characteristics of conventional linear regression analysis. See text for discussion.

plied to two random variables, either of the variables may be considered the independent variable, depending on the purpose of the calculations. However, when calibration curves are analyzed, the variables may not be interchanged; only drug concentration can be the independent variable.

As implied by the brackets of equal size along the regression line (Fig. 1), conventional linear regression calculations are based on the assumption that the standard deviation (or variance) of the dependent variable is constant. Homogeneity of variance can be tested by variance ratio or Bartlett's test. If the requirement for equal variance is not satisfied, the data may be transformed to equalize the variances, or they should be analyzed by *weighted linear regression,* in which the individual observations are weighted in proportion to the reciprocal of their variances. The assumption that the dependent variable is normally distributed at each value of the independent variable is less critical.

In complete form, regression calculations can test for deviation from linearity, usually by comparing the fit of a quadratic curve with that of the straight line. Complete calculations also provide standard errors for the slope, intercept, and assay results. These standard errors can be employed in the usual fashion to construct confidence limits or for significance tests.

Correlation Coefficient

Despite its prominent place in the historical development of statistical procedures, correlation analysis is much less useful than regression analysis. Correlation coefficient, r, is appropriate primarily as an index of the *mutual association between two random variables.* Interpretation of correlation coefficient is facilitated if it is recalled that r^2 (sometimes termed the coefficient of determination) represents the fraction of total variation in either variable that can be attributed to its relationship to the second variable.

The correlation coefficient is limited because it provides no information about the pattern of the relationship between variables. Consider, for example, a comparison of the results of two assay procedures. A value of $r = 0.95$ would seemingly suggest that the two procedures provide similar assay results. However, an equally impressive correlation coefficient would be obtained even if the assay results for one method were consistently higher or lower than those by the other method, and the correlation coefficient provides no direct evidence of the residual variation between the methods. In contrast, the slope and intercept from regression analysis provide direct evidence of the average agreement between the two methods, and the standard deviation from regression provides direct evidence of the average deviation between pairs of analyses. A simple scatter diagram greatly facilitates interpretation of both analyses, particularly to reveal whether the results are uniform over the full range of values.

Linear Regression Through the Origin

A calibration curve is often expected to be linear and to pass through the origin (0, 0). If preliminary analysis by conventional linear regression confirms that the observed intercept does not differ significantly from zero and that the relationship is linear, and if the observations are adequate to be certain that the relationship remains linear at low values, the calibration curve may be recalculated by linear regression that forces it through the origin. Linear regression through the origin is also useful for analysis of other regression relationships expected to pass through the origin, such as that between daily maintenance dosage and drug concentration during the plateau state.

The proper choice of calculations for regression through the origin depends on whether standard deviation is constant for all values of X, is proportional to X, or varies irregularly. Regression through the origin is not included in most statistical textbooks but is discussed by Snedecor and Cochran (6).

Linear Transformations

Conventional linear regression calculations should be employed only if the experimental data satisfy the requirements of linearity and homogeneous variance. If these requirements are not met, other forms of regression analysis must be used, or the data must be transformed to meet the requirements.

The use of linear transformations for regression analysis of a calibration curve is illustrated in Fig. 2. The left-hand panel depicts a calibration curve typical of many, in which standard deviation of the dependent variable varies with the independent variable. The right-hand panel illustrates the same data

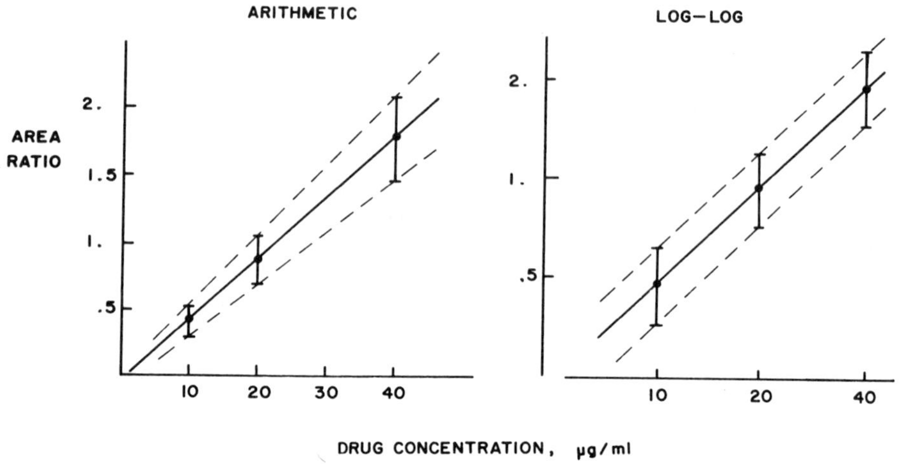

FIG. 2. An example of transformations to permit linear regression analysis of a calibration curve. See text for discussion.

after "log-log" transformation. Logarithmic transformation of the dependent variable eliminates the difference between the standard deviations but introduces curvature; logarithmic transformation of the independent variable restores linearity.

Competitive binding assays provide a more complicated example of the use of linear transformations. Several linear transformations based upon the mass-law equation may be employed for the calibration curve, or a linear relationship can usually be obtained if the assay results are converted to logits or probits and are expressed as a function of logarithm of the drug concentration. However, weighted linear regression may be required for the calculations.

Other Types of Regression Analysis

Polynomial regression, in which the regression equation takes the form

$$Y = a + b_1X + b_2X^2 + \cdots$$

is useful for description and analysis of many curves. However, it is not usually required or desired for calibration curves, since nonlinearity of a calibration curve can often be traced to some correctable flaw in the analytical procedure. As noted previously, comparison of quadratic regression with linear regression is the basis of a test for linearity, and quadratic or higher-degree polynomial regression is employed for the quench correction in liquid scintillation spectrophotometry.

Nonlinear regression technics are typically employed when experimental data can be described by a nonlinear equation, and the objective of the analysis is estimation of the parameters of the equation. Nonlinear regression is not generally required for calibration curves, but it has been employed in competitive binding assays, and is widely employed in pharmacokinetic studies.

Details of polynomial and nonlinear regression calculations have been summarized by Snedecor and Cochran (6).

EXPERIMENTAL DESIGN

Experimental design and statistical analysis are mutually related. The design of an experiment dictates the statistical analysis; conversely, and more important, principles of statistical analysis provide the basis for sound experimental design.

Details of experimental design depend on the nature and purposes of the individual experiment. However, a universal principle is that *bias must be avoided.* Bias can be excluded with certainty only if the experimental units being compared are observed *concurrently,* and if these observations are properly *randomized.* Applied to drug assays and similar analytical procedures, this principle translates into the requirement that standards for the calibration curve and one or more quality control samples be included with each series of test samples, and that the standards and controls be distributed among the test samples. In addition, the standards and controls should be the same biological matrix (e.g., serum, saliva) as the test samples, and a strong argument can also be made for analysis of all samples as unknowns. Departures from these features of sound experimental design do not always bias the assay results. Nevertheless, they should be avoided and should be suspect when an assay is unsatisfactory.

As noted previously, the regression calculations for the standards provide information for assay design. For example, when conventional linear regression is employed, the approximate standard error for an assay result ($\hat{X}$) is

$$s_{\hat{X}} = \frac{s}{b}\left(\frac{1}{r} + \frac{1}{n} + \frac{(\hat{X} - \bar{X})^2}{[\mathrm{XX}]}\right)^{1/2}$$

where s is the standard deviation of the dependent variable (assay endpoint), b is the slope of the standard curve, r is the number of replicates of the test sample, n is the number of standards, $\bar{X}$ is the mean standard concentration, and $[XX]$ is the sum of squares of deviation for the independent variable (drug concentration). This equation indicates that the inherent precision of an assay is determined by the ratio s/b. If these factors can be modified favorably, precision of an assay can be improved. The formula also illustrates the benefit of replicate determinations of a test sample and multiple standards.

SUMMARY

Drug assays must be designed to provide evidence of the precision and accuracy of the assay results.

Precision and accuracy of an assay must be assessed routinely, by analysis of internal and external quality control samples, and by maintenance of control charts. Precision of an assay can also be estimated from the calibration curve. This indirect estimate cannot replace the direct estimate of precision provided by repeated analysis of quality control samples, but it is especially useful during the development of an assay.

Common statistical procedures, including standard deviations, confidence limits, and regression analysis, provide the basis for interpretation and evaluation of an assay and the control procedures.

Dictates of sound experimental design require that standards for the calibration curve and one or more quality control samples be included in each set of test samples. Equally important, standards and control samples must be included in the assay in a manner that assures that they are representative and unbiased.

ACKNOWLEDGMENT

During preparation of this review, the author received support, in part, from U.S. Public Health Service Pharmacology Training Grant GM 00153 from the National Institutes of Health.

REFERENCES

1. Armitage, P. (1971): *Statistical Methods in Medical Research.* John Wiley & Sons, New York.
2. Barnett, R. N. (1971): *Clinical Laboratory Statistics.* Little, Brown and Company, Boston.
3. Maroude, G. R., Knapp, W. A., Lowe, R. T., and Fong, J. A. (1974): A quality control system utilizing duplicate patient specimens. *Am. J. Med. Technol.,* 40:165–168.
4. Pippenger, C. E., Penry, J. K., White, B. G., Daly, D. D., and Buddington, R. (1976): Interlaboratory variability in determination of plasma antiepileptic drug concentrations. *Arch. Neurol.,* 33:351–355.
5. Richens, A. (1975): Results of a phenytoin quality control scheme. In *Clinical Pharmacology of Anti-Epileptic Drugs,* edited by H. Schneider, D. Janz, C. Gardner-Thorpe, H. Meinardi, and A. L. Sherwin. pp. 293–303. Springer-Verlag, Berlin.
6. Snedecor, G. W., and Cochran, W. G. (1967): *Statistical Methods,* 6th ed. Iowa State University Press, Ames, Iowa.
7. Toro, G., and Ackermann, P. G. (1975): *Practical Clinical Chemistry.* Little, Brown and Company, Boston.

CLINICAL APPLICATIONS OF ANTIEPILEPTIC DRUG CONCENTRATIONS

Antiepileptic Drugs: Quantitative Analysis and Interpretation, edited by C. E. Pippenger, J. K. Penry, and H. Kutt, Raven Press, New York, © 1978.

Chapter 20

Principles of Drug Absorption, Distribution, and Metabolism

Edward Fingl

General principles of drug absorption, distribution, biotransformation, and excretion may be formulated on the basis of physicochemical, physiological, and pharmacokinetic concepts. These principles provide guidelines for drug therapy and for treatment of drug toxicity. This chapter is limited to an overview of those principles that facilitate interpretation of serum drug concentrations and their application for adjustment of drug dosage. Portions of the chapter are based on previous reviews by the author (5,6,21). The textbooks by Melmon and Morrelli (17), Levine (15), and Goldstein and co-workers (8) are recommended for more extensive review of these topics.

PERSPECTIVES

Serum drug concentrations must be interpreted with recognition that many factors modify the relationship between prescribed drug dosage and drug effects. As summarized schematically in Fig. 1, the dose-concentration rela-

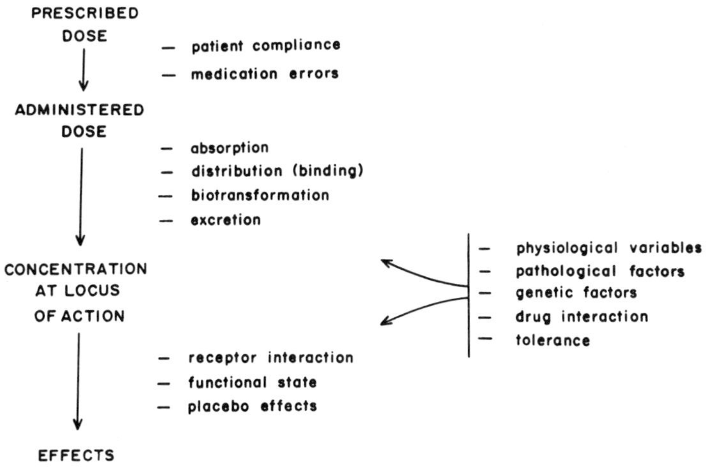

FIG. 1. Factors that determine the relationship between prescribed drug dosage and drug effects. Modified from Fingl and Woodbury (6), with permission of the editors and publisher.

tionship is influenced both by patient compliance and by drug absorption, distribution, biotransformation, and excretion. In turn, the concentration-effect relationship is determined by the multiple biochemical and physiological events that comprise the action-effects sequence. Both dose-concentration and concentration-effect relationships are modified by genetic, physiological, and pathological variables; both are also subject to drug interactions and to the development of drug tolerance.

PATIENT COMPLIANCE

Few patients comply exactly with the instructions of the physician. Some patients take drugs in excess, but most take less medication than prescribed; a significant fraction defaults completely. With appropriate allowance for variations in drug absorption, distribution, biotransformation, and excretion, monitoring of serum drug concentration can assist in detection and correction of noncompliance by the patient. Indeed, merely knowing that serum drug concentration is being monitored sometimes improves patient compliance.

Patient compliance is influenced by variables related to the physician, the patient and his illness, the particular drug and its adverse effects, and the therapeutic regimen. The most important determinant is the quality of the physician-patient relationship. Compliance can sometimes be improved by instruction of the patient about his illness and his medications, by adjustment of drug dosage to reduce adverse effects, and, when feasible, by simplification of the therapeutic regimen, as from multiple daily dosage to a single daily dose. An excellent discussion of patient compliance has been provided by Blackwell (2).

PHYSICOCHEMICAL AND PHYSIOLOGICAL PRINCIPLES

The interrelationships of drug absorption, distribution, biotransformation, and excretion are presented schematically in Fig. 2. All of these processes involve passage of the drug across cell membranes, largely by passive diffusion; hence, all are determined by the physicochemical properties of cell membranes and of the drug. Important physiological variables include cardiovascular, gastrointestinal, renal, and hepatic function.

Passive Diffusion and Influence of pH

Despite their histological diversity, the various cell membranes behave similarly as lipoid barriers to the passive diffusion of drugs. Small water-soluble molecules can traverse aqueous channels in the membrane, but diffusion of most drugs is dependent on their lipid solubility. Minimal aqueous solubility is also essential, since the drug must be in solution in the body fluids to gain access to the membrane. Diffusion is directly proportional to

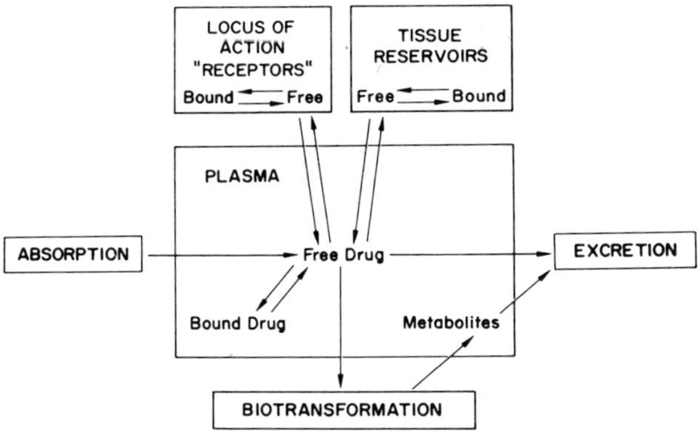

FIG. 2. Interrelationships of absorption, distribution, biotransformation, and excretion of a drug. Possible distribution and binding of metabolites are not depicted. From Fingl and Woodbury (6), with permission of the editors and publisher.

the concentration gradient of the drug and to the membrane surface area, and inversely related to the effective thickness of the membrane. Cardiac output, tissue blood flow, and gastrointestinal motility may be important, since delivery of drug to the membrane surface or its removal is sometimes limiting. In contrast with active transport, diffusion does not exhibit saturation at high concentrations and is not the basis for drug interaction.

Many drugs are weak organic acids or bases. As such, they are present in solution as both nonionized and ionized molecules. Nonionized drug is generally lipid-soluble and readily diffusible, but the ionized form usually has limited lipid solubility and, hence, is poorly diffusible. Since degree of ionization is determined by the pK_a of the drug and the pH of the solution, drug absorption and excretion may be pH-dependent. Distribution of a drug may also be influenced by pH if a pH gradient exists across the membrane. At equilibrium, concentration of readily permeant nonionized drug will be the same on the two sides of the membrane. However, since degree of ionization varies with pH, the concentration of ionized drug and, hence, concentration of total drug on the two sides of the membrane will differ.

The influence of pH, ionization, and lipid solubility on drug absorption, distribution, biotransformation, and excretion is conveniently summarized by contrasting a drug that is only partially ionized at physiological pH with one that is completely ionized. The drug that is at least in part in the lipid-soluble, nonionized form is usually adequately absorbed from the gastrointestinal tract. After absorption, it is generally widely distributed in tissues, including the central nervous system, and is significantly, if not largely, inactivated by biotransformation. Depending on its pK_a and the pH of the urine, it might be excreted in part unchanged in the urine. Absorption and distribution would also be pH dependent. In contrast, the drug that is solely in the poorly lipid-soluble, ionized form is generally slowly and erratically absorbed after oral administration. After absorption, it usually has only limited distribution in tissues and is excreted primarily unchanged in the urine, perhaps quite rapidly if it is actively transported by the renal tubules.

Active Transport

Organic anions and cations are actively transported across renal tubular cells, hepatocytes, and the choroid plexus cells between the plasma and cerebrospinal fluid. Separate membrane-carrier mechanisms exist for organic anions and organic cations. Active transport occurs against a concentration gradient and exhibits saturation as concentration is increased. Since the carrier mechanisms are relatively nonselective, many drugs are transported by these systems and may compete with each other for transport.

Plasma Protein Binding

Many drugs are bound to plasma proteins, largely plasma albumin. The extent of binding varies with the individual drug; some organic acids and bases are more than 90% bound. Only unbound drug is in equilibrium across cell membranes. Since drug effects are related to concentration of unbound drug but analytical procedures usually measure total (bound plus unbound) drug, interpretation of serum concentration of a drug that is normally highly bound must include consideration of possible changes in fractional binding. Fractional binding usually varies only slightly with drug concentration below 50 μg/ml but varies directly with albumin concentration. In addition, since binding of drugs to albumin is relatively nonselective and usually reversible, drugs and endogenous metabolites may compete with each other for these binding sites. The net effect of drug interactions involving competition for albumin binding is complex, since change in concentration of bound drug often has multiple opposing effects on drug elimination (13).

Absorption

Most drugs are absorbed from the *gastrointestinal tract* by passive diffusion. Absorption of some drugs, particularly organic acids that are largely nonionized at the low gastric pH, occurs in part through the gastric mucosa. However, because of the greater surface area of the intestinal mucosa, absorption of all drugs occurs primarily from the intestine. For this reason, drug absorption is usually delayed if gastric emptying is retarded.

Change in *gastric pH* has variable influence on drug absorption, since gastric pH may influence not only ionization of the drug but also its solubility and stability, as well as gastric emptying. Absorption from the alimentary tract is decreased if the drug binds to food or forms an insoluble complex with other ingested drugs. Serum drug concentration after oral administration may be significantly lower than that after parenteral injection, both because of the slower rate of absorption (see Fig. 4), and because orally administered drug may be metabolized in the gastrointestinal tract or in the liver before it gains access to the general circulation.

Absorption of soluble drugs from *parenteral injection* sites is generally more rapid than oral absorption and is not subject to initial passage and possible inactivation in the gastrointestinal tract and liver. However, absorption of insoluble drugs, such as phenytoin and diazepam, from intramuscular depots may be slow and erratic.

Pharmaceutical dosage forms may contain the same quantity of drug yet, upon administration by the same route, not provide similar serum drug concentrations. This biological inequivalence reflects differences in the extent and/or rate of drug absorption, and such preparations are said to differ in their *bioavailability*. These differences have been noted most frequently for oral dosage forms of drugs that have limited aqueous and/or lipid solubility. They are the result of differences in the physical form of the drug, the inert ingredients in the preparations, and/or the manufacturing process. The practical significance of differences in bioavailability of drug dosage forms has been reviewed by Koch-Weser (12).

Excretion

Most drugs and metabolites are eliminated in the *urine*. Excretion occurs by various combinations of glomerular filtration, active tubular secretion, and passive tubular reabsorption. The quantity filtered is a function of glomerular filtration rate and the fraction of the drug not bound to plasma proteins, and organic anions and cations are added to the glomerular filtrate by active transport in the proximal tubule. Ultimate disposition of filtered and secreted drug depends on its lipid solubility. If it is lipid-soluble, it is passively reabsorbed; if the drug is ionized or otherwise poorly lipid-soluble, passive reabsorption is limited and the drug is excreted in the urine. Alkalinization of the urine increases the excretion of weak organic acids, and acidification of the urine increases the excretion of weak organic bases. However, changes in renal excretion of drugs with change in urine pH is of practical importance only if the fraction of drug excreted unchanged in the urine is significant relative to that inactivated by biotransformation.

Drugs and metabolites that are lipid-soluble are excreted in the *bile* by passive diffusion, and organic anions and cations and compounds related to the steroids are excreted by active transport. Lipid-soluble drug and metabolites eliminated in the bile are subsequently reabsorbed in the intestine. Glucuronide conjugates secreted into the bile are hydrolyzed by enzymes in the intestinal mucosa and also participate in this *enterohepatic circulation*.

Excretion of drugs in saliva and milk contributes little to termination of drug effect. However, *saliva* appears to be a satisfactory alternative to serum for pharmacokinetic monitoring, and it is especially convenient when serial sampling is required. With appropriate allowance for the influence of pH on drug distribution, concentration of drug in saliva provides an estimate of the concentration of drug in serum not bound to plasma proteins (3,19). Drugs excreted in *milk* sometimes cause adverse effects in the nursing infant.

Biotransformation

Most drugs are converted to multiple metabolites. These products of biotransformation are usually less lipid-soluble than the parent drug and, hence, less able to diffuse across cell membranes, less active biologically, and more readily excreted in the urine. Thus, biotransformation commonly serves both to terminate drug effect and to facilitate drug elimination. However, some metabolites are active, and some drugs are inactive until metabolized. Activity of a metabolite may be similar to or different than that of the parent drug. The liver is the most important organ for drug biotransformation. However, other tissues, including plasma, kidney, lung, and the gastrointestinal tract, also contribute to drug metabolism.

The hepatic endoplasmic reticulum contains many enzymes that participate in drug metabolism. These enzymes are commonly termed *microsomal enzymes,* because they are recovered in the microsomal fraction when liver homogenate is fractionated. These enzymes catalyze many types of reactions, including inactivation by conjugation with glucuronic acid and numerous oxidations involving the mixed-function oxidase system and cytochrome P-450. Reactive intermediates in these oxidative reactions may cause hepatic cell necrosis and other toxic effects.

The hepatic microsomal enzymes have many unique characteristics. They are of special clinical interest because they are involved in the biotransformation of most drugs, and because activity of these enzymes may be increased, by enzyme induction, by the chronic administration of many drugs, and by exposure to a number of environmental chemicals. In man, microsomal drug-metabolizing activity may be increased as much as fourfold by administration of phenobarbital and other drugs that induce these enzymes, but the change is usually less than twofold in patients. Activity is not increased equally for all substrates. Susceptibility to induction is genetically determined; it is least for individuals with most rapid metabolism prior to induction. Drug interactions can also result in inhibition of metabolism of one drug by another. Microsomal enzyme activity is incompletely developed in the neonate but increases significantly during the initial postnatal months.

Although not involved in the biotransformation of as many drugs as are the microsomal enzymes, *nonmicrosomal enzymes* in liver and other tissues and enzymes in plasma also contribute significantly to drug metabolism. Nonmicrosomal enzymes catalyze some oxidation, reduction, and hydrolysis of drugs, as well as conjugations other than that with glucuronic acid. Several of the nonmicrosomal enzymes, including those involved in acetylation and ester hydrolysis, exhibit genetic polymorphism (distinctly slow and rapid activity in different individuals on a genetic basis). None of the nonmicrosomal enzymes is known to be inducible.

Redistribution and Tolerance

Drug effect is usually terminated by *excretion* of unchanged drug in the urine and/or by *biotransformation* to inactive metabolites. However, drug effect may also be terminated by development of drug tolerance or by redistribution of the drug from its locus of action to other tissues.

Pharmacokinetic or *drug-disposition* tolerance, such as that caused by induction of the hepatic microsomal enzymes, results in reduction of all effects of the drug without change in therapeutic index. In contrast, *pharmacodynamic* or *functional* tolerance, such as that caused by alteration of the action or effects of the drug, need not involve all effects of the drug equally; therapeutic index may increase or decrease. Both types of tolerance may develop concurrently.

Drug effect is terminated by *redistribution* of the drug primarily when a drug with high lipid solubility is injected intravenously. Administration of diazepam in the management of status epilepticus is an example. Effects of the drug on the central nervous system develop promptly, as the drug quickly reaches its locus of action in this highly perfused tissue. However, drug effect also wanes rapidly, as the drug is redistributed to muscle and other tissues that are less well perfused and equilibrate more slowly with plasma. After repeated administration of the drug, redistribution is less prominent, and drug effect is terminated primarily by biotransformation and/or excretion.

Infants and Children

Infants and children differ significantly from adults in relative sizes of the body fluid compartments, fractional binding of drugs to plasma proteins, ability of drugs to enter the central nervous system, and renal and hepatic function. The consequences of these differences on the pharmacokinetics of drugs in infants and children have been reviewed by Rane and Wilson (18).

PHARMACOKINETIC PRINCIPLES

Pharmacokinetics is concerned with the translation of the many individual factors that determine drug absorption, distribution, biotransformation, and excretion into succinct mathematical descriptions of the time course of drug concentrations in plasma (serum), other body fluids, and tissues. Discussion in this section is limited to the fundamental pharmacokinetic principles that are readily applied to therapy. A more extensive summary has been provided by Greenblatt and Koch-Weser (9); the more complex principles required for research applications have been authoritatively reviewed by Wagner (20).

Basic Concepts

For formulation of the fundamental pharmacokinetic principles, the body is viewed as a *single compartment. Distribution* of drug within this compartment is assumed to be relatively uniform, or of no practical consequence if not uniform, and to occur rapidly relative to absorption and elimination. *Volume of distribution* is that in which the drug appears to be distributed, if it exists throughout that volume at the same concentration as in plasma.

Absorption, excretion, and biotransformation of the drug are assumed to follow *exponential* (*first-order*) kinetics, in which the rate of the process increases in proportion to the concentration of the drug. The rate of an exponential process is expressed by its *rate constant, k,* the fractional change per unit of time, or by its *half-time,* $t_{1/2}$, the time required for 50% completion of the process. An exponential process is more than 90% complete after four half-times. Exponential rate constant and half-time are simply related ($kt_{1/2} = 0.693$) and may be interchanged accordingly; they are independent of drug concentration (dose). The rate constants for drug excretion and biotransformation are usually combined into a single rate constant for elimination. The single most important kinetic characteristic of a drug is its *elimination half-time.* The product of volume of distribution and elimination rate constant ($V_d k_e$) expresses the *plasma clearance* of the drug.

Zero-order elimination, in which the rate is independent of concentration, is encountered only occasionally in pharmacokinetics. Constant intravenous infusion of a drug may be viewed as zero-order absorption. Elimination of a drug by biotransformation or active transport is normally expected to exhibit *mass-law* or *saturation* kinetics, in which exponential elimination at low concentrations changes to zero-order elimination as concentration of the drug increases and the process becomes saturated. Fortuitously, because the concentration of the drug remains low relative to that required for saturation, elimination of most drugs follows the more simple exponential kinetics throughout the therapeutic range. Phenytoin is a notable exception (see page 232).

Single Doses

When a single dose of a drug is administered intravenously, serum drug concentration usually declines in two phases (Fig. 3). The initial rapid decline reflects predominately *distribution* of the drug from plasma into tissues; the subsequent slower decline, primarily *elimination* of the drug by

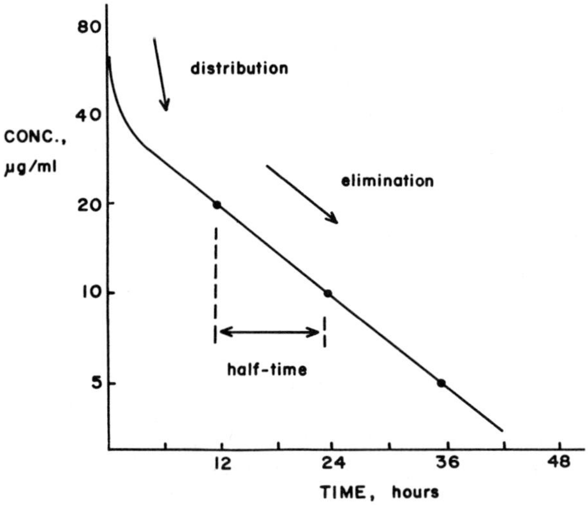

FIG. 3. Pharmacokinetic pattern after intravenous administration of a drug. Modified from Fingl and Woodbury (6), with permission of the editors and publisher.

biotransformation and/or excretion. The initial distribution phase is of practical importance with regard to termination of drug effect by redistribution (see page 227).

The influence of dosage and rates of absorption and elimination on the kinetic pattern of single doses of a drug is illustrated in Fig. 4. Differences in rate of *absorption,* particularly the large differences that result from administration of a drug by different routes, have prominent effects on the time course of drug concentration. If a drug is absorbed very slowly, effective

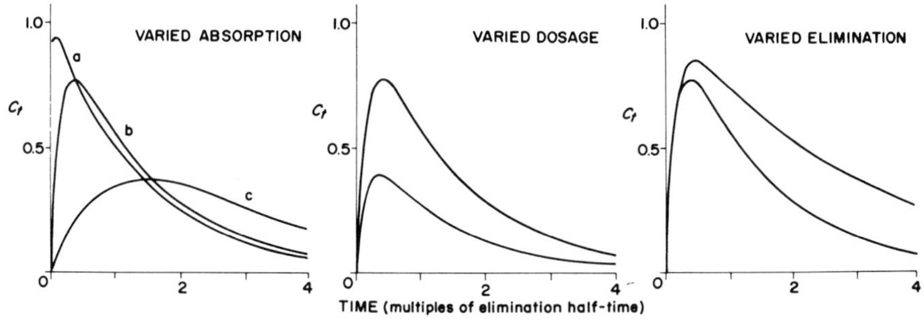

FIG. 4. Fundamental pharmacokinetic relationships for single doses of a drug. *Varied absorption:* patterns to illustrate the influence of absorption (a) 100 times as rapid as, (b) 10 times as rapid as, and (c) equal to elimination. *Varied dosage:* patterns to illustrate the influence of a twofold difference in dosage (absorption 10 times as rapid as elimination). *Varied elimination:* Patterns to illustrate influence of a twofold difference in rate of elimination (lower curve: absorption 10 times as rapid as elimination). Curves are based on the elementary one-compartment model. From Fingl and Woodbury (6), with permission of the editors and publisher.

concentrations may not be attained at its locus of action. As *dosage* is increased, the time required to attain an effective concentration is reduced without change in time of peak concentration. Duration of effective concentration is increased proportionately less than peak concentration. Therefore, increase in dosage is a suitable method for increasing duration of effect only if the drug has a wide margin of safety. Reduced drug *elimination* results in the expected prolongation of effective drug concentration but has minor effect on peak concentration if absorption of the drug is relatively rapid. In contrast, rate of drug elimination has an important effect on drug concentration during repeated administration of the agent.

Repeated Doses

When a drug that exhibits exponential elimination is administered by constant intravenous infusion, the drug accumulates until the rate of elimination equals the rate of administration (Fig. 5, smooth curve). The concentration of drug in plasma (serum) increases exponentially to a plateau, with a half-time equal to the elimination half-time; the plateau is attained after the usual

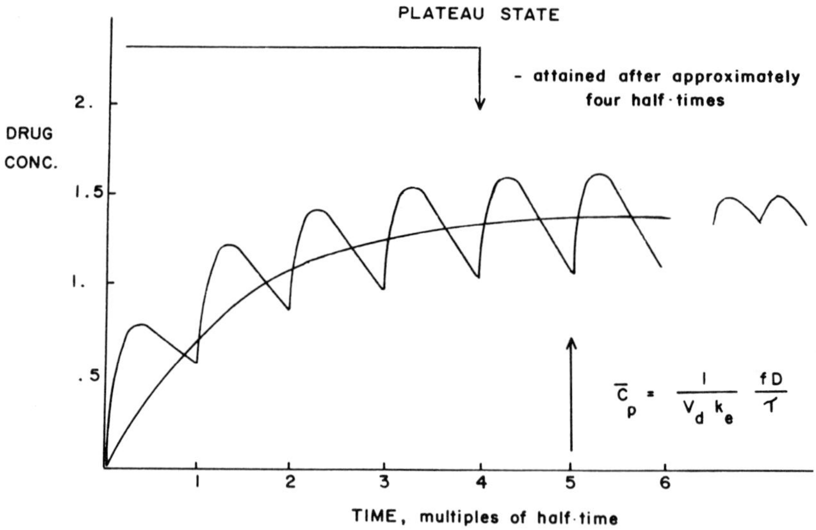

FIG. 5. Fundamental pharmacokinetic relationships for repeated administration of drugs. Irregular line depicts the pattern of drug accumulation during repeated administration of a drug at intervals equal to its elimination half-time (absorption 10 times as rapid as elimination). Curves at the extreme right are the pattern during the plateau state for half doses of the drug at half intervals. Smooth curve depicts the pattern during administration of equivalent dosage by continuous intravenous infusion. Curves are based on the elementary one-compartment model. *Formula:* $\bar{C}_p$ = average concentration during the plateau state (μg/ml), V_d = volume of distribution (liters/kg), k_e = elimination rate constant (d^{-1}), f = fractional absorption, D/τ = daily maintenance dosage (mg/kg/d). Modified from Fingl and Woodbury (6), with permission of the editors and publisher.

four half-times. This pattern of drug accumulation is termed the *plateau principle*. It applies not only when a drug is administered by intravenous infusion but also when it is administered repeatedly by any route (Fig. 5, irregular curve), and not only for the initial administration of the drug but also whenever dosage is increased or decreased.

The average drug concentration during the plateau state (see formula, Fig. 5) is linearly related to drug dosage. If maintenance dosage is doubled, plateau concentration is doubled. The factor that expresses the average relationship between plasma concentration (μg/ml) during the plateau state and daily maintenance dosage (mg/kg/d) is the reciprocal of plasma clearance ($1/V_d k_e$). Drug concentration during the plateau state is directly proportional to elimination half-time. Thus, if rates of elimination for a particular drug for two patients differ by a factor of four, daily maintenance dosage to provide the same plateau concentration for these patients will also differ by a factor of four.

Maintenance Dosage Schedule

The same average drug concentration during the plateau state can be maintained by various combinations of individual doses and dosage intervals (Fig. 5, curves at the extreme right). Half doses at half intervals provide a smoother time course than do unit doses at intervals equal to elimination half-time; double doses at double intervals would yield more extreme fluctuations. Maintenance dosage schedule should be selected primarily by consideration of these fluctuations between doses. If the dosage interval is too great and the fluctuations are excessive, peak concentration after each dose may cause needless toxicity and/or the concentration just prior to each dose may be insufficient for seizure control. A dosage interval equal to or less than the elimination half-time is usually required, but longer intervals may be satisfactory if the drug is slowly absorbed or has a wide margin of safety.

If otherwise satisfactory in terms of fluctuations, a single daily dose is often preferred for the convenience of the patient and as an aid to patient compliance. Sedation and other minor adverse effects of a drug may be less annoying to the patient if most or all of the daily dose is taken upon retiring. For other patients, daily dosage might be divided to parallel the diurnal pattern of seizures.

Initial Dosage

Antiepileptic medication is often initiated in dosage expected ultimately to be suitable for maintenance therapy. Partial effects occur promptly, but full effects for that dosage are necessarily delayed for the inevitable four half-times required for attainment of the plateau state. A dosage regimen of this type is preferred, since it provides time for adjustment of dosage for the individual patient and reduces the risk of initial adverse effects. Indeed, medications that produce prominent sedation, dizziness, or other subjective effects are sometimes intentionally started at subtherapeutic dosage; and clinically effective concentrations are attained even more slowly, with anticipation that at least partial tolerance will develop to the undesired subjective effects during the gradual increase in drug dosage.

If full therapeutic effect must be achieved promptly, medication can be initiated with a so-called *loading dose* larger than the subsequent maintenance dosage. An estimated loading dose should be administered in several divided portions, to permit some monitoring for initial adverse effects. Serum drug concentration during subsequent maintenance therapy is independent of the initial loading dose after the usual four half-times. Approximate loading dose (D^*) and maintenance dosage (D/τ) are related as follows: $D^* = 1.4 t_{1/2} D/\tau$, where $t_{1/2}$ is the elimination half-time in the same units as τ.

Adjustment for Reduced Drug Elimination

Maintenance dosage for drugs excreted largely unchanged in the urine must be adjusted for patients with impaired *renal* function. Initial estimate of the necessary adjustment can be made on the basis of the change in creatinine clearance, serum creatinine concentration, or blood urea nitrogen concentration and the fraction of the drug normally excreted unchanged in the urine (7). However, monitoring serum drug concentration is still helpful for final adjustment of dosage.

Monitoring serum drug concentration is especially helpful for adjustment of maintenance dosage for patients with *liver* disease, since drug metabolism by the liver is not consistently correlated with any of the routine hepatic function tests. However, it must also be recognized that the effects of central depressant drugs may be exaggerated in patients with liver disease, independent of changes in drug metabolism.

Since biotransformation of drugs that are rapidly cleared by the liver is influenced by changes in *cardiac output* and *hepatic blood flow,* dosage of such drugs must usually be adjusted for patients with congestive heart failure or myocardial infarction.

Dose-Dependent Elimination

The pharmacokinetic characteristics of phenytoin and other drugs that exhibit dose-dependent elimination differ significantly from those of most other drugs that exhibit exponential elimination. As drug concentration (dosage) increases, elimination does not increase proportionately. Consequently, the time required for 50% elimination of the drug and the time required to attain the plateau state are not constant but increase progressively with concentration. In addition, drug concentration during the plateau state is not linearly related to daily dosage but increases disproportionately as dosage is increased. Not unexpectedly, interindividual variation in the dose-concentration relationship is greater for drugs that exhibit dose-dependent elimination than for other drugs, and monitoring serum drug concentration is even more useful.

DRUG INTERACTIONS

The absorption, distribution, biotransformation, or excretion of a drug may be modified by prior or concurrent administration of another drug. Representative mechanisms involved in these *pharmacokinetic* drug interactions have been noted in previous sections. Depending on the nature of the interaction, serum drug concentration may be increased or decreased. Drug interactions may also result from combination of drug actions or effects. Summation of the sedative effects of two drugs is an example of such *pharmacodynamic* drug interactions.

Many reported drug interactions occur inconsistently. Some are variable because they involve several opposing mechanisms concurrently; others are a function of factors such as drug dosage, timing of the medications, or genetic factors. Nevertheless, if an unplanned interaction does occur and is not suspected and not corrected, serious toxicity or diminished drug efficacy may occur. Critical summaries of drug interactions and their potential clinical significance have been prepared by the American Pharmaceutical Association (1) and Hansten (10).

Pharmacokinetic drug interactions are only occasionally sought intentionally. Although time course of a drug may be favorably influenced, all effects are altered in parallel, without increase in therapeutic index. In contrast, pharmacodynamic drug interactions need not involve all effects of the drugs equally and may provide a valid basis for *multiple-drug therapy*. Use of several drugs concurrently is justified if therapeutic index is increased, or if the combined drugs provide greater efficacy than can be achieved with single-drug therapy without excessive toxicity.

CONCENTRATION-EFFECT RELATIONSHIP

When serum drug concentrations are employed as a guide to therapy, it must not be assumed that the concentration-effect relationships for all patients will be the same as those for the average individual. As Walter S. Loewe, one of the true pharmacologist-scholars, would have emphasized, care must be taken not to commit the "median-man fallacy."

A recommended "therapeutic" serum drug concentration is not necessarily equally satisfactory for patients with all severities, varieties, or combinations of susceptible seizures, or for all varieties of multiple-drug therapy (4,14,16). In addition, concentration-effect relationships have not been established with the desired reliability for most antiepileptic agents. For these reasons and because the concentration-effect relationship is subject to multiple sources of variation (Fig. 1), recommended serum drug concentrations must be viewed primarily as a guide for initiation of therapy. To be sure, many patients do, in fact, obtain at least partial seizure control with tolerable adverse effects when recommended serum drug concentrations are attained. However, for other patients, serial observations are required to establish the optimal dosage and optimal drug concentration for each individual. In addition, it must be recognized that a drug may be capable of only partial seizure control for a particular patient. Increase in dosage beyond that required for the ceiling effect for the individual can provide no additional benefit but can contribute further adverse effects.

MONITORING SERUM DRUG CONCENTRATIONS

The value and limitations of serum drug concentrations as a guide for therapy have been summarized for drugs in general by Koch-Weser (11) and for the antiepileptic agents by Kutt and Penry (14).

For the antiepileptic agents, monitoring of serum drug concentrations at appropriate intervals facilitates *initial* adjustment of dosage for individual differences in drug elimination and other kinetic parameters. *Subsequent* monitoring helps to minimize dose-related adverse effects and, when single-drug therapy is not completely effective, to choose between adjustment of dosage and alternative medication. *Periodic* monitoring during maintenance therapy can detect failure of the patient to take medication as prescribed, and can provide assurance for the patient with infrequent seizures that seizure control is, in fact, being maintained. During *multiple-drug therapy,* monitoring helps to identify the particular drug responsible for adverse effects, and it can guide readjustment of dosage if pharmacokinetic drug interaction occurs. Monitoring is especially helpful for patients with impaired renal or hepatic function, and whenever medication is unexpectedly ineffective or toxic. *Serial* observations are always more reliable than isolated measurements.

Application of physicochemical, physiological, and pharmacokinetic principles to interpretation of serum drug concentrations must include consideration of:

1. Reliability of the analytical procedure
2. Fractional protein binding of the drug
3. Possible active metabolites of the drug
4. Concurrent medications and possible drug interactions
5. Possible drug tolerance of either the drug disposition or functional types
6. The assumptions on which the pharmacokinetic principles are based

7. The kinetic pattern for the particular drug
8. The interval between time of sampling and the time of last drug administration
9. The plateau principle
10. Possible changes in the kinetic parameters as a result of concurrent illness
11. Interpatient variation in serum drug concentrations associated with desired and undesired drug effects

Most important, it must be recognized that monitoring serum drug concentrations leads to improvement of therapy only if the observations are interpreted in concert with other clinical monitoring, and only if drug dosage is adjusted to provide drug concentrations that are optimal for the individual patient.

SUMMARY

The pharmacological adage, "the *dose* of a drug is enough," is a succinct reminder that the dose of a drug must be adjusted for the individual patient.

Variations in patient compliance and in drug absorption, distribution, biotransformation, and excretion modify the relationship between drug dosage and serum drug concentration. Consequently, concentration-effect relationships are less variable than dose-effect relationships, and monitoring serum drug concentrations can contribute significantly to improvement of antiepileptic medication. Physicochemical, physiological, and pharmacokinetic principles greatly facilitate interpretation of serum drug concentrations for this purpose.

Nevertheless, variations in concentration-effect relationships are also clinically significant, and serum drug concentrations are a reliable guide to drug therapy only with appropriate consideration of these variations, and only in conjunction with other clinical monitoring for efficacy and safety. In brief, "the *concentration* of a drug is enough."

ACKNOWLEDGMENT

During preparation of this review, the author received support, in part, from U.S. Public Health Service Pharmacology Training Grant GM 00153 from the National Institutes of Health.

REFERENCES

1. American Pharmaceutical Association (1973): *Evaluations of Drug Interactions—1973*. American Pharmaceutical Association, Washington, D.C.
2. Blackwell, B. (1973): Patient compliance. *N. Engl. J. Med.*, 289:249–252.
3. Cook, C. E., Amerson, E., Poole, W. K., Lesser, P., and O'Tuama, L. (1975): Phenytoin and phenobarbital concentrations in saliva and plasma measured by radioimmunoassay. *Clin. Pharmacol. Ther.*, 18:742–747.

4. Feldman, R. G., and Pippenger, C. E. (1976): The relation of anticonvulsant drug levels to complete seizure control. *J. Clin. Pharmacol.,* 16:51–59.
5. Fingl, E. (1972): Absorption, distribution, and elimination: Practical pharmacokinetics. In: *Antiepileptic Drugs,* edited by D. M. Woodbury, J. K. Penry, and R. P. Schmidt, pp. 7–21. Raven Press, New York.
6. Fingl, E., and Woodbury, D. M. (1975): General principles. In: *The Pharmacological Basis of Therapeutics,* 5th ed., edited by L. S. Goodman and A. Gilman, pp. 1–46. Macmillan Company, New York.
7. Giusti, D. L., and Hayton, W. L. (1973): Dosage regimen adjustments in renal impairment. *Drug Intell. Clin. Pharm.,* 7:382–387.
8. Goldstein, A., Aronow, L., and Kalman, S. M. (1974): *Principles of Drug Action: The Basis of Pharmacology,* 2nd ed. John Wiley & Sons, New York.
9. Greenblatt, D. J., and Koch-Weser, J. (1975): Clinical pharmacokinetics. *N. Engl. J. Med.,* 293:702–705, 964–970.
10. Hansten, P. D. (1975): *Drug Interactions: Clinical Significance of Drug-Drug Interactions and Drug Effects on Clinical Laboratory Results,* 3rd ed. Lea & Febiger, Philadelphia.
11. Koch-Weser, J. (1972): Serum drug concentrations as therapeutic guides. *N. Engl. J. Med.,* 287:227–231.
12. Koch-Weser, J. (1974): Bioavailability of drugs. *N. Engl. J. Med.,* 291:233–237, 503–506.
13. Koch-Weser, J., and Sellers, E. M. (1976): Binding of drugs to serum albumin. *N. Engl. J. Med.,* 294:311–316, 526–531.
14. Kutt, H., and Penry, J. K. (1974): Usefulness of blood levels of antiepileptic drugs. *Arch. Neurol.,* 31:283–288.
15. Levine, R. R. (1973): *Pharmacology: Drug Actions and Reactions.* Little, Brown and Company, Boston.
16. Lund, L. (1974): Anticonvulsant effect of diphenylhydantoin relative to plasma levels: A prospective three-year study of ambulant patients with generalized epileptic seizures. *Arch. Neurol.,* 31:289–294.
17. Melmon, K. L., and Morrelli, H. F., editors (1972): *Clinical Pharmacology: Basic Principles in Therapeutics.* Macmillan Company, New York.
18. Rane, A., and Wilson, J. T. (1976): Clinical pharmacokinetics in infants and children. *Clin. Pharmacokinet.,* 1:2–24.
19. Schmidt, D., and Kupferberg, H. J. (1975): Diphenylhydantoin, phenobarbital, and primidone in saliva, plasma, and cerebrospinal fluid. *Epilepsia,* 16:735–741.
20. Wagner, J. G. (1975): *Fundamentals of Clinical Pharmacokinetics.* Drug Intelligence, Hamilton, Ill.
21. Woodbury, D. M., and Fingl, E. (1975): Drugs effective in the therapy of the epilepsies. In: *The Pharmacological Basis of Therapeutics,* 5th ed., edited by L. S. Goodman and A. Gilman, pp. 201–226. Macmillan Company, New York.

Antiepileptic Drugs: Quantitative Analysis and Interpretation, edited by C. E. Pippenger, J. K. Penry, and H. Kutt, Raven Press, New York, © 1978.

Chapter 21
The Pharmacokinetic Basis for Using Blood Antiepileptic Drug Levels in Monitoring and Optimizing Therapy

William H. Barr

Significant advances in methods and applications of pharmacokinetics have occurred in the last few years, providing the basis for using blood drug levels to optimize dosage regimens in patients (5,12,30,35,54,67,71). Correlations between therapeutic and adverse pharmacological responses (36,60,61), physiological variables of the patient, dose input variables, and resulting plasma drug levels now provide a systematic means of estimating and optimizing individual dosage schedules (1,5,12,30,35,50,54,56,67).

Through analog and digital computer technology (29,39), complex multicompartmental models (68,69) with nonuniform dose inputs (27,28) and nonlinear disposition characteristics can be applied to patient data. The introduction of perfusion models, based upon physiological parameters, permits correlations of plasma drug levels with known or measurable physiological variables such as cardiac output, hepatic blood flow, or glomerular filtration rate (11,55). Stochastic modeling (6,39,76) and systems analysis techniques (48,57,58,60,61) have been used to develop clinical algorithms (29,58) that maximize the use of available population and patient data. Patient variables such as age (24,57), weight, disease state, and laboratory measurements are used to estimate the initial dosing schedule (25,26,31). Blood drug level data are used to evaluate predictions, provide feedback adjustment during therapy, and periodically, to monitor drug therapy (13–16,37,39,41,56,58).

The complexity of this new applied discipline, called clinical pharmacokinetics, will probably continue to require a multidisciplinary effort not only in further scientific development of the data base and methodologies, but also, interprofessionally, to provide cost-efficient application of clinical pharmacokinetics to patient care. Nevertheless, many of the useful concepts and applications are relatively simple and can be applied by individuals with minimal training in mathematics or pharmacokinetics. The intent of this chapter is to review briefly the current status of this new field and to outline some of the basic concepts applicable to antiepileptic drug therapy. A classification of the many clinical and pharmacokinetic variables involved is suggested to allow different applications and to correlate new information.

The literature on the clinical application of blood antiepileptic drug level data is extensive. Several excellent reviews are available in the literature (13–15,29–34,47,51,54,76) and elsewhere in this volume, and no attempt is made here to give a detailed review of individual drugs. Examples were selected to illustrate general pharmacokinetic concepts rather than to document historical development. The colloquial but succinct term "(blood) drug levels" is used to refer to amounts or concentrations of drug and metabolites in body fluids, as a function of time, after single and multiple dose administration to an individual or group of individuals belonging to a population subset with particular characteristics.

PHYSIOLOGICAL BASIS FOR THE USE OF BLOOD DRUG LEVELS

A criticism, often heard, is that measurements of plasma drug concentrations are of limited usefulness in predicting pharmacological response, because response is actually a function of drug in some tissue rather than in the plasma. Since the latter is therefore only a substitute, subject to many other factors, development of methods to measure drug in tissue or to determine clinical pharmacological effect is claimed to be a more logical objective than blood drug level measurements. While there is need for objective means of measuring pharmacological response, the assumption that blood drug level data are only a convenient alternative to other intrinsically better, but inaccessible, data is a misconception that ignores the unique utility of these data. Indeed, measurements of concentration of drug in the target organ, even if routinely available, would be far less useful than measurements of drug concentration in the plasma. The great utility of plasma drug levels as a predictor of drug response is a direct consequence of the unique function that the blood circulation plays in the physiological system. The blood circulatory system has evolved to provide an internal milieu for all cells. It provides the means for transport of exogenous nutrients absorbed from the gastrointestinal tract, endogenous hormones secreted by endocrine glands, and substrates of intermediary metabolism. Thus, drug in plasma (or more correctly, the drug in serum water not bound to plasma proteins) has the potential to reach all cells. Distribution equilibrium between plasma and most tissues occurs if the plasma drug concentration is maintained. The concentration of drug in the biophase (C_b), the region considered to be immediately adjacent to the site of action (60,61), is therefore usually directly proportional to the concentration of drug in plasma or is a time-dependent function of blood drug levels. However, in a sample of tissue (e.g., brain), there is no assurance that the resultant measurement of antiepileptic drug levels represents the drug bound to receptors rather than inactive binding sites. Diffusion of drug through different tissue regions in the absence of blood flow is a very slow process, and large concentration differences in immediately adjoining tissues are possible. The concentration of phenytoin is twice as high in the white matter of a frontal lobe compared with the grey matter (59). In contrast, the plasma drug concentration is essentially homogeneous at any given time. Concentrations of drug in several regions of the brain (μg/g) show good linear correlation with plasma drug levels for phenytoin and phenobarbital (59,65). Most important is the fact that the same plasma drug level may also be used to correlate with and predict effects of the drug on other tissues. Furthermore, plasma drug levels can be used to determine the effect of the body on the drug by processes such as distribution, elimination by metabolism, or urinary excretion. Thus, the level of the drug in the blood is often the single most useful type of information for the following three functions:

1. To estimate effects of the drug on the body:
   The plasma drug concentration often closely correlates with the concentration of drug in the biophase (C_b) at one or more sites of action, which is directly related to the pharmacological response (R_i) through some response function (h_i):

$$R_i = h_i\,(C_b) \tag{1}$$

   Usually, distribution equilibrium occurs and there is a constant ratio between total plasma drug concentration (C_p), the concentration of drug in plasma water not bound to plasma proteins (C_w), and the biophase drug concentration (C_b). Thus, combining the equation for the fraction of drug unbound ($f_w = C_w/C_p$) and the equation for the fraction of drug in the biophase ($f_b = C_b/C_w$) gives $C_b = f_b \cdot f_w \cdot C_p(t)$, thereby demonstrating that the response is related to the total plasma drug concentration by

$$R_i = h_i[f_b, f_w, C_p(t)] \tag{2}$$

   where $C_p(t)$ = concentration of drug in plasma at any time (t). When steady-state plasma drug concentrations [$C_{p(ss)}$] are reached during multiple dosing, $C_p(t) = C_{p(ss)}$ and h_i, f_b, f_w are usually constant values. A given intensity or incidence of pharmacological response (R_i) will correspond to the steady-state plasma drug concentration (12,61,66).
2. To characterize and predict the effect of body processes on the drug levels: Because of the central role of the blood circulatory system, measurements of blood drug levels allow characterization of the net effects of the simultaneous processes of absorption, distribution, metabolism, and excretion of the plasma drug levels [$C_p(t)$] and the amount of drug in the body at any time [$Q_b(t)$]. The location and form of drug and metabolites can be determined by parameters of a pharmacokinetic model representing rates (k_i), volumes of distribution (V_i), and distribution ratios (K_i). Thus, the plasma or tissue concentration of drug or metabolite (C_i) is a function

(f_i) of the parameters of the model and the independent input variables of dose (D), dosage interval (Υ), and time (t), (5,12,22,23):

$$C_i(t) = f_i(K_i, k_i, V_i, D, \Upsilon, t) \tag{3}$$

3. To correlate pharmacokinetic parameters with physiological and drug variables:
   Because transport and elimination of drug generally involves either translocation by blood flow or diffusion from blood to tissue through lipid membranes, the variables $Q_b(t)$ or $C_p(t)$ can often be correlated and predicted by measurable or estimable physiological variables such as cardiac output, regional flow ($\dot{v}_i$), volumes of distribution or tissue mass (V_i), distribution ratios (K_i), and organ clearance ($\dot{V}_i$) (10,55):

$$C_i(t) = f_i(\dot{v}_i, V_i, \dot{V}_i, K_i) \tag{4}$$

   Absorption and tissue distribution can be related to *in vitro* measurements of properties of the drug such as binding constants, partition coefficients, or dissolution rates which may be a function of molecular weight, pK_a, and steric and electronic parameters of the molecule. The possibility of using *in vitro* drug parameters and physiological variables of the patient to correlate and predict drug disposition appears to be a likely future development (10,23).

USE OF RELATIONSHIPS BETWEEN PLASMA DRUG LEVELS AND PHARMACOLOGICAL RESPONSE

A time honored basis of all drug therapy (except homeopathy) is that all desired clinical effects are a function of the dose, which if increased excessively, produces a poison. Thus, the responses, therapeutic (R_T) and adverse (R_A), are

$$R_T = h_i(D) \tag{5}$$

$$R_A = h_i(D) \tag{6}$$

where h_i is some definable function. It is convenient to consider h_i as an operator which may define either a deterministic or stochastic function. The early experimental pharmacologists elucidated the relationship between the response of isolated tissue preparations and the concentration of drug in the tissue or body fluids (44,66). Intensity of response is a function of the amount of drug that occupies a fraction of the fixed number of receptors in the biophase (61,66). The reversible process follows mass law, resulting in the familiar sigmoid curve for intensity of response as a function of dose or drug concentration. The function can be linearized over most of the response range by using the log of dose as the independent variable (36). Just as individual cells or units of an isolated organ give different intensities of response which can be characterized by a log-normal frequency distribution, a similar distribution is observed for the probability of a given response when equal doses are given in any normal subset of the population.

Kalow (30) points out that one of the major conceptual advances in pharmacology was the discovery that the variability in response to a given dose of drug by different individuals could in fact be used to characterize the response through statistical methods such as probit analysis. Rather than posing insurmountable problems, the variability of individual responses to graded doses (log scale) is used to characterize the response curve. A probit plot facilitates calculation of the median dose (ED_{50}) to elicit the desired degree of response in 50% of the sample group (30). The slope of the plot provides the standard deviation of the distribution sample. This principle forms the basis of bioassays which are still used as an official compendial analytical procedure. Fingl (17) emphasizes that similar statistical methods should be used in correlations of dose with clinical response.

Pharmacokinetic optimization utilizes the same concepts in which the pharmacological response function (h_i) can be characterized by the stochastic parameters of a given frequency distribution function or statistics of the sample distribution (7,17,72). Unfortunately, the reporting of ranges of responses relative to a given dose or concentration is seldom given in statistical terms.

Use of Plasma Drug Levels as Predictors of Response

The plasma drug concentration provides a better primary estimator of probable response than the dose or estimated amount of drug in the body (total body load) through statistical parameters of this variable such as the plasma drug concentration that produces a response in 50% of individuals with a range corresponding to the 95% confidence interval (58).

This stochastic relationship provides the basis for use of individual plasma drug levels and population data to predict the probability of a therapeutic, subtherapeutic, or adverse response. When the plasma drug level is used to screen or monitor patients for potential toxicities or subtherapeutic doses, several types of statistical methods are available for determining the sensitivity and specificity of the blood drug levels, or other variables of the system, as predictors of response (39,40,48,57,58,70).

Choice of Plasma Drug Level as Therapeutic Objective

When the correlations between plasma drug levels and both therapeutic and adverse responses are known, they can be used to determine the optimum therapeutic concentration. Cost function (48,72) analysis techniques can be used to determine the ideal plasma drug concentration for a given population or as the basis of a value judgment, for a specific patient, on the appropriate target concentration that corresponds to the highest probability for therapeutic effect relative to the risk warranted for that patient.

PRIMARY PARAMETERS TO OPTIMIZE DOSE

By limiting attention to the minimum number of elements or processes necessary to describe a particular response of a system to a given input, a model system can be formulated.

The model system can be described by several possible types of mathematical models. The mathematical model is formulated in terms of dependent and independent variables, which include absolute constants (e.g., *e*, the base of natural logarithms), the space-time coordinates, and parameters which assume fixed values for a given problem but may take on different values when the system changes (e.g., the body clearance, $\dot{V}_B$, or volume of distribution, V_d, for a given drug in a particular patient or population subset). Parameters are usually independent of time but, occasionally, may be defined as a function of time. For example, the rate constant for carbamazepine metabolism (k_m) must be defined as a function of time due to an increasing rate of metabolism during multiple dosing (9, 20).

The independent variables, which vary with time, are considered external inputs to the system and are often referred to as the forcing functions [e.g., a single i.v. dose or multiple oral doses (D) at periodic constant time intervals (Υ)] (53).

Because of the many possible factors that can affect drug response, the concepts of state variables and primary parameters are useful. State variables are any group of dependent (output) variables of the system [e.g., $C_p(t)$, $Q_b(t)$, $C_i(t)$] that, when known, completely define a particular performance or state of the system with a minimum redundancy of information (58,60). The choice of state variables can be quite arbitrary, depending on the problem being solved. For example, the variables defining drug in tissue or metabolites in plasma may not be essential in defining problems requiring only the relationship between the dose administered and the resulting serum concentration of unchanged drug. However, when the pharmacological effect is a function of tissue levels or an active metabolite, additional state variables are required. The mathematical model therefore involves additional parameters requiring additional data.

The dependent variables may be observed directly [e.g., $C_p(t)$] or may have to be estimated from the model, such as the amount of drug in tissue [$Q_t(t)$].

The application of pharmacokinetics to optimize individual dosage regimens involves different limitations than in research studies where many data points can be taken to characterize equations involving several parameters. In the clinical situation, it is usually possible to obtain only a few blood samples. Therefore, it is essential to use the simplest model with the minimum number of variables and parameters. When the number of parameters is too large relative to the number of blood samples, errors will occur in the estimation of parameters. The number of samples must exceed the number of parameters. The simplest system is to use plasma drug levels as both the therapeutic objective and the observed system output variable to monitor response to a given drug dosage input (D/Υ). Alternatively, $Q_b(t)$ (total body load) may be selected as the primary state response variable when plasma drug levels are not available (58).

The response of a system is usually described by a differential equation in which the constant coefficients are parameters defining relationships between the elements of the system and the output variable of the system. To solve the equation, it is necessary to specify the initial condition (C_O) and the input or forcing function [$f(Q)$], which is considered to be from outside the system and thus has an opposite sign. The relationship between the response variables [$C_p(t)$] and dose input when the parameters of the system are defined as the volume of the body (V_d) and the total body clearance (V_B) is described by

$$V_d \cdot dC_p(t)/dt + \dot{V}_B C_p(t) - f(Q) = 0 \tag{7}$$

If the input function is a continuous dose rate [$f(Q) = D/\Upsilon$], after some time, steady-state is reached where $dC_p(t)/dt = 0$ and thus $C_p(t)$ equals the mean steady-state plasma drug concentration [$C_{p(ss)}$]. The relationship reduces to

$$D/\Upsilon = \dot{V}_B \cdot C_{p(ss)} \tag{8}$$

The mean whole body clearance ($\dot{V}_B$) is the only parameter needed to calculate the dose rate (input variable) required to reach a given steady-state plasma drug level (system output variable). Furthermore, $\dot{V}_B$ is an experimentally obtained value and therefore model "independent." At any time before steady-state is reached, the mean concentration can be obtained if one additional parameter is known. The general differential equation above can be solved for $C_p(t)$ as a function of time, giving

$$D/\Upsilon = \dot{V}_B C_{p(ss)}(1 - e^{-\beta t}) \tag{9}$$

where β is an experimentally derived overall first order rate constant, obtained from the terminal log-linear slope of the plasma time curve after dosing stops. Like the clearance term, β is independent of the number of compartments of a compartmental model. It can be considered equivalent to the first order elimination rate constant of the one-compartment model (K) and directly related to the biological half-life:

$$t_{1/2} = 0.693/\beta \tag{10}$$

Thus, the time required to reach steady-state is completely determined by the value of β or the corresponding half-life ($t_{1/2}$). After dosing for an interval equal to one half-life, the mean plasma drug level will have reached

50% of the ultimate steady-state level. When the dosing period equals $3.3 \cdot t_{1/2}$, C_p will be 90% of the ultimate steady-state concentration. A similar expression can be derived if $Q_b(t)$ is used as the output variable:

$$Q_b(t) = Q_{b(ss)}/\beta\,(1 - e^{-\beta t}) \tag{11}$$

Therefore, $Q_{b(ss)}$ is related to $C_{p(ss)}$ by a volume parameter, $V_{d(ss)}$. Both $\dot{V}_B$, the mean total body clearance, and β apply to single or multiple compartment systems with constant rate input, including oral or i.v. multiple dosing where D/Υ is a finite dose given every time interval and $C_{p(ss)}$ is defined as the mean plasma drug concentration at steady-state. The same equation was also described by Orr et al. (43) in different terms in which the reciprocal of total body clearance was called the "occupancy." A further variation was given by Bergner et al. (6) who derived the equation by considering the system as a purely stochastic process.

The parameters β and $\dot{V}_B$ for an individual may be estimated using average values which characterize the particular population subset assumed to contain the patient. These estimates may be a function of such patient variables as weight, age, sex, race, disease state, or concomitant drug therapy (18,24–26,42,47). Any change in these variables will be reflected in a change in either the mean value or standard deviation about the sample mean, or both. The average values of $\dot{V}_B$ and β for different populations have been obtained for several antiepileptic drugs, where it is assumed that body weight can be used to normalize individual values. Normalizing patient parameters for individual subjects by dividing by body weight can be misleading (17). Correlations with age, sex, and weight should also be examined by covariance or multiple regression techniques (70).

Relationships between patient variables and parameters describing the primary variables are often very useful for estimating the patient parameters before the initial dose and dosage regimen reach a given level (45,63).

A basic assumption in the dose-response analysis by probits is that the distribution curve is unimodal, characteristic of multifactorial traits. Genetic differences in metabolism or response may result in a bimodal frequency distribution which is not characterized by the probit plot for either of the two populations (17). For example, a genetic deficiency in parahydroxylation of phenytoin has been reported (46), but there is presently no additional information on the incidence of this genetic trait in the general population. A single plasma drug level is often useful in screening patients to detect or confirm potentially toxic or subtherapeutic levels. When a low level is found it often requires a more complex model and additional types of data to determine the cause of anomalous values (31,34). Characterization of the patient's disposition parameters may often be accomplished by simultaneous measurements of both free drug and metabolites in plasma and/or urine to determine if low plasma drug levels are due to poor compliance, decreased absorption, or rapid elimination (41,46,53,56,62–64).

Primary and Secondary Parameters to Characterize Kinetics of Drug Absorption, Distribution, Metabolism, and Excretion

The concentration of drug in plasma at the biophase as a function of time is the net result of several sequential and parallel rate processes of absorption, distribution, tissue and plasma binding, metabolism (e.g., hepatic), and excretion (renal and biliary), which may be considered sequential and parallel elements of the system. Each of these disposition processes can be characterized by one or more parameters which may be related to a specific model (volume terms and rate constants, V_i, k_i) or may be model independent and derived directly from the plasma levels of drug or metabolites following single or multiple i.v. or oral doses.

The relationship between plasma drug levels as a function of time and dose input variables can be defined by individual clearance terms, which are model-independent. These parameters can be obtained directly from single dose concentration-time curves of drug or metabolites in plasma and/or urine by the following relationships:

$$\dot{V}_B = FD/\mathrm{AUC} \tag{12}$$

$$\dot{V}_r = (dQ_u/dt)/C_p(t) \tag{13}$$

$$\dot{V}_m = \dot{V}_B - \dot{V}_r \tag{14}$$

where F is the fraction of the dose absorbed, AUC is the area under the plasma time curve, dQ_u/dt is the rate of urinary excretion, $\dot{V}_r$ and $\dot{V}_m$ are renal and metabolic clearances, and k_r and k_m are first order rate constants for excretion and metabolism.

Total body clearance ($\dot{V}_B$) can be divided into individual rate constants and volumes which are model-dependent, where $\dot{V}_r + \dot{V}_m = V_d k_r + V_d k_m$ and $K = k_r + k_m$, or clearance terms for each elimination process. These parameters can often be estimated by secondary physiological variables such as creatinine renal clearance (39) and hepatic blood flow (55) or modified by extraneous variables such as induction or inhibition of metabolism by barbiturates or change in plasma protein binding due to hepatic or renal disease. For example, the fraction of phenytoin that is protein-bound is usually relatively constant in a given individual and has a narrow distribution range in the normal population (42). Therefore, it is not usually necessary to routinely determine this parameter. Reduction of albumin concentration in uremic patients significantly decreases the mean fraction of bound drug (42). It also greatly alters the variability about the mean in this population, requiring individual assessment. Since the reduction alters distribution of drug to receptors and metabolizing sites, a change downward in the target plasma drug levels and alteration of dose to adjust for clearance changes may be required. It is not essential to perform lengthy protein binding studies; however, as direct estimates of albumin concentrations (8,42) and measurements of the ratio of the drug in plasma and red blood cells, both correlate quite well with changes in the fraction bound.

Nonlinear Metabolism

The nonlinear kinetics of some drugs can be characterized quite well by using a single nonlinear "Michaelis-Menten" term to describe metabolism (4,49,62). The usual equation is thus given by:

$$V_d \cdot dC_p/dt + V_d \cdot V_{\max} \cdot C_p/K_m + C_p - D/\Upsilon = 0 \quad (15)$$

Application of this model to fit plasma drug levels using nonlinear computer programs such as Metzler's "NONLIN" has been used by a number of authors to explain blood drug level curves after overdoses (1,3,4,19,21), to estimate the relative bioavailability of different phenytoin products, or to determine the effect of differences in rate of dosage and absorption on steady-state levels (73–75).

The use of steady-state plasma drug levels to optimize dose input presents significant problems when the system is nonlinear. The most important distinction is that if the maximum rate of metabolism (V_{max}) is exceeded by the dose input (D/Υ), steady-state does not occur and excessive accumulation occurs.

A nomogram has been constructed by Richens and Dunlop (52) which uses population values of V_{max} and K_m (Michaelis constant) and a single plasma point to adjust the dose of phenytoin in order to reach the target level of 10 to 20 mg/liter. Although this method provides an initial means of adjustment, individual K_m and V_{max} values vary considerably. Additional steady-state plasma drug levels obtained with different doses can be used to determine individual V_{max} and K_m parameter values as suggested by Ludden et al. (37). This requires several weeks because of the time required to reach steady-state.

The use of analog and digital computers to estimate disposition parameters during multiple dosing before steady-state is reached would probably represent the best approach. Attempts to use computer estimates of V_{max} and K_m after a single dose were not found practical by Mawer et al. (39,40).

SUMMARY

The concepts of systems analysis and pharmacokinetic modeling provide a systematic means of identifying, classifying, and correlating the numerous variables that can be determinates of drug effect and determining which should be used for different purposes. The basic objective is to develop procedures that provide the most effective means of determining the optimum dosage regimens for individual patients. Blood drug levels serve as the primary (observable) dependent variable relative to independent dose input variables. Plasma drug levels also can be used to obtain parameter values which characterize other significant processes and variables. The choice of variables and parameters to characterize the system is arbitrary and depends on the requirements of the problem to be solved. A minimum number of terms should be used for the purpose of determining the drug input variables, which include the loading dose (D^*), maintenance (D), dose interval (Υ), and number of doses (n) given by a particular route of administration.

The unique properties of the blood circulation allow blood drug level measurements alone to be used (a) to correlate with and predict the probability of therapeutic and adverse pharmacological response, (b) to characterize the disposition processes of absorption, distribution, metabolism, and excretion, and (c) to correlate with secondary variables related to the properties of the drug and with physiological variables related to the patient and disease state. Secondary variables may change mean values of parameters or response functions and/or the distribution frequency about the mean. When these effects are known and characterized, these variables can be used as initial estimators of system parameters prior to dosing. When the relationships are not characterized, these variables are extraneous modifiers of system parameters, resulting in greater variability of the system. It is important, therefore, to design systems that will permit systematic accumulation of data which will allow further retrospective correlations between secondary variables and system parameters. Because blood drug level data can be used to estimate the probability of both therapeutic and adverse effects, a given plasma drug level or range can be used as a therapeutic objective to adjust dosages. Blood concentrations of the drug may be considered the system output and thus the means of monitoring the effectiveness of a particular dosage regimen in achieving the particular therapeutic objective. The collection of data on the level of drug in the blood during the monitoring phase permits further refinement or estimate of system parameters and the development of improved models which better characterize mechanisms of drug disposition and response. Reliable estimates of pharmacokinetic models can often provide the basis for explanation of apparent anomalous responses. Understanding the pharmacokinetic models for specific drugs allows more efficient use of data and rational approaches to problem solving, for example, the use of alternate fluids for sampling, the use of metabolites in urine to distinguish between malabsorption, rapid elimination, or poor compliance, or the use of salivary drug levels to characterize changes in protein binding. Probably, the ideal procedure is provided when the blood drug levels are correlated with a careful record of seizure rate. The data of Lund (38) and Feldman and Pippenger (16) show that plasma drug levels which correspond to therapeutic effect can be precisely determined for a particular individual, thus providing the ideal therapeutic objective if dosage readjustment is required. Accumulating evidence also strongly indicates the need not only periodically to monitor plasma drug levels to assure therapeutic levels but to better understand and prevent a variety of chronic adverse effects which may be both dose- and time-dependent (2,11,14,45).

REFERENCES

1. Albert, K. S., Sakmar, E., Hallmark, M. R., Weidler, D. J., and Wagner, J. G. (1974): Bioavailability of diphenylhydantoin. *Clin. Pharmacol. Ther.,* 16:727–729.
2. Andreasen, P. B., Lyngbye, J., and Trolle, E. (1973): Abnormalities in liver function tests during long-term diphenylhydantoin therapy in epileptic out-patients. *Acta Med. Scand.,* 194:261–264.
3. Arnold, K., and Gerber, N. (1969): The rate of decline of diphenylhydantoin in human plasma. *Clin. Pharmacol. Ther.,* 11:121–134.
4. Atkinson, A. J., and Shaw J. M. (1973): Pharmacokinetic study of a patient with diphenylhydantoin toxicity. *Clin. Pharmacol. Ther.,* 14:521–528.
5. Benet, L. Z. (1972): General treatment of linear mammillary models with elimination from any compartment as used in pharmacokinetics. *J. Pharm. Sci.,* 61:536–541.
6. Bergner, P. E. E., Birniker, K., Cooper, T. B., Cradigan, J. R., and Simpson, G. M. (1973): Lithium kinetics in man: Effect of variation in dosage pattern. *Br. J. Pharmacol.,* 49:328–339.
7. Bliss, C. I. (1968): Experimental design: Its use and misuse. In: *Importance of Fundamental Principles in Drug Evaluation,* edited by D. H. Tedeschi and R. E. Tedeschi. Raven Press, New York.
8. Boston Collaborative Drug Surveillance Program, (1973): Diphenylhydantoin side effects and serum albumin levels. *Clin. Pharmacol. Ther.,* 14:529–532.
9. Boxenbaum, H. G., Geitner, K. A., Jack, M. L., Dixon, W. R., Spegel, H. E., Symington, J., Christian, R., Moore, J. D., Weissman, L., and Kaplan, S. A. (1977): Pharmacokinetic and biopharmaceutic profile of chlordiazepoxide HC1 in healthy subjects: Single-dose studies by the intravenous, intramuscular, and oral routes. *J. Pharmacokinet. Biopharm.,* 5:3–24.
10. Bungay, P. M., Dedrick, R. L., and Guarino, A. M. (1976): Pharmacokinetic modeling of dogfish shark (Squalus acanthias): Distribution of urinary and biliary excretion of phenol red and its glucuronide. *J. Pharmacokinet. Biopharm.,* 4:377–94.
11. Conrad, G. J., Jeffay, H., Boshes, L., and Steinberg, A. (1974): Levels of 5,5-diphenylhydantoin and its major metabolites in human serum, saliva, and hyperplastic gingiva. *J. Dent. Res.,* 53:1323–1329.
12. Dettli, L. (1973): Translation of pharmacokinetics to clinical medicine. *J. Pharmacokinet. Biopharm.,* 1:403–418.
13. Eadie, M. J. (1974): Laboratory control of anticonvulsant dosage. *Drugs,* 8:386–397.
14. Eadie, M. J. (1976): Plasma level monitoring of anticonvulsants. *Clin. Pharmacol.,* 1:52–66.
15. Eadie, M. J., and Tyrer, J. H. (1973): Plasma levels of anticonvulsants. *Aust. NZ J. Med.,* 3:290–303.
16. Feldman, R. G., and Pippenger, C. E. (1976): The relation of anticonvulsant drug levels to complete seizure control. *J. Clin. Pharmacol.,* 16:51–58.
17. Fingl, E. (1968): Drug dosage, time of observation, and duration of medication as factors in drug evaluation. In: *Importance of Fundamental Principles in Drug Evaluation,* edited by D. H. Tedeschi and R. E. Tedeschi. Raven Press, New York.
18. Garrettson, L. (1972): Pharmacology of anticonvulsants. *Pediatr. Clin. N. Am.,* 19:179–191.
19. Garrettson, L. K., and Jusko, W. J. (1975): Diphenlyhydantoin elimination kinetics in overdosed children. *Clin. Pharmacol. Ther.,* 17:481–491.
20. Gerardin, A. P., Abradie, F. V., Campestrini, J. A., and Theobald T. (1976): Pharmacokinetics of carbamazepine in normal humans after single and repeated doses. *J. Pharmacokinet. Biopharm.,* 4:521–535.
21. Gerber, N., and Wagner, J. G. (1972): Explanation of dose-dependent decline of diphenylhydantoin plasma levels by fitting to the integrated form of the Michaelis-Menten equation. *Res. Commun. Chem. Path. Pharmacol.,* 3:455–466.

22. Gibaldi, M., Nagashima, R., and Levy, G. (1969): Relationship between drug concentration in plasma or serum and amount of drug in the body. *J. Pharm. Sci.*, 58: 193.
23. Glazko, J. (1975): Antiepileptic drugs: Biotransformation, metabolism, and serum half-life. *Epilepsia* 16:367–391.
24. Hayes, M. J., Langman, M. J., and Short, A. H. (1975): Changes in drug metabolism with increasing age: a. Phenytoin clearance and protein binding. *Br. J. Clin. Pharmacol.*, 2:73–79.
25. Hooper, W. D., Bochner, F., Eadie, M. J., and Tyrer, J. H. (1974): Plasma protein binding of diphenylhydantoin. Effects of sex hormones, renal and hepatic disease. *Clin. Pharmacol. Ther.*, 15:276–282.
26. Houghton, G. W., and Richens, A. (1976): Effect of age, height, weight and sex on serum phenytoin concentration in epileptic patients. *Br. J. Clin. Pharmacol.*, 2: 251–256.
27. Howell, J. R. (1975): Mathematical formulation for non-uniform multiple dosing. *J. Pharm. Sci.*, 64:464–466.
28. Jelliffe, R. W., Buell, J., and Kalaba, R. (1972): Reduction of digitalis toxicity by computer assisted glycoside dosage regimens. *Ann. Int. Med.*, 77:891–907.
29. Jusko, W. J., Koup, J. R., and Alvan, G. (1976): Nonlinear assessment of phenytoin bioavailability. *J. Pharmacokinet. Biopharm.*, 4:327–336.
30. Kalow, W. (1965): Dose-response relationships and genetic variation. *Ann. NY Acad. Sci.*, 123:212–218.
31. Kutt, H. (1974): Pharmacodynamic and pharmacokinetic measurements of antiepileptic drugs. *Clin. Pharmacol. Ther.*, 16:243–250.
32. Kutt, H., and McDowell, F. (1968): Management of epilepsy with diphenylhydantoin sodium. *JAMA* 203:167–170.
33. Kutt, H., and Penry, J. K. (1974): Usefulness of blood levels of antiepileptic drugs. *Arch. Neurol.*, 31:283–288.
34. Kutt, H., Winters, W., and Sherman, R. (1964): Diphenylhydantoin and phenobarbital toxicity. The role of liver disease. *Arch. Neurol.*, 11:649–656.
35. Levy, G., editor (1974): Clinical pharmacokinetics. *Symposium Proceedings.* American Pharmaceutical Association: Washington, D.C.
36. Levy, G., Gibaldi, M., and Jusko, W. J. (1969): Multicompartmental pharmacokinetic models and pharmacologic effects. *J. Pharm. Sci.*, 58:422–424.
37. Ludden, T. M., Hawkins, D. W., Allen, J. P., and Hoffman, S. F. (1976): Optimum phenytoin dosage regimens. *Lancet* 1:307–308.
38. Lund, L. (1974): Anticonvulsant effect of diphenylhydantoin relative to plasma levels. *Arch. Neurol.*, 31:289–294.
39. Mawer, G. E. (1976): Computer assisted prescribing of drugs. *Clin. Pharmacol.*, 1:67–78.
40. Mawer, G. E., Mullen, P. W., Rogers, E. M., and Robins, A. J. (1974): Phenytoin dose adjustment in epileptic patients. *Br. J. Clin. Pharmacol.*, 1:163–168.
41. Medwin, D. G. (1973): Why should we measure serum levels of anticonvulsant drugs for epilepsy? *Clin. Electroencephalogr.*, 4:132–134.
42. Odar-Cederloff, J., and Borga, O. (1974): Kinetic diphenylhydantoin in uraemic patients: Consequences of decreased plasma protein binding. *Eur. J. Clin. Pharmacol.*, 7:31–37.
43. Orr, J. W., Shimmins, J., and Spiers, C. F. (1969): Method for estimating individual drug dosage regimens. *Lancet* 2:771–773.
44. Paton, W. D. M., and Waud, D. R. (1964): A quantitative investigation of the relationship between rate of access of a drug to a receptor and the rate of onset or offset of action. *Naunyn Schmiedebergs Arch. Pharmacol.*, 248:124–143.
45. Pelkonen, R., Fogelholm, R., and Nikkila, E. A. (1975): Increase in serum cholesterol during phenytoin treatment. *Br. Med. J.*, 1:85.
46. Pruitt, A. W., Zwiren, G. T., Patterson, J. H., Dayton, P. C., Cook, C. E., and Wall, M. E. (1975): A complex pattern of disposition of phenytoin in severe intoxication. *Clin. Pharmacol. Ther.*, 18:112–120.
47. Rane, A., and Wilson, J. T. (1976): Clinical pharmacokinetics in infants and children. *Clin. Pharmacokinet.*, 1:2–24.

48. Ranjbaran, E., and McLaren, R. W. (1976): Modeling, testing, simulation and optimization of digitalis pharmacokinetics. Adv. Prog. IEEE, 1976 International Conference of Cybernetics Society, Washington, D.C.
49. Remmer, H., Hirschmann, J., and Greiner, I. (1969): Diphenylhydantoin. *Dtsch. Med. Wochenschr.,* 94:1265–1272.
50. Reuning, R. H., Sams, R. A., and Notari, R. E. (1973): Role of Pharmacokinetics in drug dosage adjustment. I. Pharmacologic effect, kinetics, and apparent volume of distribution of digoxin. *J. Clin. Pharmacol.,* 13:127–141.
51. Reynolds, E. H. (1975): Chronic antiepileptic toxicity. A review. *Epilepsia,* 16:319–352.
52. Richens, A., and Dunlop, A. (1975): Serum-phenytoin levels in management of epilepsy. *Lancet* 2:247–248.
53. Robinson, J. D., Morris, B. A., Aherne, G. W., and Marks, V. (1975): Pharmacokinetics of a single dose of phenytoin in man measured by radioimmunoassay. *Br. J. Clin. Pharmacol.,* 2:345–349.
54. Rose, S. W., Smith, L. D., and Penry, J. K. (1971): Blood Level Determinations of Antiepileptic Drugs: Clinical Value and Methods. National Institutes of Health, Bethesda, Maryland.
55. Rowland, M., Benet, L. Z., and Graham, G. (1973): Clearance concepts in pharmacokinetics. *J. Pharmacokinet. Biopharm.,* 1:123–136.
56. Rowland, M., and Matin, S. B. (1973): Kinetics of drug-drug interactions. *J. Pharmacokinet. Biopharm.,* 1:553–567.
57. Sheiner, L. B., Melmon, K. L., and Rosenburg, B. (1975): Instructional goals for physicians in the use of blood level data and the contribution of computers. *Clin. Pharmacol. Ther.,* 16:260–271.
58. Sheiner, L. B., Rosenburg, B., and Melmon, K. L. (1972): Modeling of individual pharmacokinetics for computer-aided drug dosage. *Comput. Biomed. Res.,* 5:441–459.
59. Sherwin, A. L., Eisen, A. A., and Sokolowski, C. D. (1973): Anticonvulsant drugs in human epileptogenic brain. *Arch. Neurol.,* 29:73–77.
60. Smolen, V. F. (1976): Theoretical and computational basis for drug bioavailability determinations using pharmacological data. II. Drug input response relationships. *J. Pharmacokinet. Biopharm.,* 4:355–375.
61. Smolen, V. F., Turrie, B. D., and Weigand, W. (1972): Dose input optimization time optimal control of simultaneously occurring multiple pharmacological effects and their inter-relationships. *J. Pharm. Sci.,* 61:1941–1952.
62. Svensmark, O., Schiller, P. J., and Buchthal, F. (1960): 5,5-diphenylhydantoin (Dilantin) blood levels after oral intravenous dosage in man. *Acta Pharmacol. Toxicol.,* 16:331–346.
63. Travers, R. D., Reynolds, E. H., and Gallagher, B. B. (1972): Variation in response to anticonvulsants in a group of epileptic patients. *Arch. Neurol.,* 27:29–33.
64. Troupin, A. S., and Ogemann, L. M. (1975): Paradoxical intoxication: a complication of anticonvulsant administration. *Epilepsia,* 16:753–758.
65. Vajda, F., Williams, F. M., Davidson, S., Falconer, M. A., and Breckenridge, A. (1974): Human brain, cerebrospinal fluid, and plasma concentrations of diphenylhydantoin and phenobarbital. *Clin. Pharmacol. Ther.,* 15:597–602.
66. Van Rossum, J. M. (1963): Cumulative dose-response curves. II. Techniques for the making of dose-response curves in isolated organs and the evaluation of drug parameters. *Arch. Int. Pharmacodyn.,* 143:299–330.
67. Vessell, E. S., and Passananti, G. T. (1971): Utility of clinical chemical determinations of drug concentrations in biological fluids. *Clin. Chem.,* 17:851–866.
68. Wagner, J. G. (1976): Linear pharmacokinetics models and vanishing exponential terms: Implications in pharmacokinetics. *J. Pharmacokinet. Biopharm.,* 4:395–425.
69. Wagner, J. G. (1976): Scientific Commentary: Linear pharmacokinetic equations allowing direct calculation of many needed pharmacokinetic parameters from the coefficients and exponents of polyexponential equations which have been fitted to the data. *J. Pharmacokinet. Biopharm.,* 4:443–467.
70. Wagner, J. G., Yates, J. D., Wills, P. W., Sakmar, E., and Stoll, R. G. (1974):

Correlation of plasma levels of digoxin in cardiac patients with dose and measures of renal function. *Clin. Pharmacol. Ther.*, 15:291–301.
71. Westlake, W. J. (1971): Problems associated with analysis of pharmacokinetic models. *J. Pharm. Sci.*, 60:882–885.
72. Wheeler, L. A., and Sheiner, L. B. (1976): A general method for optimal drug dose computation. *J. Pharmacokinet. Biopharm.*, 4:487–497.
73. Wilder, B. J., and Ramsay, R. E. (1975): Oral and intramuscular phenytoin. *Clin. Pharmacol. Ther.*, 19:360–364.
74. Wilder, B. J., Serrano, E. E., and Ramsay, R. E. (1973): Plasma diphenylhydantoin levels after loading and maintenance doses. *Clin. Pharmacol. Ther.*, 14:797–801.
75. Wilson, J. T., Höjer, B., and Rane, A. (1976): Loading and conventional dose therapy with phenytoin in children: Kinetic profile of parent drug and main metabolite in plasma. *Clin. Pharmacol. Ther.*, 20:48–58.
76. Woodbury, D. M., Penry, J. K., and Schmidt, R. P., editors. (1972): *Antiepileptic Drugs*. Raven Press, New York.

Antiepileptic Drugs: Quantitative Analysis and Interpretation, edited by C. E. Pippenger, J. K. Penry, and H. Kutt, Raven Press, New York, © 1978.

Chapter 22
Clinical Use and Interpretation of Serum Phenytoin Levels

Harold E. Booker

The value of phenobarbital as the first modern antiepileptic drug was determined empirically in the second decade of this century. Its clinical usefulness was limited, however, by its hypnotic effect. Based on the assumption that the hypnotic and anticonvulsant effects might be unrelated, Merritt and Putnam set out to test drugs that were poor sedatives for possible anticonvulsant effects. Phenytoin was supplied to these workers by Parke-Davis Laboratories, where it had been screened for hypnotic activity. Of the many drugs tested by Merritt and Putnam, phenytoin was the most effective in preventing convulsions induced by electroshock in cats. Successful clinical trials soon followed, and in 1938, phenytoin was introduced into clinical use as the first antiepileptic drug based on theory and preclinical animal testing (3,4). Since then, it has become one of the most widely studied drugs, and a complete bibliography would contain several thousand entries. Its success stimulated the search for other chemically related drugs that might have high anticonvulsant and low hypnotic activity. The majority of the currently available antiepileptic drugs are the result of that search.

Although it has demonstrable effects on many tissues and organs, the major clinical use of phenytoin is in the control of epilepsy. The chemistry and pharmacology of phenytoin relevant to its use in epilepsy have been extensively reviewed (7,8). Treatment with phenytoin (or with any of the other antiepileptic drugs) does not cure the epilepsy, but it does suppress or prevent the recurrence of seizures. The exact mechanism of the anticonvulsant effect is unknown, but it is most probably related to the ability of phenytoin to prevent the spread of abnormal or excessive neuronal discharge in the central nervous system (7). Phenytoin is generally ineffective in controlling minor generalized seizures (absence attacks or petit mal epilepsy). It is more effective against the partial epilepsies (psychomotor or temporal lobe seizures; focal motor or Jacksonian seizures), and is most effective against major generalized attacks (tonic-clonic convulsions or grand mal seizures). In these latter situations it is one of the most effective and extensively used drugs.

The aim of treatment of epilepsy with drugs is to prevent seizures from occurring without causing significant side effects. Sensitivity to both the therapeutic and the toxic effects of the antiepileptic drugs varies among patients, and may vary at different times in the same patient. Thus, the determination of the optimum dose for each patient must be based on the patient's clinical response. For each individual, the serum level of phenytoin and the degree of clinical response are directly related. This relationship is consistent enough among patients that general population values for the optimal therapeutic and potentially toxic ranges of serum levels can be defined. Most patients will continue to have some seizures when the serum level is below 10 μg/ml. Most will obtain maximum seizure control when the serum level is between 10 and 20 μg/ml. The frequency and severity of dose-dependent toxic effects (nystagmus, ataxia, and slurred speech) increase as the serum level rises progressively above 20 μg/ml (8). This relationship is shown diagrammatically in Fig. 1.

Although the correlation between serum level and clinical response is high, the correlation between dose and serum level is very low, not only among subjects but also in the same subject under different situations. For these reasons, problems in the clinical use of phenytoin are better understood by referring to the serum level rather than the dose. Since the serum level cannot usually be predicted from the dose, the use of serum level determina-

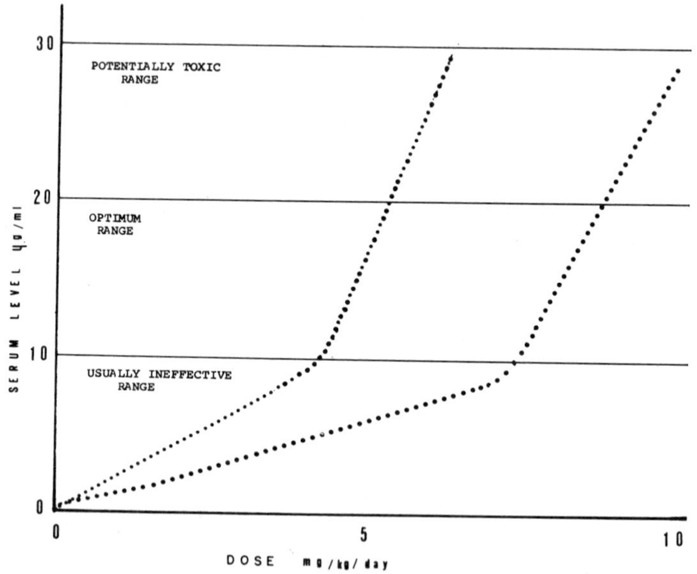

FIG. 1. Dose response relationship of phenytoin. The two curves represent the extremes of the relationship between dose and serum level in subjects when absorption is complete or metabolism is impaired or inefficient (to the left) or when absorption is incomplete or metabolism is efficient (to the right). The change in slope of the curves near the lower end of the optimum range of serum levels reflects the dose-dependent kinetics of phenytoin.

tions in the clinic is becoming more important and is invaluable if not imperative. We first discuss those features of the absorption and biotransformation of phenytoin that account for this, and then discuss the use and interpretation of serum levels in the clinical situation.

ABSORPTION

Phenytoin is a weak acid and should be absorbed from the stomach. Because of its low solubility, however, absorption is delayed until the drug reaches the small intestine. Even there, absorption is slow and may be incomplete, and the fraction of dose absorbed varies. The time of peak serum level after a single oral dose ranges from 4 to 12 hr. Reentry of drug into the gastrointestinal tract by biliary secretion further prolongs the absorption of phenytoin. Thus, with chronic daily administration of divided doses, the absorption of phenytoin at steady state approaches that of a continuous steady infusion. Consequently, the serum level is reasonably stable and independent of the time of last dose, so that a random specimen obtained at any time gives a reasonable estimate of the overall situation.

The slow absorption is a disadvantage when it is desirable to obtain high serum levels rapidly. This can be done by starting with a large dose (10 to 15 mg/kg) the first day, half of that the second day, and continuing with more usual doses (5 mg/kg) thereafter. When it is necessary to obtain high serum levels very rapidly (as in status epilepticus), phenytoin may be given intravenously. Infusion rate should not exceed 50 mg/min, as rates above this may cause cardiac and respiratory depression. Absorption after intramuscular administration is less complete and slower than after oral administration of similar doses. Intramuscular use should be avoided whenever possible. When it is necessary, the serum levels should be monitored frequently so that appropriate adjustment in doses can be effected (6).

DISTRIBUTION

Phenytoin is widely distributed throughout the body and accumulates in most tissues in greater concentration than in serum. It binds heavily to serum proteins, primarily albumin, but to a lesser extent to globulins. It competes with thyroxin for binding to thyroglobulin, which causes a low protein-bound iodine level in patients taking phenytoin. Such patients are euthyroid, however, as phenytoin does not interfere with thyroid function. In the concentrations usually encountered in clinical experience, approximately 90% of the total drug in serum is bound to protein. The usual analytical procedures determine the total level rather than the free or unbound level. Since pharmacologic effect and biotransformation are related to the concentration of free rather than to bound drug, variations in binding could account for changes in the kinetics and clinical effect of phenytoin. Free drug concentration may be determined by such techniques as dialysis or ultrafiltration, but a practical method in the clinic is to determine the concentration of phenytoin in saliva, as this concentration is equivalent to the free level in serum. Individual variations in the degree of protein binding are related primarily to the concentration of serum albumin and may have clinical significance (2). Several drugs are known that may interfere with the protein binding of phenytoin *in vitro,* but this is seldom a problem *in vivo.*

BIOTRANSFORMATION

The major step in the biotransformation of phenytoin consists of the hydroxylation of one of the phenyl substituents. Although several other metabolites are known, the hydroxylated derivative (5-*p*-hydroxyphenyl-5-phenylhydantoin or HPPH) accounts for 60 to 70% of phenytoin elimination. The reaction is carried out by the microsomal mixed function oxidase system of the liver. The affinity for the enzyme is low so that saturation of the system occurs as the serum level rises (5). Metabolism of phenytoin can also be inhibited by a variety of other commonly prescribed drugs (see Table 1). HPPH itself may inhibit the reaction (end product inhibition) and further limits the ability of the liver to metabolize phenytoin.

TABLE 1. *Some drugs that may inhibit phenytoin metabolism*

Disulfiram
Isoniazid
Sulthiame
Bishydroxycoumarin
Phenyramidol
Phenylbutazone
Chloramphenicol
Chlorpromazine
Prochlorperazine
Estrogens
Propoxyphene
Benzodiazepines

Listed in decreasing order of probability of causing significant clinical effects. Those below phenylbutazone rarely cause problems.

ELIMINATION

Metabolism to HPPH and subsequent renal excretion of the HPPH (conjugated with glucuronic acid) accounts for the major pathway for elimination, as less than 5% of the unchanged drug is excreted in the urine. At steady state, the 24-hr urine output of HPPH accounts for 60 to 70% of the daily phenytoin dose. Gas-liquid chromatographic procedures for determination of HPPH concentration in urine are available and can be utilized in the study of unusual situations in individual patients.

KINETICS

Under the usual clinical condition of chronic daily doses, the serum level will change after each change in phenytoin dose but will eventually stabilize at a new maximum or minimum. The full therapeutic and toxic potential of each dosage schedule cannot be determined until this steady state is reached. The rate at which it is reached will be determined by the rate of elimination of the drug. The most convenient measure of the rate of elimination is the serum half-life of a drug, that is, the time required (after absorption is complete) for the process of elimination to reduce the serum level to one-half of its initial value. Generally, a steady state will be reached in four to five half-lives of a drug. For many drugs, the half-life is constant and independent of the dose. The average half-life of phenytoin is around 24 hr, but may vary from 10 to 45 hr. Not only is there considerable interindividual variation in the half-life of phenytoin, but the half-life will change in the same subject at different dosage levels. At low doses (and low serum levels) the rate of metabolism is proportional to the serum level and the half-life is constant (first-order kinetics). However, as the dosage and serum level increase, the biotransformation system becomes saturated and no further increases in the rate of elimination occur (zero-order kinetics). At this stage, the half-life becomes a direct function of the serum level. Thus, longer times are required to reach steady state at higher doses than at low doses, and phenytoin is said to exhibit "dose-dependent" kinetics. Therefore, it is difficult to predict the rates at which the serum level of phenytoin will change unless the change is monitored by serum-level determinations.

The dose-dependent kinetics of phenytoin are the reason why the relationship between dose and serum level in individual subjects is nonlinear (see Fig. 1). The dose-serum level relationship is a family of curves generally isomorphic to the two dashed curves representing the extremes. The greater the fraction of dose absorbed or the more inefficient the metabolic process, the more the curve for an individual will be displaced toward the left. The lower the fraction of dose absorbed, or the more efficient the metabolism, the more the curve for the individual will be toward the right.

Even at constant doses, the serum level will stay at steady state only so long as the patient remains in a steady state. Since epilepsy is a chronic disorder, and many of its victims are forced to take phenytoin for many years, it is highly probable that major changes in the biology of the host will occur. The serum half-life of phenytoin is influenced by age, being much shorter in children than in adults. Because of the long periods at risk, patients taking phenytoin have a high probability of suffering other intercurrent illnesses. Thus, the probability of conjoint administration of other drugs that may interfere with phenytoin metabolism is also great. Any change in gastrointestinal motility or absorption could change the fraction of dose absorbed. Intercurrent illness may also change the kinetics of phenytoin by changes in the concentration of serum albumin or by the occurrence of renal disease and uremia. The degree of protein binding of phenytoin is decreased under both of these conditions, with a resultant change in the kinetics of phenytoin. Thus, the dose-serum level curve for individual subjects is not fixed, but may be shifted to the right or the left for a variety of reasons, and the shift may be temporary or permanent. In some situations the shift may be anticipated, as in aging or administration of other drugs known to inhibit phenytoin metabolism. All too often, however, the change is first suspected after it has occurred. The usual consequence is that the patient suffers more seizures, or becomes markedly intoxicated. Monitoring of the serum level is necessary to detect these changes early, and to allow for appropriate adjustments in dose.

CLINICAL USE AND INTERPRETATION OF SERUM PHENYTOIN LEVELS

Of major importance in the process of treatment with phenytoin is the fact that as the serum level approaches the lower limits of the optimum therapeutic range, the slope of the dose-serum level curve changes markedly. This change reflects the "dose-dependent" kinetics of phenytoin and occurs when elimination changes from "first order" to "zero order." At the point of change, small increases in dose result in large increases in the serum level. If the conventional practice of increasing doses by the size of the available commercial preparations (usually 50 to 100 mg) is followed, the serum level frequently rises rapidly. We have seen patients in whom an increase in dose from 200 to 300 mg/day caused a rise in the serum level from a steady state around 5 μg/ml to a new steady state above 30 μg/ml. This results in significant "overkill" in which the patient is exposed to potentially severe toxicity. In addition, the patient and/or physician may conclude that phenytoin is an ineffective drug based on their observations that the previous dose did not control seizures whereas the "next" dose caused significant toxicity. To obtain maximum efficiency and benefit from treatment with phenytoin, it is necessary to monitor serum levels frequently in the beginning stages of treatment. When the serum level begins to approach the lower end of the optimum therapeutic range, progressively smaller increases in dose should be prescribed.

After the optimal dose and serum level have been determined for each patient, it is important to monitor the serum levels periodically. The recurrence of seizures can be disastrous, particularly for the patient who has experienced previous periods of seizure control. Periodic monitoring of the serum level can help detect the changes in kinetics of phenytoin associated with age, drug interactions, and other illnesses described above. It is also important in the patient who experiences none of these problems. Often the patient who is doing well becomes complacent about his problem and compliance in adhering to his prescribed doses declines. If such a patient's optimum serum level is near the break in the dose-serum level curve (as is frequently the case), even a few missed doses, as little as one dose every other day or so, can result in a drop of the serum level below the therapeutic range. Noncompliance is a major problem in the seizure clinic and can best be suspected on the basis of serum-level determinations that show either a very low phenytoin level for dose or a decreasing level on stable dose. In some patients, continued seizures and low serum levels are due not to poor compliance but to poor absorption of phenytoin. Recognition of the low serum level and its correction by altering dose often resolve the problem. In other cases, therapeutic failure will be associated with very high, potentially toxic serum levels of phenytoin. Since too much phenytoin may actually aggravate seizures, these patients frequently benefit from lowering the dose and bringing the serum level into the optimum therapeutic range. Finally, some patients will be refractory to the therapeutic effects of phenytoin and seizures will continue whatever the serum level. In any case, the first and most important step in evaluating causes of therapeutic failure with phenytoin is to determine the serum level.

Determination of the serum level is invaluable in cases of toxic reactions. This is particularly true when the patient is taking more than one antiepileptic drug. It has been our experience that, for practical purposes, it is impossible to separate the various side effects of the antiepileptic drugs in patients taking more than one drug. In these situations determination of the offending drug (or drugs) is for practical purposes impossible unless the serum levels are determined. Determination of the serum levels is particularly valuable in recognizing unusual or atypical side effects. We have seen patients whose clinical picture showed none of the classical features of phenytoin intoxication (nystagmus, slurred speech, and ataxia) but whose clinical presentation were indistinguishable from those produced by vascular or demyelinating disease in the brainstem. In other cases the clinical picture was that of an acute hysterical reaction (1). Although we might have ultimately uncovered the cause of the problem without serum-level determinations, their availability greatly facilitated the process and significantly reduced morbidity for the patient.

SUMMARY

Phenytoin is one of the oldest, most effective, and most extensively prescribed antiepileptic drugs. It was the first such drug introduced in clinical use after animal experimentation and was the prototype for the majority of the currently used antiepileptic drugs.

Despite its clinical efficacy, there are several problems involved in the management of epilepsy with phenytoin. The optimum dose and serum level must be determined in each patient on the basis of the clinical response. It is pointless in the patient who is doing well clinically (free of both seizures and side effects) to change dosage schedules because the serum level does not fall within the optimum therapeutic range for the general population. Nevertheless, the majority of patients will obtain the optimum clinical response when the serum level is maintained between 10 and 20 μg/ml. The probability of toxic overdose effects increases as the serum level rises above this, and approaches certainty when the serum level is above 30 μg/ml.

Because of individual differences in the fraction of the dose absorbed, the interindividual correlation between dose and serum level is low. Because of the dose-dependent kinetics and nonlinear relationship of the serum level to dose within the individual subject, it is difficult to predict the serum level at steady state in a given patient for any dosage schedule. Thus, serum-level determinations are invaluable if not imperative in initiating therapy and in chronic maintenance therapy. They are also invaluable in evaluating toxicity, particularly in patients taking more than one antiepileptic drug or when unusual or atypical toxic reactions are present. Serum-level determinations must be reliable and accurate, however, as it is better not to have serum-level determinations than to have inaccurate ones. The availability of the methods for reliable determination of serum phenytoin levels in more clinical laboratories and their more frequent intelligent use by the clinician should increase the benefits that phenytoin can provide to many patients with epilepsy.

REFERENCES

1. Booker, H. E. (1975): Management of the difficult patient with complex partial seizures. In: *Complex Partial Seizures and Their Treatment, Advances in Neurology, Vol. 11,* edited by J. K. Penry and D. D. Daly, pp. 369–382. Raven Press, New York.
2. Booker, H. E., and Darcey, B. (1973): Serum concentrations of free diphenylhydantoin and their relationship to clinical intoxication. *Epilepsia,* 14:177–184.
3. Merritt, H. H., and Putnam, T. J. (1938): A new series of anticonvulsant drugs tested by experiments on animals. *Arch. Neurol. Psychiatr.,* 39:1003–1015.
4. Merritt, H. H., and Putnam, T. J. (1938): Sodium diphenyl hydantoinate in the treatment of convulsive disorders. *JAMA,* 111:1068–1073.
5. Richens, A. (1975): A study of the pharmacokinetics of phenytoin (diphenylhydantoin) in epileptic patients, and the development of a nomogram for making dose increments. *Epilepsia,* 16:627–646.
6. Serrano, E. E., Roye, D. B., Hammer, R. H., and Wilder, B. J. (1973): Plasma diphenylhydantoin values after oral and intramuscular administration of diphenylhydantoin. *Neurology* (Minneap.), 23:311–317.
7. Woodbury, D. M. (1969): Mechanisms of action of anticonvulsants. In: *Basic Mechanisms of the Epilepsies,* edited by H. H. Jasper, A. A. Ward, Jr., and A. Pope, pp. 647–681. Little, Brown and Company, Boston.
8. Woodbury, D. M., Penry, J. K., and Schmidt, R. P., editors (1972): *Antiepileptic Drugs.* Raven Press, New York.

Antiepileptic Drugs: Quantitative Analysis and Interpretation, edited by C. E. Pippenger, J. K. Penry, and H. Kutt, Raven Press, New York, © 1978.

Chapter 23
Some Quantitative Aspects of the Pharmacology of Phenobarbital

Thomas C. Butler

In 1911 phenobarbital was synthesized by Hörlein of the Bayer dye works and submitted for clinical trials. The reports of these trials, which appeared in the following year, included a recognition of the efficacy of the new drug in epilepsy (12). Phenobarbital was the second derivative of barbituric acid to have been introduced into medical use. Barbital had been introduced in 1903 as a result of the study of a series of barbituric acid derivatives by Fischer and von Mering (10). In more recent years, large numbers of barbituric acid derivatives have been synthesized and tested, and more than a score of them are or have been in medicinal use.

In animal tests, phenobarbital has been found to have much greater anticonvulsant activity relative to hypnotic activity than barbituric acids having only alkyl or alkenyl substituents in the 5-position. It has been generally accepted that this relationship applies as well to antiepileptic effects in man, but clinical experience with 5,5-disubstituted barbituric acids other than phenobarbital in human epilepsy has been meager.

ACIDIC PROPERTY

An important difference between phenobarbital and the other barbiturates in medicinal use is that it is a considerably stronger acid. The electron-attracting force of the phenyl group favors the dissociation of a proton from nitrogen and results in a lower ionization exponent than if only alkyl or alkenyl groups are substituents in the 5-position. The pK' of phenobarbital at 37°C and an ionic strength of 0.16 is 7.2, whereas that of pentobarbital, for instance, is 7.9. This is of importance in relation to the distribution and excretion of the drug and the ways in which these can be influenced.

The plasma membranes of cells in general behave as if freely permeable to the undissociated forms of weak organic acids and bases but impermeable or relatively impermeable to the ionized forms. This is shown in Fig. 1. The undissociated form is in equal concentration on both sides of the membrane, but the concentration of the ionized form depends on pH and will be unequal on the two sides if the two pH values differ. The total concentration will be higher on the side of higher pH. If the pH on one side is changed without

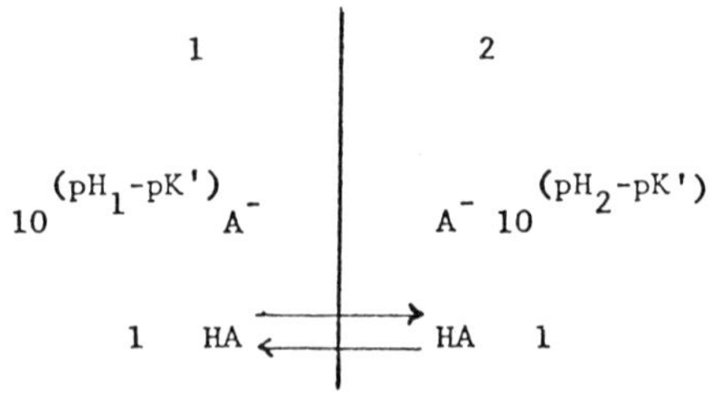

FIG. 1. Solutions of a weak acid separated by a semipermeable membrane.

$$\frac{C_1}{C_2} = \frac{10^{(pH_1 - pK')} + 1}{10^{(pH_2 - pK')} + 1}$$

changing the other side, there will be a shift of the compound across the membrane from one compartment to the other. These effects of change of pH are of importance in causing shifts of the drug between the intracellular and extracellular compartments and in changing the rate of excretion of the drug by the kidney, where only the undissociated species is reabsorbed by passive diffusion through the epithelium of the renal tubule.

The effects of change of pH on the distribution of a weak acid across a semipermeable membrane are greater the lower the pK' of the acid. Figure 2 shows the rate of change of the extracellular:intracellular concentration ratio of an acid with change of extracellular pH as a function of the pK' of

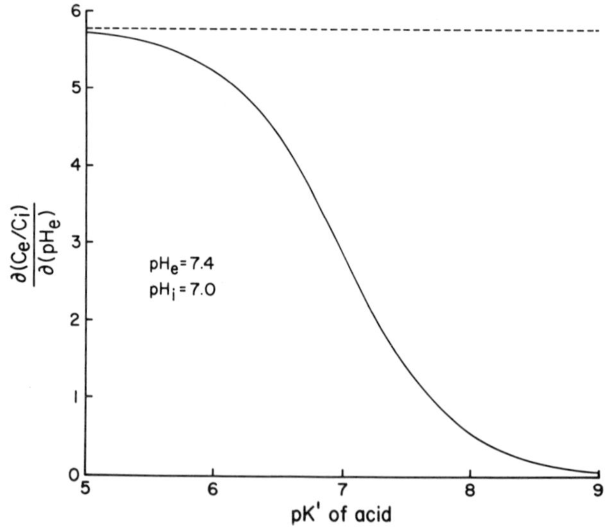

FIG. 2. The partial derivative of the extracellular: intracellular concentration ratio (C_e/C_i) with respect to extracellular pH (pH_e) as a function of the pK' of a weak acid.

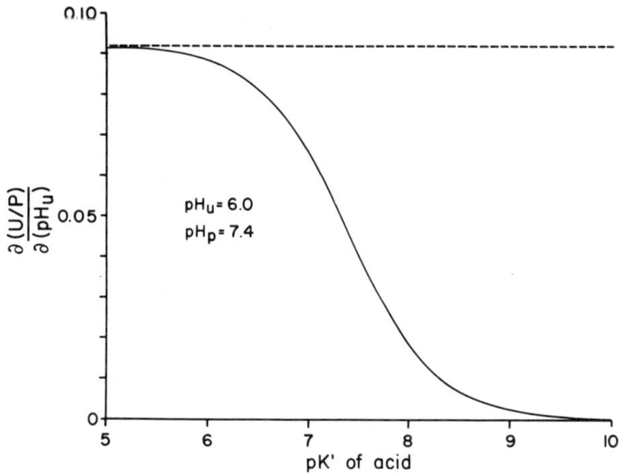

FIG. 3. The partial derivative of the urine: plasma concentration ratio (U/P) with respect to urinary pH (pH_u) as a function of the p*K*′ of a weak acid. Complete equilibration between tubular urine and plasma is assumed.

the acid. This value is 3.5 times as high for an acid with the p*K*′ of phenobarbital as for an acid with the p*K*′ of pentobarbital.

In the renal tubule only the undissociated form of a weak acid can penetrate the epithelium of the tubule and be reabsorbed by passive diffusion as water is reabsorbed. The concentration of the undissociated form in tubular urine approaches equality with the concentration of the undissociated drug in plasma water, although this equilibrium is seldom actually attained. On the assumption of complete equilibration between tubular urine and plasma, Fig. 3 shows the rate of change of the urine:plasma concentration ratio with change of urinary pH as a function of the p*K*′ of a weak acid. The value is higher the lower the p*K*′ of the acid. That is, the stronger the acid, the greater the effect of change of urinary pH on the rate of its excretion. The value is 2.6 times as high for an acid with the p*K*′ of phenobarbital as for an acid with the p*K*′ of pentobarbital.

BINDING TO ALBUMIN

In 4% (w/v) solutions of human and bovine serum albumin and in human and dog plasma, about 40% of phenobarbital was found to be bound (23). The percentage bound was little influenced by the concentration of phenobarbital in the therapeutic range or by pH. In a group of 20 epileptic patients, Lous (18) found that 41 to 56% (average 47%) of the phenobarbital in serum was bound. The concentration in cerebrospinal fluid was equal to that in an ultrafiltrate of serum. The amount of phenobarbital bound to plasma albumin is only about 2% of the total amount in the body. Displacement of bound phenobarbital by another drug would accordingly have little effect on tissue concentrations.

DISTRIBUTION

The apparent volume of distribution [total amount in body (mg/kg)/ concentration in plasma (mg/liter)] was found to be 0.75 liter/kg in the dog (6) and 0.89 liter/kg in the rat (8). In infants given single intramuscular doses of phenobarbital, Jalling (15) found volumes of distribution ranging from 0.50 to 0.76 liter/kg. I am not aware of a similar direct determination in adult patients. Using the value of 0.75 liter/kg from the dog and the elimination rate determined after withdrawal of the drug, Butler et al. (9) calculated the equilibrium plasma concentration that would be attained on a long-continued chronic dosage schedule. In 4 of 6 patients, the calculated value differed from the observed value by no more than 10%. Svensmark and Buchthal (21), using a similar calculation with the volume of distribution taken as 0.6 liter/kg, found good agreement between calculated and observed courses of accumulation on chronic schedules in 5 of 6 subjects.

Tissue analyses (23) showed that, at normal values of blood pH, the concentration of phenobarbital in brain is about equal to that in plasma, whereas that in muscle is lower. The concentration in liver is higher than in the other tissues.

As discussed above, the p*K'* of phenobarbital is such that a change of extracellular pH (pH_e) without a corresponding change of intracellular pH (pH_i) will cause a shift of the drug from one compartment to the other. When pH_e is changed without change of pCO_2, there is relatively little change of pH_i. When pCO_2 is changed, there are larger changes in pH_i but not sufficient to prevent a shift of an acidic drug (24). Metabolic and respiratory alkalosis and acidosis cause important shifts of phenobarbital between the extracellular and intracellular compartments. This was shown in experiments in dogs anesthetized with phenobarbital, in which intravenous $NaHCO_3$ increased the plasma concentration of phenobarbital by withdrawing the drug from tissues and in which inhalation of CO_2 decreased the plasma concentration by forcing the drug into tissues (23). That this interpretation is correct was shown by analyses of tissues.

The withdrawal of phenobarbital from brain by production of alkalosis lightens depression. The median anesthetic dose of phenobarbital in mice is increased 21% by administration of $NaHCO_3$ (23). Intravenous infusion of $NaHCO_3$ has proved of practical value in the treatment of phenobarbital poisoning. It has a dual beneficial effect, that of decreasing the concentration of drug in the brain and that of increasing renal excretion, to be discussed below. On the other hand, hypercapnia increases the concentration of phenobarbital in brain and deepens depression. The hypercapnia consequent to respiratory depression in phenobarbital poisoning establishes a vicious circle, and its correction will of itself lighten depression.

RENAL EXCRETION

The p*K*′ of phenobarbital is such that a large effect of change of urinary pH on renal clearance is to be expected. This has been found to be the case, the clearance being much higher when urine is alkaline than when it is acid. The clearance has also been found to increase with increasing rate of urine flow. These effects have been demonstrated in the dog and in man (23).

As might be expected, in patients with uncontrolled water intake and diet, the rate of renal excretion of unchanged phenobarbital varies considerably. Under ordinary circumstances, about 25% of a dose will be excreted unchanged. However, it is possible by induction of diuresis and alkalosis to increase this proportion considerably. These are measures that have proved of practical value in the treatment of phenobarbital poisoning.

METABOLISM

The first major metabolite of phenobarbital to be recognized was 5-ethyl-5-(*p*-hydroxyphenyl)-barbituric acid (7). This metabolite is excreted in the urine partly free and partly conjugated with glucuronic acid. The major part is conjugated. The total *p*-hydroxyphenobarbital found in urine is usually somewhat less than the amount of unchanged phenobarbital, but in any individual patient on any one day it may be greater or less.

Other metabolites of phenobarbital that have been identified by gas chromatography-mass spectrometry (13) are 5-ethyl-5-(3,4-dihydroxy-1,5-cyclohexadien-1-yl)-barbituric acid, 5-ethyl-5-(3,4-dihydroxyphenyl)-barbituric acid, and 5-(1-hydroxyethyl)-5-phenyl-barbituric acid. No quantitative assessment of the amounts of these metabolites has been made, but it appears that they must account for only a very minor proportion of the metabolism of phenobarbital.

It had been found that the sum of the amounts of unchanged phenobarbital and of free and conjugated *p*-hydroxyphenobarbital appearing in urine did not nearly account for all of an administered dose (e.g., 25). Clearly a major pathway of metabolic inactivation of phenobarbital was still unrecognized. Recently Tang et al. (22) identified N-hydroxyphenobarbital as a major metabolite in man. It was present in urine in larger amounts than the *p*-hydroxy derivative and accounted for 31% of a dose of phenobarbital.

The hydroxylation of phenobarbital on the phenyl ring and presumably also on nitrogen is brought about by the mixed-function oxidases located in the endoplasmic reticulum of the liver. Phenobarbital causes a proliferation of the hepatic endoplasmic reticulum with an increase in the amounts of drug-metabolizing enzymes and can thus bring about an increase in the rate of its own metabolism. There are many other drugs that also cause an induction of drug-metabolizing enzymes. Such drugs used concomitantly with phenobarbital can also accelerate its metabolism.

RATE OF ELIMINATION

In the elimination of phenobarbital, renal excretion and metabolism are both processes of major importance. In view of the diverse factors that can influence the rates of both of these processes, it is understandable that there may be considerable variation in overall elimination rate from patient to patient and in the same patient from day to day. Phenobarbital is by far the most persistent of any of the barbiturates in medicinal use. For instance, the proportion of phenobarbital eliminated in 24 hr is only about the same as that of pentobarbital eliminated in 1 hr. The persistence of phenobarbital is an advantageous property in the treatment of epilepsy but makes it unsuitable for use as a hypnotic in ambulatory patients and makes the treatment of phenobarbital poisoning especially difficult.

Despite the complexity of the processes responsible for its elimination, the disappearance of phenobarbital from plasma after cessation of dosage is ordinarily approximately exponential, and the elimination rate is commonly expressed as a half-life (see Chapter 20). Reported half-lives of phenobarbital in adults have ranged from 2 days to nearly 8 days (e.g., 1,3,9, 17,20). This corresponds to the daily elimination of 9 to 29% of the amount present in the body at the time. The half-life is reported to be shorter in children than in adults (11) and longer in patients with cirrhosis of the liver than in normal subjects (1). In view of the extremely slow elimination of phenobarbital, dosage schedules often advocated in the past are clearly at unnecessarily frequent intervals. Probably in most epileptic patients the drug level can be kept within acceptable limits with one dose a day. A sustained-release preparation is an obvious absurdity.

ACCUMULATION

When a drug is administered at intervals such that it is not completely eliminated between doses, accumulation will occur. With a drug eliminated as slowly as phenobarbital, administration at daily or more frequent intervals will lead to pronounced accumulation. The calculated course of accumulation of phenobarbital administered once a day is shown in Fig. 4. Actually, the course of accumulation is not predictable with any great precision. The induction of drug-metabolizing enzymes might increase the elimination rate after a few days, and other factors might cause renal excretion to vary somewhat from day to day.

Accumulation will continue until the rate of elimination equals the rate of intake. For instance, if one-fifth of the amount in the body is eliminated

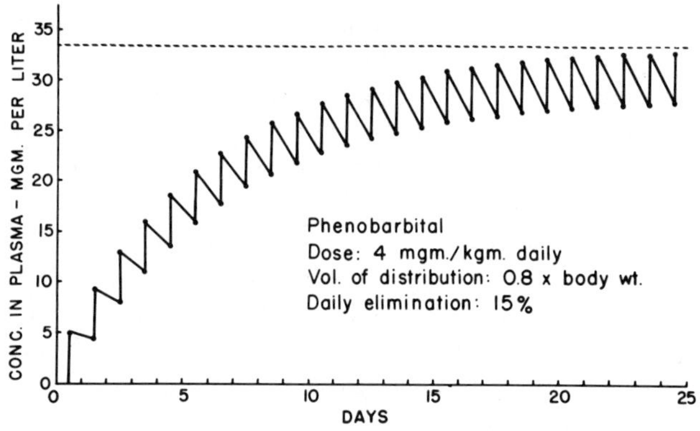

FIG. 4. Calculated course of accumulation of phenobarbital with one dose a day and a constant elimination rate.

daily, the level finally reached will be five times that attained during the first day. The time required for the accumulated level to reach 90% of its final value is 3.3 half-lives and to reach 95% of its final value, 4.3 half-lives.

TOLERANCE

A marked degree of tolerance develops to the hypnotic effects of phenobarbital. In an experiment by Butler et al. (9) in which 5 men were given daily doses of 2 mg/kg or 4 mg/kg, all complained during the first 3 days of drowsiness so severe as to interfere seriously with their usual activities. Thereafter these symptoms rapidly disappeared, and at the end of the experiment on the 12th day when the plasma concentrations were five times as high as on the first day, there were no subjective effects. This is a true tolerance unrelated to any development of more rapid metabolism of the drug. It is not unusual for epileptic patients treated with phenobarbital to be asymptomatic with plasma concentrations that would cause coma in cases of acute poisoning. Tolerance more than keeps pace with cumulation and completely obscures any symptomatic evidence of cumulation.

Phenobarbital has traditionally been used to produce long-term sedative effects. Physicians have taken for granted that phenobarbital should be useful for this purpose and that they were accomplishing their end in prescribing it. However, in view of the striking tolerance that is developed to the hypnotic effects of phenobarbital in the first few days, it may well be questioned whether long-term sedation is actually an effect that can be achieved with phenobarbital.

Although tolerance to light hypnotic effects is conspicuous, it is uncertain how much tolerance is developed to concentrations in the lethal range. Certainly the tolerance to phenobarbital is of a limited degree and not comparable to that which can develop toward morphine. In the small number of cases of acute poisoning studied by Lous (19), patients who had previously been on chronic phenobarbital dosage aroused from coma at serum concentrations in the same range as patients with no previous experience with the drug. Yet some epileptic patients are asymptomatic with concentrations this high or nearly this high.

Although there is mention of tolerance to the antiepileptic effect of phenobarbital in the clinical literature, evidence that such a phenomenon actually occurs is not convincing. It is the usual experience that a patient's seizures can be controlled with undiminishing effectiveness over a period of years without increasing the dosage of the drug. In ordinary clinical practice, recognition of the development of any limited degree of tolerance to antiepileptic effects that might be taking place in the first few days would be impossible. If there is any tolerance whatever to antiepileptic effects, it cannot be of any great magnitude or progress over any long period of time.

PENETRATION INTO BRAIN

A feature of the pharmacology of phenobarbital noted in the first study (14) but still not always appreciated is that there is a lag in the onset of its action after intravenous administration of a solution of the sodium salt. Among the derivatives of barbituric acid, there are some with essentially immediate onset of action after intravenous injection and others, including phenobarbital, showing a pronounced delay (4). In the dog, it may be as much as an hour before the full depressant effect of an intravenous dose of phenobarbital is seen. With barbital, which has an even longer lag than phenobarbital, it was shown that the drug enters the brain slowly after intravenous injection (5). The delay in onset of action of phenobarbital is also undoubtedly due to slow penetration from blood to brain. Whenever phenobarbital is to be used intravenously, it should be kept in mind that the depressant effects will continue to increase for some time after the injection is ended.

EFFECTIVE PLASMA CONCENTRATIONS

The plasma concentrations required for antiepileptic effects are generally in the range of 15 to 40 μg/ml. In Lous' (19) cases of acute poisoning, awakening occurred at concentrations in the range of 50 to 100 μg/ml. Yet a patient on chronic dosage has been described as asymptomatic with a concentration of 70 μg/ml (2). The concentration required to kill undoubtedly depends on the length of time that the patient is subjected to the high level. Poisoned patients who reach a hospital alive and have their plasma concentrations measured are likely to survive. Patients with concentrations above 250 μg/ml have survived, but they were treated with measures to accelerate the elimination of the drug.

INTERACTIONS

When phenobarbital is used together with other drugs, interactions may be conspicuous and clinically important. Phenobarbital induces the hepatic microsomal enzymes that are responsible for the metabolic inactivation of a great many drugs. Phenobarbital can thus increase the rate of metabolism of a variety of drugs, decreasing the concentrations attained with a given dosage. On the other hand, phenobarbital may inhibit the metabolism of another drug. Both of these effects may be seen when phenobarbital and phenytoin are used together. Phenytoin undergoes metabolic hydroxylation of one phenyl ring in the para position, a reaction analogous to that undergone by phenobarbital. Phenobarbital induces the enzymes that hydroxylate phenytoin and at the same time acts as a competitive inhibitor of the reaction. When phenobarbital is added to the medication of a patient being treated with phenytoin, the net effect on the plasma phenytoin level depends on the balance between these opposing effects. The level of phenytoin may fall or rise or be unchanged. Usually the change is not large enough in either direction to be of importance. The interactions between phenobarbital and phenytoin have been reviewed by Kutt (16).

Although phenobarbital is one of the most potent enzyme inducers and the best recognized one, it is by no means unique in this action. Enzyme induction has been demonstrated with a large number of drugs of diverse structure. Any of these used together with phenobarbital might add to the enzyme induction produced by phenobarbital itself and further accelerate its metabolism. The complexity and unpredictability of potential drug interactions are such as to indicate the advisability of avoiding unnecessary use of multiple drug therapy.

CONCLUSIONS

Phenobarbital had been in use for many years before analytical methods were developed that made possible a more rational and scientific use of the drug. It is not surprising that unscientific and antiquated uses of phenobarbital persist along with the antiquated apothecary system in which the dosage forms are still provided. A sustained-release form of phenobarbital and numerous preparations combining small doses of phenobarbital with such drugs as antispasmodics, bronchodilators, and coronary dilators are all still marketed, presumably profitably, a fact doing little to encourage an optimistic view of the impact of science on the practice of medicine. If a drug is to be used irrationally, there can be little enthusiasm for applying quantitative methods to the quantitation of irrationality. However, in its use as an anticonvulsant, the one application in which phenobarbital is unquestionably an effective and useful drug, quantitative measurement of concentrations in plasma has much to offer in improving the empiricism practiced before the days of adequate analytical methodology. Accurate monitoring of plasma concentrations of phenobarbital has great potential for improvement of seizure control, prevention of toxicity, and avoidance of unnecessary multiple-drug therapy.

ACKNOWLEDGMENTS

Some of the work by the author and his colleagues included in this discussion was supported by National Institutes of Health Grants M-393 and B-384. The author is recipient of U.S. Public Health Service Research Career Program Award 5 KO6 GM19, 429 from the National Institute of General Medical Sciences.

REFERENCES

1. Alvin, J., McHorse, T., Hoyumpa, A., Bush, M. T., and Schenker, S. (1975): The effect of liver disease in man on the disposition of phenobarbital. *J. Pharmacol. Exp. Ther.*, 192:224–235.
2. Atkinson, A. J., Jr. (1974): Individualization of anticonvulsant therapy. *Med. Clin. North Am.*, 58:1037–1049.
3. Bloomer, H. A. (1966): A critical evaluation in the treatment of barbiturate intoxication. *J. Lab. Clin. Med.*, 67:898–905.
4. Butler, T. C. (1942): The delay in onset of action of intravenously injected anesthetics. *J. Pharmacol. Exp. Ther.*, 74:118–128.
5. Butler, T. C. (1950): The rate of penetration of barbituric acid derivatives into the brain. *J. Pharmacol. Exp. Ther.*, 100:219–226.
6. Butler, T. C. (1952): Quantitative studies of the metabolic fate of mephobarbital (N-methyl phenobarbital). *J. Pharmacol. Exp. Ther.*, 106:235–245.
7. Butler, T. C. (1956): The metabolic hydroxylation of phenobarbital. *J. Pharmacol. Exp. Ther.*, 116:326–336.
8. Butler, T. C., Mahaffee, D., and Mahaffee, C. (1952): The role of the liver in the metabolic disposition of mephobarbital. *J. Pharmacol. Exp. Ther.*, 106:364–369.
9. Butler, T. C., Mahaffee, C., and Waddell, W. J. (1954): Phenobarbital: Studies of elimination, accumulation, tolerance, and dosage schedules. *J. Pharmacol. Exp. Ther.*, 111:425–435.
10. Fischer, E., and von Mering, J. (1903): Ueber eine neue Klasse von Schlafmitteln. *Therapie der Gegenwart*, 44:97–101.
11. Garrettson, L. K., and Dayton, P. G. (1970): Disappearance of phenobarbital and diphenylhydantoin from serum of children. *Clin. Pharmacol. Ther.*, 11:674–679.
12. Hauptmann, A. (1972): Luminal bei Epilepsie. *Münch. Med. Wochenschr.*, 59: 1907–1909.
13. Horning, M. G., Butler, C. M., Nowlin, J., and Hill, R. M. (1975): Drug metabolism in the human neonate. *Life Sci.*, 16:651–672.
14. Impens, E. (1912): Pharmakologisches über Luminal oder Phenyläthylbarbitursäure. *Dtsch. Med. Wochenschr.*, 38:945–947.
15. Jalling, B. (1974): Plasma and cerebrospinal fluid concentrations of phenobarbital in infants given single doses. *Develop. Med. Child Neurol.*, 16:781–793.
16. Kutt, H. (1975): Interactions of antiepileptic drugs. *Epilepsia*, 16:393–402.
17. Lous, P. (1954): Plasma levels and urinary excretion of three barbituric acids after oral administration to man. *Acta Pharmacol. Toxicol.*, 10:147–165.

18. Lous, P. (1954): Blood serum and cerebrospinal fluid levels and renal clearance of phenemal in treated epileptics. *Acta Pharmacol. Toxicol.,* 10:166–177.
19. Lous, P. (1954): Barbituric acid concentration in serum from patients with severe acute poisoning. *Acta Pharmacol. Toxicol.,* 10:261–280.
20. Morselli, P. L., Rizzo, M., and Garattini, S. (1971): Interaction between phenobarbital and diphenylhydantoin in animals and in epileptic patients. *Ann. N.Y. Acad. Sci.,* 179:88–107.
21. Svensmark, O., and Buchthal, F. (1963): Accumulation of phenobarbital in man. *Epilepsia,* 4:199–206.
22. Tang, B. K., Inaba, T., and Kalow, W. (1977): N-hydroxyphenobarbital—The major metabolite of phenobarbital in man. *Fed. Proc.,* 36:966.
23. Waddell, W. J., and Butler, T. C. (1957): The distribution and excretion of phenobarbital. *J. Clin. Invest.,* 36:1217–1226.
24. Waddell, W. J., and Butler, T. C. (1959): Calculation of intracellular pH from the distribution of 5,5-dimethyl-2,4-oxazolidinedione (DMO). Application to skeletal muscle of the dog. *J. Clin. Invest.,* 38:720–729.
25. Whyte, M. (1976): Phenobarbital (PB) disposition in man: Presumptive evidence for several metabolites. *Fed. Proc.,* 35:565.

Antiepileptic Drugs: Quantitative Analysis and Interpretation, edited by C. E. Pippenger, J. K. Penry, and H. Kutt, Raven Press, New York, © 1978.

Chapter 24
Clinical Application of Serum Primidone Levels

Dorothy D. Schottelius and R. W. Fincham

Primidone (2-deoxyphenobarbital or 5-ethyl-5-phenyldihydro-4,6-(1H,5H)-pyrimidinedione), synthesized by Bogue and Carrington in 1949, is a white crystalline substance with a molecular weight of 218.25. It is sparingly soluble in water and most organic solvents. The early clinical and laboratory evaluations of this compound were reported by Handley and Stewart (20), Bogue and Carrington (4) and Goodman et al. (19). Several clinical studies were performed between 1952 and 1956 to demonstrate the effectiveness of primidone as an anticonvulsant, and these have been reviewed by Booker (5). These studies in man and experimental animals were done prior to the time that the conversion of primidone to phenobarbital was published (8). Several additional clinical studies were published between 1956 and 1970 in which serum levels of primidone were not determined.

This chapter emphasizes the investigations of primidone as an antiepileptic drug and the relationship of serum level to dose and clinical control of seizures.

TYPES OF SEIZURES—USE OF PRIMIDONE

Clinically, primidone has been used in the treatment of tonic-clonic generalized seizures (grand mal) and partial seizures with complex symptomatology (psychomotor). The drug is usually prescribed after the patient has been unsuccessfully treated with phenytoin or phenytoin plus phenobarbital. Prior to the introduction of carbamazepine, primidone was the drug of choice in treatment of complex partial seizures and was usually administered in combination with phenytoin.

The generalized tonic-clonic seizure may or may not be preceded by an aura followed by a sudden loss of consciousness. A tonic spasm of the body takes place immediately after or coincident with the loss of consciousness. All voluntary muscles participate in the spasm, and occasionally these are violent enough to result in dislocation of joints or fractures of bones. As the tonic muscular spasm relaxes, clonic movements appear. All degrees of events may occur in the generalized seizure. Consciousness usually returns in a few minutes, and the individual then may lapse into a heavy sleep.

The complex partial seizure may consist of complex and essentially psychic symptoms such as mental confusion or illusions and, therefore, may be thought of as consisting of an alteration in the content of consciousness that may be manifested as unresponsiveness, confusion and amnesia. More complete descriptions of the clinical and electroencephalographic events have been provided by others (18,26).

PRIMIDONE METABOLISM

Biotransformation

In man, primidone is converted into two major metabolites, phenylethylmalonamide (PEMA) and phenobarbital, as illustrated in Fig. 1. The importance of the conversion of primidone to phenobarbital in man was emphasized by two studies (8,25) in which therapeutic doses of primidone in man resulted in plasma phenobarbital levels capable of exerting a significant anticonvulsant effect. The same conversion has been reported in dogs (8), rats (2), and rabbits (13). We consider this conversion of primidone to two active antiepileptic compounds in a later section dealing with clinical application of primidone levels. This conversion, however, also may influence all aspects of primidone metabolism.

Absorption

Peak serum concentrations of primidone have been determined utilizing 500- and 750-mg doses in two separate studies (6,16) and averaged approximately 3.0 hr. The range of peak absorption times was quite large, from 0.5

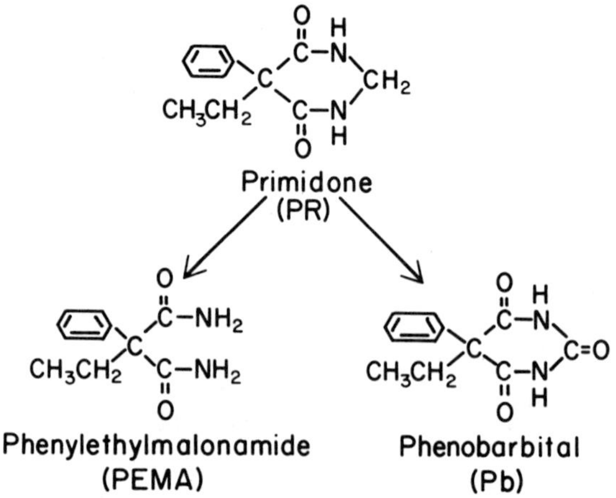

FIG. 1. Metabolic pathways of primidone.

to 7.3 hr, and there seemed to be some prolongation of peak values with repeated administration. The peak absorption time did not seem to be altered by the different doses; however, much of these data were obtained following a single morning dose in the fasting state. The individual variability in absorption rates and conditions that may alter this parameter should be considered in future studies utilizing this drug. Additional studies on the absorption of primidone are warranted.

Distribution

Several studies have been reported concerning the distribution of primidone and phenobarbital derived from primidone in the cerebrospinal fluid with a wide range of CSF/serum ratios recorded (30). Values of CSF/serum ratios have ranged from 0.53 to 1.13; from this information it has often been inferred that primidone is not protein bound. Our study has indicated that this ratio will vary with the dose-sample time interval. When this interval was 2 to 4 hr we obtained a CSF/serum ratio of 0.60; when it was 7 hr the ratio was 0.997. There was some indication that co-medication with phenytoin also may influence this distribution. We found no difference in the distribution of derived phenobarbital when compared to phenobarbital (ratio 0.48); this was not unexpected.

Primidone has been measured in saliva and the saliva/plasma level ratio was 0.73 (23). This value also indicates that there is significant protein binding of primidone.

Relatively little information has been published citing brain tissue levels of primidone. Houghton et al. (21) found a significant correlation between brain and plasma primidone concentration with a brain/plasma ratio of 0.87. They also reported a CSF/plasma ratio of 0.81, indicating protein binding of this drug. This study was done with a relatively small number of patients, and because of the treatment schedule individuals may not have been in steady state and treatment was discontinued 1 day prior to obtaining the various samples.

Primidone can reach the fetus during pregnancy by transplacental passage (24), although no constant ratio was found between maternal and cord blood. We also have found primidone in cord blood, and we are currently collecting samples to further establish maternal-fetal relationships.

Disposal and Excretion

The apparent half-life of primidone is short and appears to range from 3 to 12 hr (6,14). The half-life of primidone appears to be highly individualized and may be influenced by other anticonvulsant drugs.

Primidone excretion occurs by its conversion to phenobarbital and excretion of that compound by the usual pathways; its conversion to PEMA, which may be excreted unchanged; and by the excretion of primidone itself. Crystalluria has been found in cases associated with acute primidone intoxication (1,6,9), and these crystals have been identified as primidone itself. Additional experimental studies should be performed on the disposition and excretion of this anticonvulsant drug, and the effect of other drugs on this excretion.

MECHANISM OF ACTION

It is difficult to evaluate the early studies on the mechanism of action of primidone (4,19), since they failed to take into account the possible effects of its metabolites. The only data from those trials that may be valid would be those obtained on tests undertaken shortly after dosing with primidone—it has been demonstrated that low levels of phenobarbital are present in rats up to 6 hr after a single intragastric administration of primidone (17). In retrospect, therefore, the data presented concerning electrically induced seizures in rats (4,19) obtained at 3 hr may indicate an independent action of primidone. Data presented by Gallagher et al. (17) would also indicate some effect of primidone in raising the tonic-clonic threshold in rats.

Few, if any, detailed *in vitro* electrophysiological studies have been reported utilizing primidone or PEMA, and these studies should be encouraged. The mechanism of action in man has not been clarified, and the presence of two active metabolites makes this a difficult task.

DRUG INTERACTIONS WITH PRIMIDONE

Interactions among primidone, PEMA, and phenobarbital have been investigated in animals and were summarized by Gallagher and Baumel (15). These studies indicated a synergistic action of PEMA and primidone.

The effect of phenytoin on the conversion of primidone to phenobarbital in humans has been reported (11,27) and is illustrated in Fig. 2. This figure compares the serum concentration of phenobarbital as a function of the serum concentration of primidone in 43 patients taking primidone only and 127 patients taking primidone and phenytoin. All of these individuals were in a steady state, having been on the same dosage of medication for at least 3 weeks. All blood samples were collected between 2 and 4 hr after the last dose of primidone. The correlation coefficients are indicated on the figure and the linear regression equations are as follows: primidone only, serum phenobarbital level = 5.9 + 0.97 serum primidone level; primidone + phenytoin, serum phenobarbital level = 13.6 + 1.7 serum primidone level. The variability of the data is clearly apparent. Table 1 indicates that the average dose of primidone and the range of doses were similar in the two groups—however, the serum level of primidone was higher and the phenobarbital level was lower in the primidone-only group. The Pb/Pr ratio is significantly lower

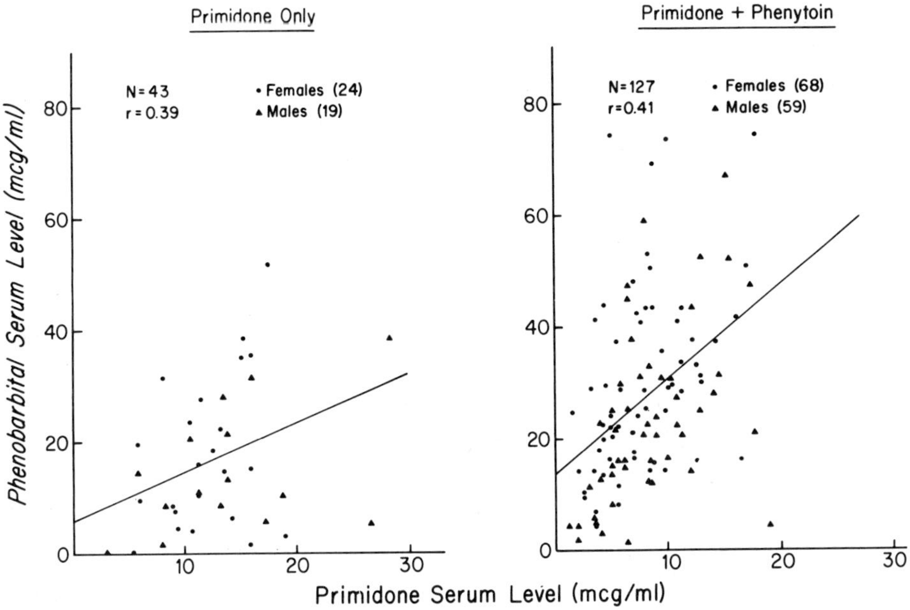

FIG. 2. Serum phenobarbital levels as a function of serum primidone levels in patients taking only primidone and patients taking primidone and phenytoin.

in the primidone-only group, but it should be noted that there is some overlap in the range. Even though there is definitely an increase in the conversion of primidone to phenobarbital when phenytoin is a co-medication, the range of values indicates the individual variability in both groups and therefore the importance of determining the serum primidone level as well as the serum phenobarbital level.

TABLE 1. *Effect of Phenytoin on Primidone Metabolism*

	Primidone	Primidone + phenytoin
N	43	127
Pr dose (mg/kg)	10.9 ± 0.67[a] (2.3–21.5)	10.6 ± 0.42 (3.3–22.0)
DPH dose (mg/kg)	—	4.8 ± 0.14 (1.4–9.2)
DPH serum level (μg/ml)	—	12.06 ± 0.09 (1.8–46.1)
Pr serum level (μg/ml)	13.15 ± 0.86 (3.0–28.4)	8.1 ± 0.36 (1.9–17.8)
PB serum level (μg/ml)	17.34 ± 1.9 (0.0–51.5)	27.20 ± 1.4 (2.1–74.6)
Pb/Pr	1.35 ± 0.14 (0.0–3.89)	3.82 ± 0.24 (1.01–16.5)

[a] Mean ± standard error; ( ) range.

A preliminary report (10) indicates that carbamazepine may increase primidone and phenobarbital levels in some patients, but the carbamazepine therapy was not continued long enough and the number of patients were too few to draw firm conclusions. It indicates, however, that the possible interaction of these two drugs warrants close observation.

Isoniazid has been reported to inhibit the metabolism of primidone in one patient with focal seizures (31). In this instance the half-life of primidone was 1.6 times as long with isoniazid therapy (14 hr versus 8.7 hr).

CLINICAL UTILIZATION OF SERUM PRIMIDONE LEVELS

Even though primidone has been used extensively as an anticonvulsant for more than 20 years, controversy still continues as to whether or not primidone itself has any anticonvulsant activity apart from the derived phenobarbital. Several reasons may be cited that have contributed to this problem: (a) clinical evaluations of the drug prior to 1956 have questionable validity because of the lack of knowledge of the conversion of primidone to phenobarbital; (b) evaluations of the drug from 1956 to 1970 were done without the utilization of reliable serum levels; (c) there have been insufficient clinical trials utilizing available information concerning the pharmacodynamics of primidone; and (d) there are still insufficient pharmacokinetic data available to us for all of the antiepileptic drugs. Until such time as all of these questions are answered, we should critically evaluate the information available.

Various animal studies have demonstrated protection against induced seizures prior to the conversion to phenobarbital (3,17) and when comparisons were made between primidone and phenobarbital in mice and dogs (12).

Several reports have appeared in the literature that both support and deny the anticonvulsant activity of primidone (6,16,25,28,32), but these are difficult to evaluate in some cases because of the presence of co-medications, lack of serum primidone levels, and necessity of blood sampling at specific times after dose, among other factors.

Recently discussion has also taken place regarding the usefulness of serum primidone levels in addition to derived serum phenobarbital levels (29), and even in this area there is a division of opinion. We have been determining serum levels of primidone in our laboratory and utilizing these levels clinically for approximately 5 years.

Figure 3 illustrates the data collected from the patients referred to earlier (Table 1) and demonstrates the variability found in both primidone and derived phenobarbital levels as a function of dose of primidone. It should be emphasized again that all of these patients were in steady state and that the blood samples were collected between 2 and 4 hr after primidone dose. The correlation of serum primidone level with dose in those individuals on only primidone is not very good—the regression line parameters were serum

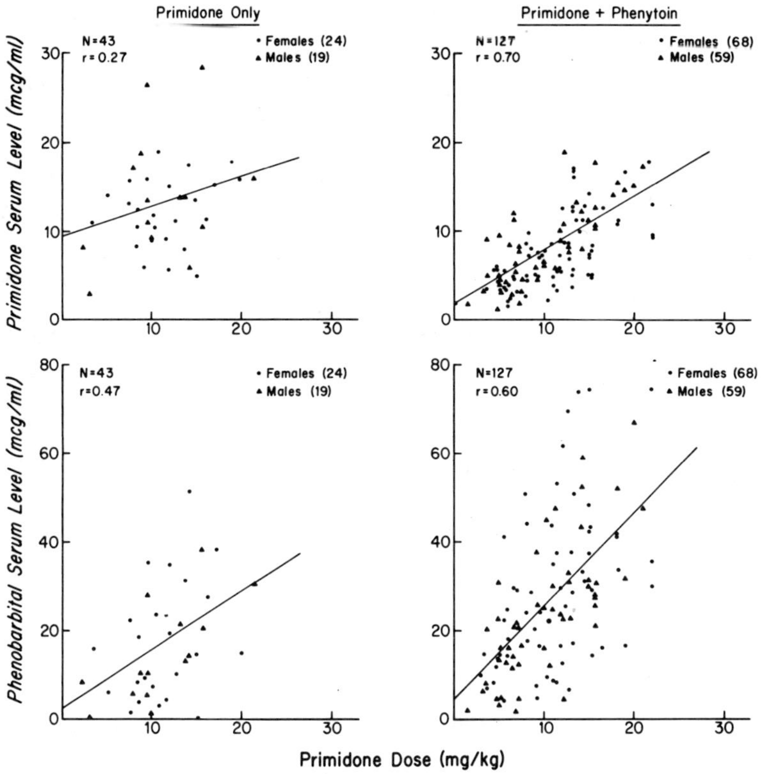

FIG. 3. Serum primidone and phenobarbital levels as a function of primidone dose in patients taking only primidone and patients taking primidone and phenytoin.

primidone level = 9.4 + 0.34 primidone dose (mg/kg). The derived phenobarbital-primidone dose correlation is somewhat better—serum phenobarbital level = 2.5 + 1.35 primidone dose (mg/kg)—but again we see a great deal of variability. Twenty-three of the patients on primidone only had derived phenobarbital levels less than 15 μg/ml. The average phenobarbital level was 7.6 μg/ml (range 0 to 15; SE 0.96); The average primidone level for this same group was 12.08 μg/ml (range 3.0 to 26.5; SE 1.17). The phenobarbital/primidone ratio for these 23 patients was 0.7 $\pm$ 0.12 (range 0.0 to 2.42). When one considers the ranges of values just cited and shown in Table 1, there appears to be no predictable relationship to adjust the primidone dosage on an individual basis if one has only the derived phenobarbital in the patients who are taking only primidone.

The data on the 127 individuals who were on the co-medications primidone and phenytoin are also shown in Fig. 3. There seems to be a better correlation in these individuals between primidone dose and serum level; the regression line parameters: serum primidone level = 1.6 $\pm$ 0.60 primidone dose, $r = 0.70$. The derived phenobarbital-primidone dose correlation is also better in this group than in the group taking only primidone, and the parameters are serum phenobarbital level = 4.9 + 2.07 primidone dose, $r = 0.60$. These data along with those in Table 1 again show a great deal of individual variability.

In the primidone plus phenytoin group there were 25% of the individuals (32) whose derived phenobarbital level was below 15 μg/ml—these individuals had a lower average primidone level (5.1 ± 0.63; range 1.2 to 19.0) than the primidone only group; a somewhat higher derived phenobarbital level (9.7 ± 0.81; range 1.7 to 15.0) and their conversion ratio was 2.43 ± 0.28 (range 0.23 to 6.86), approximately 3.5 times that of the primidone-only group. The ranges in these data are also quite broad, making it difficult to predict primidone dose from only the derived phenobarbital level.

From this information and several individual instances of alteration in the conversion ratio of individuals taking primidone, we believe that the determination of serum levels of primidone in addition to the derived phenobarbital is a clinically useful procedure. The variability that is exemplified in the data clearly indicates the necessity of determining this level in the adjustment of dosage. Because of the variability in half-life of this drug, it is also clearly evident that the time the sample is obtained in relation to dose is clearly an important measurement, and if dose adjustments are being made the best procedure is to determine the levels at the same time of day as well as at a constant dose-sample time.

The establishment of a definitive therapeutic range for this drug still presents a problem (22), but we believe that the upper limit can probably be extended to 12 μg/ml for primidone. Of course, this is dependent on the amount of derived phenobarbital. We are currently working on correlations between clinical control and primidone and phenobarbital levels. Obviously our data would be greatly enhanced by the determination of PEMA levels as well, but we do not believe at this time that the routine determination of PEMA levels is necessary.

SUMMARY

Primidone has been used as an antiepileptic drug for the treatment of generalized and partial seizures with elementary and complex symptomatology. In man it is metabolized to two metabolites, phenylethylmalonamide and phenobarbital, both of which have antiepileptic activity. The degree to which primidone is converted to phenobarbital varies among individuals, thus making the serum level of both drugs necessary for proper adjustment of dosage. Other drugs, in particular phenytoin, and metabolic changes can alter the rate and extent of the conversion of primidone to phenobarbital, and these factors also render necessary the determination of serum primidone levels.

The drug has a variable but short half-life (3 to 10 hr), and peak serum levels are usually attained approximately 3 hr after dose. These two factors indicate that it is necessary to administer multiple daily doses and to obtain blood samples for quantitation within a specified time after dose. Because of the variability in half-life and absorption, it is probably best to obtain the samples at the same time of day when dose adjustments are made. In the patient with intractable epilepsy, a distinct benefit may be gained in determination of an individual half-life.

The therapeutic range with this drug has not been established with certainty, and some controversy still exists as to whether or not primidone itself has antiepileptic activity. Clinically we feel that it has been of benefit in many patients, and we have several examples of good clinical control of seizures when adequate primidone levels are present in conjunction with little or no derived phenobarbital. We feel that the upper limit of the therapeutic range of primidone should be approximately 12 μg/ml. We have not encountered indications of clinical toxicity in patients until serum primidone levels have exceeded this value by 2 to 3 μg/ml as long as their derived phenobarbital levels had not exceeded 35 to 40 μg/ml.

A great deal of investigation is still indicated into the metabolism, mechanism of action, and clinical usefulness of this compound before we can properly define its role in the armamentarium of antiepileptic drugs.

REFERENCES

1. Bailey, D. N., and Jatlow, P. I. (1972): Chemical analysis of massive crystalluria following primidone overdose. *Am. J. Clin. Pathol.,* 58:583–589.
2. Baumel, I. P., Gallagher, B. B., DiMicco, J., and Goico, H. (1973): Metabolism and anticonvulsant properties of primidone in the rat. *J. Pharmacol. Exp. Ther.,* 186:305–314.
3. Baumel, I. P., Gallagher, B. B., and Mattson, R. H. (1972): Phenylethylmalomide (PEMA). An important metabolite of primidone. *Arch. Neurol.,* 27:34–41.
4. Bogue, J. Y., and Carrington, H. C. (1953): The evaluation of "Mysoline" a new anticonvulsant drug. *Br. J. Pharmacol.,* 8:230–236.
5. Booker, H. E. (1972):Primidone: Relation of plasma levels to clinical control. In: *Antiepileptic Drugs,* edited by D. M. Woodbury, J. K. Penry, and R. P. Schmidt, pp. 373–376. Raven Press, New York.
6. Booker, H. E., Hosokowa, K., Burdette, R. D., and Darcey, B. (1970): A clinical study of serum primidone levels. *Epilepsia,* 11:395–402.
7. Brillman, J., Gallagher, B. B., and Mattson, R. H. (1974): Acute primidone intoxication. *Arch. Neurol.,* 30:255–258.
8. Butler, T. C., and Waddell, W. J. (1956): Metabolic conversion of primidone (Mysoline) to phenobarbital. *Proc. Soc. Exp. Biol. Med.,* 93:544–546.
9. Cate, J. C., and Tenser, R. (1975): Acute primidone overdosage with massive crystalluria. *Clin. Toxicol.,* 8:385–389.
10. Cereghino, J. J., Van Meter, J. C., Brock, J. T., Penry, J. K., Smith, L. D., and White, B. G. (1973): Preliminary observations of serum carbamazepine concentration in epileptic patients. *Neurology,* 23:357–366.

11. Fincham, R. W., Schottelius, D. D., and Sahs, A. L. (1974): The influence of diphenylhydantoin on primidone metabolism. *Arch. Neurol.,* 30:259–262.
12. Frey, H. H., and Hahn, I. (1960): Untersuchungen über die Bedeutung des durch Biotransformation gebildeten Phenobarbital für die antikonvulsive Wirkung von Primidon. *Arch. Int. Pharmacodyn. Ther.,* 128:281–290.
13. Fujimoto, J. M., Mason, W. H., and Murphy, M. (1968): Urinary excretion of primidone and its metabolites in rabbits. *J. Pharmacol. Exp. Ther.,* 159:379–388.
14. Gallagher, B. B., and Baumel, I. P. (1972): Primidone biotransformation. In: *Antiepileptic Drugs,* edited by D. M. Woodbury, J. K. Penry, and R. P. Schmidt, pp. 361–366. Raven Press, New York.
15. Gallagher, B. B., and Baumel, I. P. (1972): Primidone—interaction with other drugs. In: *Antiepileptic Drugs,* edited by D. M. Woodbury, J. K. Penry, and R. P. Schmidt, pp. 367–371. Raven Press, New York.
16. Gallagher, B. B., Baumel, I. P., and Mattson, R. H. (1972): Metabolic disposition of primidone and its metabolites in epileptic subjects after single and repeated administration. *Neurology* (Minneap.), 22:1186–1192.
17. Gallagher, B. B., Smith, D. B., and Mattson, R. H. (1970): The relationship of the anticonvulsant properties of primidone to phenobarbital. *Epilepsia,* 11:239–301.
18. Gastaut, H., Broughton, R., Roger, J., and Tassinari, C. A. (1974): Generalized convulsive seizures without local onset. In: *The Epilepsies, Handbook of Clinical Neurology,* Vol. 15, edited by O. Magnus and A. M. Lorentz de Haas. American Elsevier Publishing Co., New York.
19. Goodman, L. S., Swinyard, E. A., Brown, W. C., Schiffman, D. O., Grewal, M. S., and Bliss, E. L. (1953): Anticonvulsant properties of 5-phenyl-5-ethylhexahydropyrimidine-4-6-dione (Mysoline), A new antiepileptic. *J. Pharmacol. Exp. Ther.,* 108:428–436.
20. Handley, R., and Steward, A. S. R. (1952): Mysoline®: A new drug in the treatment of epilepsy. *Lancet,* 262:742–744.
21. Houghton, G. W., Richens, A., Toseland, P. A., Davidson, S., and Falconer, M. A. (1975): Brain concentrations of phenytoin, phenobarbitone and primidone in epileptic patients. *Eur. J. Clin. Pharmacol.,* 9:73–78.
22. Kutt, H. (1974): Pharmacodynamic and pharmacokinetic measurements of antiepileptic drugs. *Clin. Pharmacol. Ther.,* 16:243–250.
23. McAuliffe, J. J., Sherwin, A. L., Leppick, I, E., Fayle, S. A., and Pippenger, C. E. (1977): Salivary levels of anticonvulsants: A practical approach to drug monitoring. *Neurology* (Minneap.), 27:409–413.
24. Martinez, G., and Snyder, R. D. (1973): Transplacental passage of primidone. *Neurology* (Minneap.), 23:381–383.
25. Olesen, O. V., and Dam, M. (1967): The metabolic conversion of primidone to phenobarbitone in patients under long term treatment. *Arch. Neurol. Scand.,* 43:348–356.
26. Penry, J. K., and Daly, D. D., Editors (1975): *Complex Partial Seizures and Their Treatment,* Advances in Neurology, Vol. 11. Raven Press, New York.
27. Reynolds, E. H., Fenton, G., Penwick, P., Johnson, A. L., and Laundy, M. (1975): Interaction of phenytoin and primidone. *Br. Med. J.,* 2:594–595.
28. Rodin, E. A., Choon, S. R., Kitano, H., Lewis, R., and Rennick, P. M. (1976): A comparison of the effectiveness of primidone versus carbamazepine in epileptic outpatients. *J. Nerv. Ment. Dis.,* 163:41–45.
29. Schneider, H. Janz, D., Gardner-Thorpe, C., Meinardi, H., and Sherwin, A. L., Editors (1975): *Clinical Pharmacology of Antiepileptic Drugs.* Springer-Verlag, Berlin.
30. Schottelius, D. D., and Fincham, R. W. (1977): Cerebrospinal fluid/serum ratios of primidone—inferences to protein binding. *Epilepsia,* 18:291 (abst.).
31. Sutton, G., and Kupferberg, H. J. (1975): Isoniazid as an inhibitor of primidone metabolism. *Neurology* (Minneap.), 25:1179–1181.
32. White, P. T., Plott, D., and Norton, J. (1966): Relative anticonvulsant potency of primidone. *Arch. Neurol.,* 14:31–35.

Antiepileptic Drugs: Quantitative Analysis and Interpretation, edited by C. E. Pippenger, J. K. Penry, and H. Kutt, Raven Press, New York, © 1978.

Chapter 25
Clinical Pharmacology of Ethosuximide

Allan L. Sherwin

Epilepsy is as old as the race, older perhaps. As long as there is brain action, epilepsy will appear from time to time, presenting problems forever difficult and yet revealing.

Wilder Penfield
(1891–1976)

ABSENCE SEIZURES

Absence (petit mal) seizures are characterized by brief episodes of transient loss of awareness without gross convulsive movements. There may be blinking of the eyes or other minor movements, simple automatisms, or other postural changes. The attacks usually last a few seconds, seldom more than 15 sec, and occur without warning or after effect. The seizures almost always begin in childhood, usually occur many times a day, and can frequently be elicited by prolonged hyperventilation. There is a rather characteristic electroencephalographic abnormality in which bursts of high-voltage spikes followed by dome-shaped waves are recorded simultaneously over both cerebral hemispheres with a frequency of approximately 3 cps (21,30).

Clinically well-defined absence seizures can also be observed in patients with a variety of underlying disorders, thus a uniform etiology has not been established. They are classified as a subgroup of the generalized epilepsies, being bilaterally symmetrical without local onset (18). Other related seizure patterns included in this group are myoclonic seizures (symmetrical jerking of the limbs), drop attacks (a sudden decrease in postural tone), and a number of other types (19). Episodes of prolonged confusion, even stupor, can result from continuous epileptic activity of the spike-wave variety (absence status). Tonic-clonic convulsive seizures (grand mal) are also classified as generalized epilepsies. Indeed, many patients with absence seizures also exhibit tonic-clonic seizures at some time or other during the course of the illness. Occasionally, a series of absence attacks may be observed to precede a tonic-clonic seizure.

Ethosuximide is specifically indicated for the control of absence seizures; should the patient also have tonic-clonic seizures, simultaneous therapy with other agents is required. For appropriate drug selection, it is particularly essential to distinguish the absence seizures of generalized epilepsy from complex partial (psychomotor) seizures. The clouding of consciousness observed during the latter attacks—also referred to as "absences"—results from localized discharge in the temporal lobe(s) (38). Complex partial seizures are treated with drugs such as carbamazepine or phenytoin rather than with ethosuximide.

Despite their brief duration, frequent absence attacks require treatment because of their disruptive effect on the patient's normal activities. Often they lead to embarrassment at school or interfere with work, and the possibility of accidental injury is always present. Moreover, psychological functions are impaired during brief bursts of spike-wave discharge (2,44).

BASIC PHARMACOLOGY

Structure-Activity Relationships

Phenytoin was shown by Merritt and Putnam in 1938 (39,40) to prevent electrically induced convulsions in animals. In the dramatic clinical studies that followed, approximately two-thirds of the patients treated with this new agent were helped. However, phenytoin failed to control absence seizures, in fact, in some patients the attacks increased in frequency and severity. Effective therapy for this group of patients only became available 7 years later when Lennox (34), testing a potential new anticonvulsant trimethadione, found that the compound did not prevent tonic-clonic or partial seizures, but was strikingly beneficial in controlling absence attacks. These and other advances in therapy were made possible by painstaking research in which a knowledge of the chemical structure of potential agents was coupled with pharmacological screening by means of two main test systems: protection against electrically induced seizures (54), and convulsions provoked by pentylenetetrazol (Metrazol) (52). The success of Everett and Richards (16) in identifying trimethadione showed that protection against pentylenetetrazol seizures was a practical means of testing drugs likely to be effective in preventing absence attacks. However, from the point of view of mechanisms of action, it is of interest that initiation of treatment with trimethadione occasionally precipitated grand mal seizures.

Ethosuximide evolved from a structure-activity research program initiated by Miller and Long (41) designed to develop a drug effective against absence (petit mal) seizures, but with a low incidence of harmful side effects. The careful screening program carried out by Chen et al. (10,11) is a superb demonstration of the differential effects on various types of seizures by a variety of substitutions on a heterocyclic molecule. Succinimide itself has no anticonvulsant properties, but the presence of an alkyl grouping at the C-2 position resulted in a drug (i.e., ethosuximide) that was remarkably effective in controlling absence seizures (Fig. 1). The presence of a single phenyl ring in this position resulted in a drug (i.e., methsuximide) that was

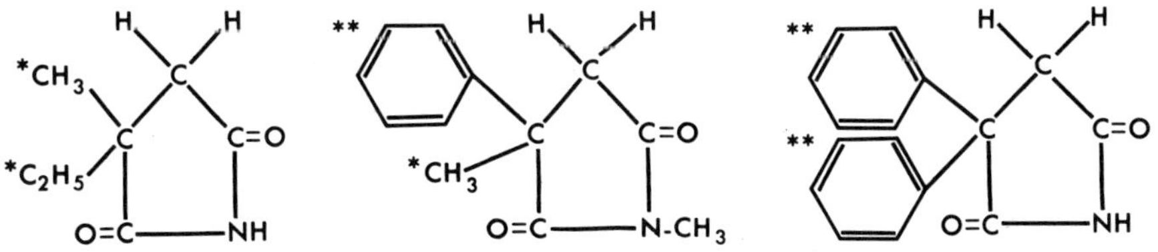

	2-ethyl, 2-methyl (Ethosuximide)	2-methyl, 2-phenyl, N-methyl (Methsuximide)	2, 2 diphenyl (Resembles phenytoin)
PTZ	++	+	0
MES	0	+	++

* Alkyl grouping is anti-clonic, anti-petit mal
** Phenyl groups protect against tonic seizures

FIG. 1. Effects of various substitutions at the carbon-2 position of succinimide on the anticonvulsant activity in the pentylenetetrazol (PTZ) and maximal electroshock seizure (MES) tests in rodents. Ethosuximide proved to be the most effective derivative for the treatment of patients with absence seizures. Taken from data of Chen et al. (10).

less effective than phenytoin, but because of the presence of the phenyl group, did not appear to have the same tendency to provoke or exacerbate grand mal seizures (53). The 2,2′-diphenyl derivative resembles phenytoin and may be a useful anticonvulsant for tonic-clonic or partial seizures. Support for this view comes from a study of a similar diphenyl derivitive of trimethadione, Epidon®, which, in a limited clinical trial, was shown to be effective against grand mal, but not against petit mal (14).

The structure of ethosuximide, especially the striking influence of the C-2 alkyl groupings in producing anticlonic and anti-petit mal effects, may provide some insight into the mechanisms of action of this drug and its putative receptor sites. Such investigations are particularly opportune in view of the identification of specific stereospecific opiate receptor binding sites in brain (43). Seeman et al. (47) have demonstrated brain receptors for antipsychotic drugs and utilize direct binding assays to screen potentially useful neuroleptic drugs.

Mechanisms of Action

A clinical model of absence seizures can be produced in cats by intramuscular administration of large doses of penicillin (22). For a period of approximately 6 hr the animals exhibit brief episodes of staring, unresponsiveness, blinking of the eyes, and slight myoclonus of the face; electroencephalograms show generalized epileptiform discharges, often assuming a spike-wave form, which at times are virtually indistinguishable from those recorded from patients with absence seizures. We recently showed that the frequency of epileptic bursts was significantly reduced when the animals were pretreated with ethosuximide so as to achieve plasma levels similar to those effective in patients (26). There was a significant linear correlation ($p < 0.001$) between the plasma drug level and antiepileptic effect. Ethosuximide has also been shown to be effective in abolishing estrogen-induced electrographic spike-wave discharges (31).

Lockard and Levy (36) studied the effects of ethosuximide on chronic focal motor and secondarily generalized tonic-clonic seizures induced in monkeys. The drug had a variable influence on the experimental seizure disorder, increasing paroxysms in certain animals but favorably affecting the seizures in others, which was also found in earlier studies of cobalt foci (12). Interestingly, these experimental observations are compatible with clinical reports that ethosuximide was useful as an adjunctive agent in patients with various other refractory seizure disorders (46).

The basic mechanisms underlying the action of ethosuximide in controlling absence seizures are best illustrated by the use of more discrete physiological test systems. Although they appear far removed from clinical epilepsy, these models enable us to scrutinize the action of the drug at the synaptic level. Capek and Esplin (7) recently showed that ethosuximide deepened the decline of the amplitude of the monosynaptic response evoked by trains of low-frequency stimuli to a motor nerve without affecting the transmission of single impulses. Indeed, they were able to demonstrate significant effects on release of synaptic transmitters. Ethosuximide increased the fractional release of apparent transmitter stores in the presynaptic terminals without a consistent effect on the rate of replacement. This may account for the preferential depression of abnormal showers of impulses, whereas the transmission of impulses required for normal physiological processes remains unimpaired.

It appears that absence seizures involve epileptiform activity that is reinforced and spread by low-frequency repetitive discharges from the cerebral cortex to subcortical structures (22). The elegant studies of Fromm and Kohli (17) have demonstrated that ethosuximide has the ability to suppress the activities of certain inhibitory pathways, a phenomenon not shared by drugs effective against tonic-clonic convulsive seizures (42). Drugs effective against absence seizures, such as ethosuximide, act on low-frequency inhibitory pathways (15), in contrast to drugs such as phenytoin, which are particularly effective in preventing the spread of high-frequency discharges from epileptic neurons (42,55). Hence, studies of the mechanism of action of ethosuximide reveal that it is a drug with distinct properties separate from and often antagonistic to those of drugs effective in grand mal seizures—observations that are quite compatible with the hypothesis that absence attacks constitute a distinct clinical entity.

PHARMACOKINETICS

Absorption

Ethosuximide is rapidly absorbed from the gastrointestinal tract; clinically significant plasma concentrations are achieved within 1 hr following a single dose, whereas peak levels occur within 3 to 7 hr. The syrup is absorbed more rapidly than the capsules, but Buchanan et al. (4) carried out a comparative study in children that showed that both formulations have equivalent total absorption. Hence, patients can be switched from one form to the other, and dosage schedules remain unchanged, without concern over loss of seizure control. The drug appears to be completely absorbed (9), and in adults steady-state plasma levels and urinary throughput are proportional to dose, being comparable when the drug is given as a single or divided dose (25).

Distribution

In experimental studies in the rat, ethosuximide was distributed rather uniformly throughout the tissues apart from adipose tissue, in which levels were lower than elsewhere (9). The apparent volume of distribution was found to be 0.69 liter/kg in children under 10 years of age (4) and 0.62 liter/kg in adults (5). This suggests that the distribution of the drug conforms to that of total body water. The degree of protein binding is negligible, and we observed no significant differences among ethosuximide levels in plasma dialysates, cerebrospinal fluid, or saliva (Chapter 9; 37). Horning et al. (28) demonstrated placental transfer of unchanged ethosuximide and a number of metabolites in samples of urine collected from a newborn infant whose mother was maintained on ethosuximide. Similarly, Hill et al. (27) identified unchanged ethosuximide in a mother's breast milk by which route the drug had gained access to her nursing infant.

Biotransformation and Excretion

Ethosuximide is extensively metabolized during chronic administration, probably mainly in the liver (8). Free as well as conjugated metabolites are excreted in urine, and four monohydroxy metabolites have been identified in urine by gas chromatography-mass spectrometry-computer techniques (28). Hydroxylation of the ethyl and methyl side chain at the C-2 ring carbon appears to be the primary metabolic pathway. In addition, Chang et al. (8) have identified a ketone derivative, 2-acetyl-2-methylsuccinimide, in urine from patients receiving multiple doses of ethosuximide. The presence of the hydroxyl group in the metabolites permits conjugation with glucuronic acid so that most of the metabolites in human urine are present in conjugated form (8). The drug does not contain a carbon-carbon double bond, and it is not metabolized by epoxidation (28). The synthetic ethosuximide administered to patients in clinical practice has an asymmetric carbon atom and consists of an equal mixture of two isomers. Chang et al. (8) found the optical rotation of the excreted drug to be zero in rat urine, suggesting that the isomers were metabolized at the same rate. This is in contrast to studies of the metabolism of phensuximide by Dudley et al. (13), where different pathways appear to be involved. None of the metabolites of ethosuximide have been reported as having significant anticonvulsant properties (8).

In our studies, the elimination half-life of ethosuximide in plasma following cessation of chronic therapy ranged from 18 to 72 hr (mean, 38.8 hr, $n = 13$), with a significant trend correlating plasma half-life with body weight ($p < 0.05$) (48). Buchanan et al. (6) observed a mean plasma half-life of 29 hr in 9 patients (median age, 16.5 years; median weight, 35.0 kg), whereas in another study (25) a mean plasma half-life of 52 hr was found in 20 healthy male volunteers (mean age, 26.7 years; mean weight, 74.3 kg). Browne et al. (1) found that half-life did not vary significantly with age over 5 to 15 years or with increasing plasma concentration or dose. The prolonged half-life, together with our previous finding of minimal diurnal variation (50), suggests and, indeed, Buchanan et al. (6) demonstrated, that once daily dosage is feasible, transfering patients from multiple to single daily doses of ethosuximide does not reduce seizure control.

Dose-Plasma Level Relationships

In order to compare the effects of age and sex on plasma levels, 245 patients (115 males and 130 females) receiving stable doses of ethosuximide were monitored regularly by our laboratory. The patients were arbitrarily divided into three age groups: 2 to 10, 11 to 15, and 16 to 45 years. In each successive age group the average plasma levels achieved using a mean dose of 22.6 mg/kg were significantly higher. We had previously demonstrated this age-dependent effect on plasma phenytoin levels (49). No significant difference was demonstrated between the plasma levels of either sex in any age group.

Regression lines with 95% tolerance limits from a study of plasma ethosuximide levels are shown in Fig. 2. Plasma levels were obtained on single blood samples from patients known to be receiving constant dosages of ethosuximide either alone or in combination with other anticonvulsants. The slope of the linear regression line of ethosuximide dose to plasma level is significantly less ($p < 0.01$) in children from 3 to 10 years than in patients 11 years of age and older, in agreement with the data of Browne et al. (1). In previous studies (48), we have found the use of such regression lines to be helpful in evaluating adequacy of dosage and compliance with therapy.

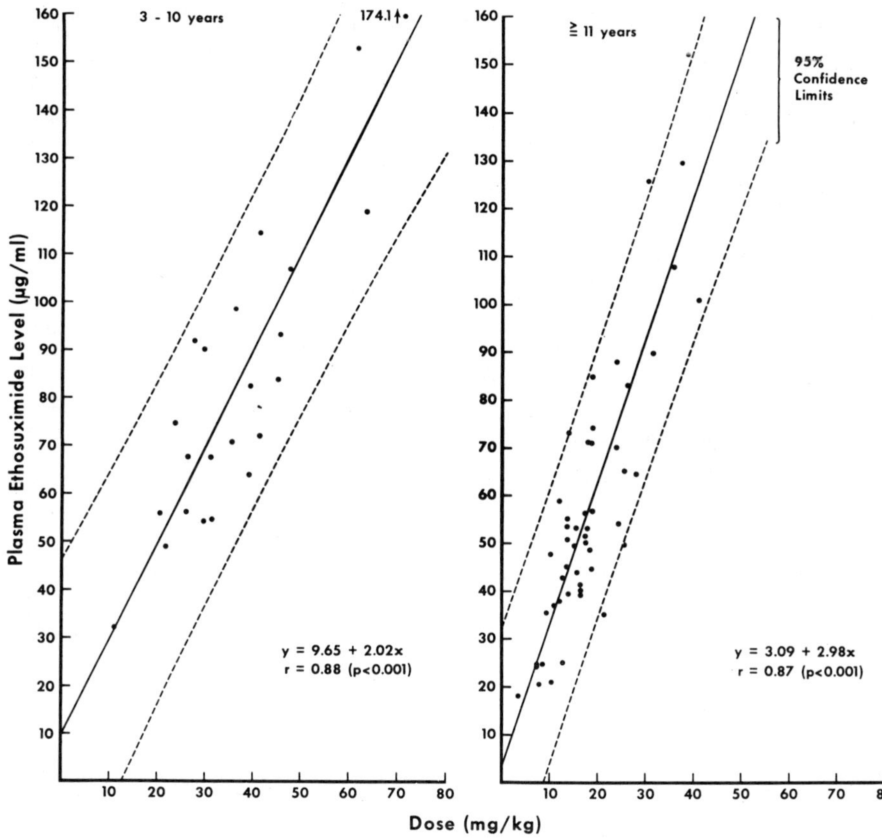

FIG. 2. Relationship of plasma ethosuximide level to dose in hospitalized patients at steady state. The slope of the regression line for patients ranging in age from 2 to 10 years ($n = 23$) is significantly less than that for patients 11 years of age and older ($n = 49$) ($p < 0.01$).

At the very least, it enables one to decide which patients require additional plasma-level monitoring.

ADVERSE REACTIONS

There is a significant correlation between dose and plasma ethosuximide level (1,51). The drug is well tolerated, however, and adverse reactions do not necessarily correlate with higher plasma levels. In this respect, ethosuximide differs from phenytoin, where a striking correlation can be demonstrated between plasma levels and toxic manifestations (32). Nausea is the most common side effect observed following initiation of ethosuximide therapy and appears to be dose related (1). Therapy can be continued, however, by allowing the patient to develop tolerance to the drug by gradual increments of dosage or by reducing dosage.

Headaches, frequently in the occipital region, may be noted at the onset of therapy but often disappear with time, as do fatigue, lethargy, dizziness, hiccoughs, and euphoria (3). Rarer symptoms, including behavioral abnormalities and even transient psychotic disturbances, may occur (45). Many of these patients were in the older age group and had had a prior history of psychiatric disturbance. Photophobia and basal ganglia dysfunction have also been reported (23).

Leukopenia has been reported in a number of patients shortly after the onset of ethosuximide administration (1). Most of the patients had also been receiving other anticonvulsants. However, in the cases reviewed, the white blood cell count recovered following the reduction or withdrawal of ethosuximide. Other idiosyncratic side effects include pancytopenia, and a few fatalities have been reported (3). Thus the physician must be advised to pertorm periodic blood cell counts in patients receiving ethosuximide and to be alert to signs and symptoms of bone marrow depression of any type. Fortunately, such tests can be done at the time of periodic plasma level monitoring. When the EMIT® technique is employed, a single fingerprick sample is sufficient for both types of analyses. As with many anticonvulsant drugs, cases of systemic lupus erythematosis have been reported following ethosuximide therapy. Nonspecific skin rashes and erythema multiforme bullosa (Stevens-Johnson syndrome) have also been described (3).

Several investigators (24,45) have found impaired performance in various test situations to be correlated with frequency of spike-wave discharges. To test the effectiveness of a drug such as ethosuximide it is thus essential to monitor plasma ethosuximide levels and the frequency and duration of spike-wave discharges in order to arrive at a more accurate assessment. The study of Browne et al. (1), which fulfills these criteria, showed no significant deterioration in psychometric performance during 8 weeks of ethosuximide treatment. On the contrary, the performance of many of the patients improved significantly, and only one of the 39 patients performed less well after taking the drug. An important point raised by the latter study was that patients with clinical evidence of structural central nervous system abnormalities also responded very well to treatment with ethosuximide.

In general, adverse reactions to ethosuximide are usually of a minor nature, dose related, and can be minimized by careful adjustments of the dosage in small increments over a period of time. The main long-term effect is a mild degree of anorexia which, however, does not usually contribute to a significant weight loss. Acute overdose would be expected to produce central nervous system depression (35). Since the drug undergoes extensive metabolism in the liver, it should not be administered to patients with severe hepatic dysfunction. As a number of anticonvulsant drugs have been suspected of having teratogenic potentialities, ethosuximide should be avoided from the onset of pregnancy. Owing to the prolonged plasma half-life, an adequate period should be allowed for complete elimination of the drug.

CLINICAL EFFECTIVENESS

Ethosuximide has been shown to be an effective agent for the control of absence seizures (56). Goldensohn et al. (23) were able to obtain complete control in 48% of patients. In a similar series studied by Dr. J. P. Robb, we were able to demonstrate that regular monitoring of plasma levels resulted in 61% of the patients attaining complete control of absence attacks. As shown in Fig. 3, there was a significant difference in the degree of seizure control after 2½ and 5 years of therapy. The striking feature of these pie diagrams is the reduction in the number of patients with frequent attacks in the first 2½ year period. During this time the mean plasma ethosuximide level in the newly controlled patients rose from 57.2 μg/ml to 76.1 μg/ml, a significant increase ($p < 0.05$), which was not observed in those patients who continued to have frequent attacks.

It is well known that patients with absence seizures tend to cease having attacks with advancing age (33), although some studies have reported a more guarded prognosis (20). The rate of spontaneous improvement observed by Janz (29) in his long-term study of petit mal epilepsy suggests that this could not in itself account for the increase in the number of controlled patients observed in our study. The improvement is the result of ethosuximide therapy adjusted according to the results of plasma-level determinations.

Although control of absence attacks is often attained at plasma levels above 40 μg/ml (Fig. 4), an average therapeutic range of 40 to 100 μg/ml is likely more appropriate. A degree of interindividual variability exists in the plasma concentration required to achieve maximal seizure control. In

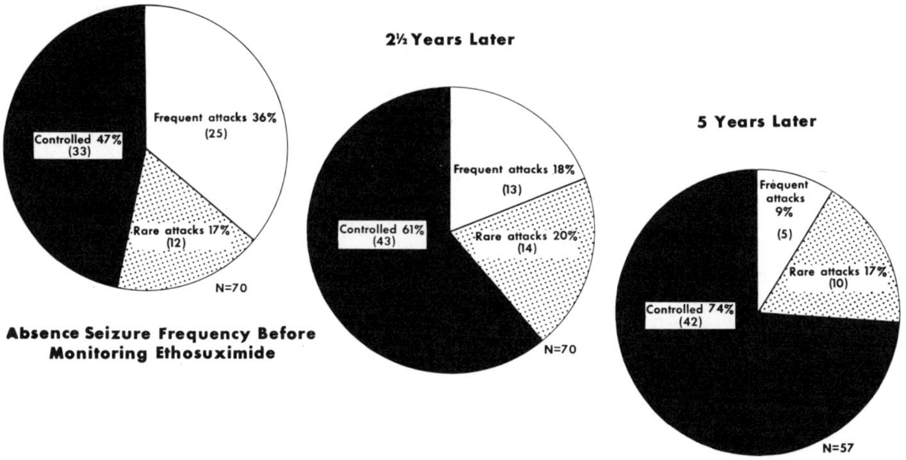

FIG. 3. Control of absence attacks before and after commencing regular plasma-level monitoring with titration of ethosuximide dosage. There is a highly significant alteration in the distribution of clinical control (χ^2 test, $p < 0.005$).

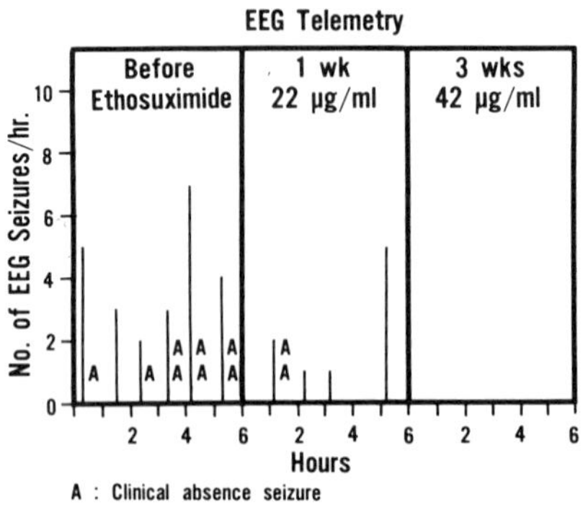

FIG. 4. Titration of ethosuximide dosage to achieve a minimal effective level (42 μg/ml) as determined by EEG telemetry and clinical observation. Seizure control was maintained in this patient over the subsequent 5-year period at plasma levels ranging from 40 to 100 μg/ml. (Courtesy Dr. J. Woods, Professor P. Gloor, and Mrs. J. Ives.)

order to obtain the "fine tuning" required in some patients with refractory seizures, ethosuximide levels as high as 150 μg/ml may prove useful. Regular monitoring enables the physician to maintain adequate drug levels during maturation, especially at puberty when changes in body weight, hormonal balance, and drug metabolism occur. This role of drug monitoring appears to be of equal importance in children to that of maintenance of the patient's compliance with ethosuximide therapy.

ACKNOWLEDGMENTS

This work would not have been possible without the encouragement and wholehearted support of Dr. J. Preston Robb, Professor of Neurology at McGill University. Professor M. Yalovsky kindly provided advice on the statistical analysis of the data, and Mrs. J. Loynd, Miss C. Cotter, and Mrs. S. Charlton provided technical assistance. This work was supported by the Medical Research Council of Canada and the Savoy Foundation.

REFERENCES

1. Browne, T. R., Dreifuss, F. E., Dyken, P. R., Goode, D. J., Penry, J. K., Porter, R. J., White, B. G., and White, P. T. (1975): Ethosuximide in the treatment of absence (petit mal) seizures. *Neurology* (Minneap.), 25:515–524.
2. Browne, T. R., Penry, J. K., Porter, R. J., and Dreifuss, F. E. (1974): Responsiveness before, during and after spike-wave paroxysms. *Neurology* (Minneap.), 24:659–665.
3. Buchanan, R. A. (1972): Ethosuximide: Toxicity. In: *Antiepileptic Drugs,* edited by D. M. Woodbury, J. K. Penry, and R. P. Schmidt, pp. 449–454. Raven Press, New York.
4. Buchanan, R. A., Fernandez, L., and Kinkel, A. W. (1969): Absorption and elimination of ethosuximide in children. *J. Clin. Pharmacol.,* 9:393–398.
5. Buchanan, R. A., Kinkel, A. W., and Smith, T. C. (1973): The absorption and excretion of ethosuximide. *Int. J. Clin. Pharmacol., Ther. Toxicol.,* 7:213–218.
6. Buchanan, R. A., Kinkel, A. W., Turner, J. L., and Heffelinger, J. C. (1976): Ethosuximide dosage regimens. *Clin. Pharmacol. Ther.,* 19:143–147.
7. Capek, R., and Esplin, B. (1977): Effects of ethosuximide on transmission of repeti-

tive impulses and apparent rates of transmitter turnover in the spinal monosynaptic pathway. *J. Pharmacol. Exp. Ther.,* 201:320–325.
8. Chang, T., Burkett, A. R., and Glazko, A. J. (1972): Ethosuximide: Biotransformation. In: *Antiepileptic Drugs,* edited by D. M. Woodbury, J. K. Penry, and R. P. Schmidt, pp. 425–429. Raven Press, New York.
9. Chang, T., Dill, W. A., and Glazko, A. J. (1972): Ethosuximide: Absorption, distribution, and excretion. In: *Antiepileptic Drugs,* edited by D. M. Woodbury, J. K. Penry, and R. P. Schmidt. Raven Press, New York, pp. 417–423.
10. Chen, G., Portman, R., Ensor, C. R., and Bratton, A. C. (1951): The anticonvulsant activity of α-phenylsuccinimides. *J. Pharmacol. Exp. Ther.,* 103:54–61.
11. Chen, G., Weston, J. K., and Bratton, A. C. (1963): Anticonvulsant activity and toxicity of phensuximide, methsuximide and ethosuximide. *Epilepsia,* 4:66–76.
12. Dow, R. C., McQueen, J. K., and Townsend, H. R. A. (1972): The production and detection of epileptogenic lesions in rat cerebral cortex. *Epilepsia,* 13:459–465.
13. Dudley, K. H., Bius, D. L., and Grace, M. E. (1972): Metabolic fates of N-methyl-α-phenylsuccinimide (phensuximide, milontin) and of α-phenylsuccinimide in the dog. *J. Pharmacol. Exp. Ther.,* 180:167–179.
14. Ellerman, M. (1947): Experimental and clinical studies on the anticonvulsant properties of Epidon (5,5-diphenyl-2-4-dioxazolidine). *J. Nerv. Ment. Dis.,* 106:369–383.
15. Englander, R. N., Johnson, R. N., Brickley, J. J., and Hanna, G. R. (1977): Effects of antiepileptic drugs on thalamocortical excitability. *Neurology* (Minneap.) (*in press*).
16. Everett, G. M., and Richards, R. (1944): Comparative anticonvulsive action of 3,5,5-trimethaloxalidine 2–4 dione (Tridione®), Dilantin® and phenobarbital. *J. Pharmacol. Exp. Ther.,* 81:402–407.
17. Fromm, G. H., and Kohli, C. M. (1972): The role of inhibitory pathways in petit mal epilepsy. *Neurology* (Minneap.), 22:1012–1020.
18. Gastaut, H. (1973): *Dictionary of Epilepsy. Part I: Definitions.* World Health Organization, Geneva.
19. Gastaut, H., and Broughton, R. (1973): Epileptic seizures: Their clinical nature, pathophysiology and differential diagnosis. In: *International Encyclopedia of Pharmacology and Therapeutics, Section 19. Vol. 1: Anticonvulsant Drugs,* edited by J. Mercier, pp. 3–44. Pergamon Press, Oxford.
20. Gibberd, F. B. (1966): The prognosis of petit mal. *Brain,* 89:531–538.
21. Gibbs, F. A., Davis, H. A., and Lennox, W. G. (1935): The electroencephalogram in epilepsy and in conditions of impaired consciousness. *Arch. Neurol. Psychiatr.,* 34:1133–1148.
22. Gloor, P., and Testa, G. (1974): Generalized penicillin epilepsy in the cat: Effects of intracarotid and intravertebral pentelenetetrazol and amobarbital injections. *Electroencephalogr. Clin. Neurophysiol.,* 36:499–515.
23. Goldensohn, E. S., Hardie, J., and Borea, E. D. (1962): Ethosuximide in the treatment of epilepsy. *JAMA,* 180:840–842.
24. Goode, D. J., Penry, J. K., and Dreifuss, F. E. (1970): Effects of paroxysmal spike-wave on continuous visual-motor performance. *Epilepsia,* 11:241–254.
25. Goulet, J. R., Kinkel, A. W., and Smith, T. C. (1976): Metabolism of ethosuximide. *Clin. Pharmacol. Ther.,* 20:213–218.
26. Guberman, A.. Gloor, P., and Sherwin, A. L. (1975): Response of generalized penicillin epilepsy in the cat to ethosuximide and diphenylhydantoin. *Neurology* (Minneap.), 25:758–764.
27. Hill, R., Horning, M., and Horning, E. (1973): Identification of transplacentally acquired anticonvulsant agents in the neonate. In: *Methods of Analysis of Anti-Epileptic Drugs,* edited by J. W. A. Meijer, H. Meinardi, C. Gardner-Thorpe, and E. van der Kleijn, pp. 146–147. American Elsevier, New York.
28. Horning, M. G., Stratton, C., Nowlin, J., Harvey, D. J., and Hill, R. M. (1973): Metabolism of 2-ethyl-2-methyl succinimide in the rat and human. *Drug Metab. Dispos.,* 1:569–576.
29. Janz, D. (1969): *Die Epilepsien-Spezielle Pathologie und Therapie,* p. 94. Stuttgart, Georg Thieme.

30. Jasper, H. (1954): Centrencephalic seizures—primary bilateral synchrony. In: *Epilepsy and the Functional Anatomy of the Human Brain,* by W. Penfield and H. Jasper, pp. 623–645. Little, Brown and Company, Boston.
31. Julien, R. M., Fowler, G. W., and Danielson, M. G. (1975): The effects of anti-epileptic drugs on estrogen-induced electrographic spike-wave discharge. *J. Pharmacol. Exp. Ther.,* 193:645–656.
32. Kutt, H., and McDowell, F. (1968): Management of epilepsy with diphenylhydantoin sodium. *JAMA,* 203:969–972.
33. Lees, F., and Liversedge, L. A. (1962): The prognosis of "petit mal" and minor epilepsy. *Lancet,* 2:797–799.
34. Lennox, W. G. (1945): The petit mal epilepsies: Their treatment with tridione. *JAMA,* 129:1069–1074.
35. Livingston, S. (1972): *Comprehensive Management of Epilepsy in Infancy, Childhood and Adolescence,* p. 240. Charles C Thomas, Springfield, Ill.
36. Lockard, J. S., and Levy, R. H. (1977): Efficacy testing of valproic acid compared to ethosuximide in monkey model: II. Seizure, EEG, and diurnal variations. *Epilepsia,* 18:205–224.
37. McAuliffe, J. J., Sherwin, A. L., Leppik, I. E., Fayle, S. A., and Pippenger, C. E. (1977): Salivary levels of anticonvulsants: A practical approach to drug monitoring. *Neurology* (Minneap.), 27:409–413.
38. McNaughton, F. L. (1954): Observations on diagnosis and medical treatment. In: *Epilepsy and the Functional Anatomy of the Human Brain,* by W. Penfield and H. Jasper, pp. 540–568. Little, Brown and Company, Boston.
39. Merritt, H. H., and Putnam, T. J. (1938): A new series of anticonvulsant drugs tested by experiments on animals. *Arch. Neurol. Psychiatr.,* 39:1003–1015.
40. Merritt, H. H., and Putnam, T. J. (1938): Sodium diphenyl hydantoinate in the treatment of convulsive disorders. *JAMA,* 111:1068.
41. Miller, C. A., and Long, L. M. (1953): Anticonvulsants. IV. An investigation of α-(substituted phenyl)-succinimides. *J. Am. Chem. Soc.,* 75:6256–6258.
42. Morrell, F., Bradley, W., and Ptashne, M. (1959): Effect of drugs on discharge characteristics of chronic epileptogenic lesions. *Neurology* (Minneap.), 7:492–498.
43. Pert, C. B., and Snyder, S. H. (1975): Opiate receptor: Demonstration in nervous tissue. *Science,* 179:1011–1014.
44. Porter, R. J., Penry, J. K., and Dreifuss, F. E. (1973): Responsiveness at the onset of spike-wave bursts. *Electroencephalogr. Clin. Neurophysiol.,* 34:239–245.
45. Roger, J., Grangeon, H., Guey, J., and Lob, H. (1968): Psychiatric and physiological effects of ethosuximide treatment in epileptics. *Encephale,* 57:407–438.
46. Scholl, M. L., and Schwab, R. S. (1971): The triggering of grand mal and psychomotor spells by spike-wave discharges. *Electroencephalogr. Clin. Neurophysiol.,* 31:419 (Abst.).
47. Seeman, P., Chau-Wong, M., Tedesco, J., and Wong, K. (1975): Brain receptors for antipsychotic drugs and dopamine: Direct binding assays. *Proc. Natl. Acad. Sci. USA,* 72:4376–4380.
48. Sherwin, A. (1973): Does monitoring of anti-epileptic drugs lead to improved seizure control? Ethosuximide levels in absence of attacks. In: *Methods of Analysis of Anti-Epileptic Drugs,* edited by J. W. A. Meijer, H. Meinardi, C. Gardner-Thorpe, and E. van der Kleijn, pp. 1–5. American Elsevier, New York.
49. Sherwin, A. L., Loynd, J. S., Bock, G. W., and Sokolowski, C. D. (1974): Effect of age, sex, obesity, and pregnancy on plasma diphenylhydantoin levels. *Epilepsia,* 15:507–521.
50. Sherwin, A. L., and Robb, J. P. (1972): Ethosuximide: Relation of plasma levels to clinical control. In: *Antiepileptic Drugs,* edited by D. M. Woodbury, J. K. Penry, and R. P. Schmidt, pp. 443–448. Raven Press, New York.
51. Sherwin, A. L., Robb, J. P., and Lechter, M. (1973): Improved control of epilepsy by monitoring plasma ethosuximide. *Arch. Neurol.* (Chicago), 28:178–181.
52. Stone, W. E. (1972): Systemic chemical convulsants and metabolic derangements. In: *Experimental Models of Epilepsy,* edited by D. P. Purpura, J. K.

Penry, D. Tower, D. M. Woodbury, and R. Walters, pp. 407–432. Raven Press, New York.
53. Sutherland, J. M., Tait, H., and Eadie, M. J. (1974): *The Epilepsies: Modern Diagnosis and Treatment,* p. 109. Churchill Livingstone, Edinburgh.
54. Swinyard, E. A. (1972): Electrically induced convulsions. In: *Experimental Models of Epilepsy,* edited by D. P. Purpura, J. K. Penry, D. Tower, D. M. Woodbury, and R. Walter, pp. 432–458. Raven Press, New York.
55. Ward, A. A. (1969): The epileptic neuron: Chronic foci in animals and man. In: *Basic Mechanisms of the Epilepsies,* edited by H. H. Jasper, A. A. Ward, and A. Pope, pp. 263–288. Little, Brown and Company, Boston.
56. Zimmerman, F. T., and Burgemeister, B. B. (1958): A new drug for petit mal epilepsy. *Neurology* (Minneap.), 8:769–775.

Antiepileptic Drugs: Quantitative Analysis and Interpretation, edited by C. E. Pippenger, J. K. Penry, and H. Kutt, Raven Press, New York, © 1978.

Chapter 26
Clinical Pharmacology of Carbamazepine

Henn Kutt

Carbamazepine is chemically related to the tricyclic antidepressants. It was developed in the Geigy Laboratories in Basel in the late 1950s to early 1960s from a tricyclic nucleus iminodibenzyl. The anticonvulsant properties of carbamazepine were demonstrated by Theobald and Kunz (24), who reported protection in rats against electroshock seizures with low doses, whereas considerably higher doses were needed for protection against pentylenetetrazole. The mechanism of action of carbamazepine is not yet clearly understood. It reduces posttetanic potentiation (like phenytoin) (14), increases the threshold for electrically induced cortical afterdischarges, and reduces synaptic transmission in the trigeminal system as well as the penicillin-induced afterdischarges (13).

Numerous clinical trials have demonstrated effectiveness of carbamazepine in patients with partial seizures with complex symptomatology (psychomotor seizures) and generalized tonic-clonic seizures (grand mal), while being relatively ineffective against absence seizures (petit mal). For literature reviews, see Parsonage (20) and Cereghino et al. (4). Carbamazepine is also effective in alleviating the symptoms of trigeminal neuralgia (tic doloreaux) (2). A psychotropic effect, mentioned in some clinical reports, is generally rarely seen in patients taking carbamazepine.

The clinically used doses have ranged from 200 to 2,400 mg daily, the most common being 600 to 1,200 mg. This is usually divided into two or three daily doses.

Carbamazepine, 5-carbamyl-5H dibenzo[b,f]azepine, carbamyliminostilbene, Tegretol® (Ciba), is a white crystalline substance marketed in the United States as scored round 200-mg tablets. Its structure is shown in Fig. 1A. It is very poorly soluble in water but dissolves in organic solvents. Aqueous solutions can be prepared with the aid of propylene gycol or ethanol. Methods for determination of carbamazepine concentration have been recently reviewed (15).

ABSORPTION

Absorption of carbamazepine from the intestinal tract is generally slow. Peak plasma level following an oral dose is usually seen in 6 hr or later (range 2 to 12 hr) (19). The absorption may not be complete, as up to

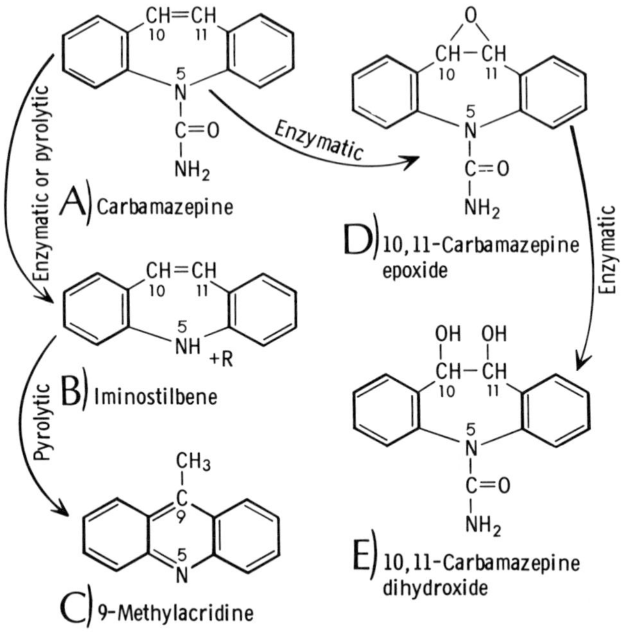

FIG. 1. Carbamazepine and its major metabolic and pyrolytic products. From Kutt (15).

15% of the ingested dose may be found in the form of unchanged parent drug in the feces (9). Some improvement of the absorption may be seen when the drug is ingested with a meal, presumably from the increased secretion of digestive fluids (17).

DISTRIBUTION

Following absorption, carbamazepine is distributed to all tissues. In animal experiments highest concentrations were found in the liver and kidneys, followed by plasma, heart, and lungs, whereas the brain concentration equalled that of the plasma. In man the brain concentration has been found also to equal or be even higher than that of plasma (19).

Carbamazepine passes the placenta. Cord blood from babies born to mothers who had been receiving the drug contained carbamazepine in concentrations approximately equal to those of the mothers (21).

BIOTRANSFORMATION

Carbamazepine is metabolized extensively (see Fig. 1), presumably by the hepatic mixed function oxidase system. The most important metabolite of carbamazepine is its 10,11-epoxide (Fig. 1D), which is quite stable, pharmacologically active, and found in the plasma and tissues in fair amounts (on the average one-third of that of the parent compound). The potency of 10,11-epoxide in protection against electroshock and pentylenetetrazole convulsions in mice was nearly equal to that of the parent compound (10). Eventually, the 10,11-epoxide is metabolized further, mostly to 10,11-dihydroxide (Fig. 1E) and eliminated in the urine in part free (two-thirds), in part conjugated (one-third) to glucuronic acid (1). A minor metabolite of carbamazepine found in the urine is iminostilbene (Fig. 1B), formed by cleaving off the carbamyl group (10). This cleavage also takes place pyrolytically at high temperatures in the gas chromatograph and is the main reason for difficulties with gas chromatographic determinations of carbamazepine concentrations. The endproduct of pyrolytic breakdown of carbamazepine is 9-methyl-acridine (Fig. 1C).

Carbamazepine appears to induce its own metabolism during chronic administration. This was observed in laboratory animals, evidenced by a shortening of the apparent plasma half-life (19), as well as in man, evidenced by some decline of plasma levels while receiving chronically the same dosage (8). Other antiepileptic drugs such as phenytoin, phenobarbital, and primidone also seem to induce carbamazepine metabolism (5,22).

ELIMINATION

Data about elimination of carbamazepine are still incomplete. In the urine, up to 1% of the dose appears as the parent compound, 1 to 2% as 10,11-epoxide, approximately 20% as the 10,11-dihydroxy compound, and traces (less than 1%) as iminostilbene. Another 10 to 20% of the dose may be found in the feces, part as the parent drug, part as the metabolites. Apparently, enterohepatic cycling takes place (19).

PLASMA PROTEIN BINDING

Several authors have reported that approximately 70 to 80%, average 75%, of carbamazepine in the plasma is protein bound, mostly to the albumin (12). CSF and saliva concentrations, which may be considered as ultrafiltrates of plasma, are about 25% of that of plasma, generally agreeing with the results of the *in vitro* binding studies obtained by dialysis or ultrafiltration experiments (19,23). The 10,11-epoxide is bound to protein in a lesser extent; values between 50 and 60% have been reported (7).

APPARENT PLASMA HALF-LIFE

Apparent plasma half-life of carbamazepine has been reported to range from 8 to 60 hr. The lowest values, 8 to 20 hr, were observed in newborn babies born to mothers receiving carbamazepine (21). The high values,

30 to 60 hr, were seen mostly in studies where volunteers received a single dose of carbamazepine; and shorter times, 15 to 40 hr, were observed in the same individuals after they had been given the drug chronically (8,19). It has also been observed that the apparent plasma half-life of carbamazepine is shorter in patients who are receiving other antiepileptic drugs, such as phenytoin, phenobarbital, or primidone, than in patients taking carbamazepine alone. Thus the state of induction of carbamazepine metabolism seems to play an important role in the outcome of a half-life study. Carbamazepine plasma half-life did not appear to be dose dependent when low test doses, 3 or 6 or 9 mg/kg, were used (17). Quotable figures for carbamazepine plasma half-life as population average probably would be 30 hr for unconditioned individuals and 20 hr for patients receiving the drug chronically. The plasma half-life of 10,11-epoxide is shorter than that of the parent compound; values of 5 to 16 hr have been reported (8,19).

TIME TO REACH STEADY-STATE PLASMA LEVEL

The time to reach steady-state plasma concentration with a given dose appears to be 2 to 4 days. There are diurnal variations of the plasma level to some extent (20 to 50%); therefore, for a serial followup the blood samples should be drawn at the same time of the day relative to the dosing (8,25).

DOSE AND PLASMA-LEVEL RELATIONS

Generally, low doses produce low plasma levels and higher doses result in higher levels of both the parent compound and the 10,11-epoxide metabolite. The plasma concentration of the latter is usually lower than that of the unchanged drug, ranging from 10 to 50%, average 30%. There are marked interindividual variations in the ratio of dose to plasma level (4,7,16,19,22,25). The reason for the interindividual variations are not clear but may include genetic and environmental factors influencing the rate and completeness of carbamazepine absorption and biotransformation. The plasma levels with a given dose tend to be higher when carbamazepine alone is used, whereas coadministration of other antiepileptic drugs, particularly phenytoin and/or phenobarbital or primidone, usually results in lower plasma levels of the parent compound. The 10,11-epoxide plasma concentration usually makes up a larger percentage of the total circulating compounds in patients on multiple drugs than in those patients taking carbamazepine alone (6,22).

On the average, doses of 200 to 600 mg daily are expected to produce plasma levels of carbamazepine ranging from 1 to 6 μg/ml, and doses of 600 to 1,200 mg daily render values of 3 to 16 μg/ml (Fig. 2). With doses of 1,600 mg or more, plasma concentrations up to 20 μg/ml and higher may be seen. When values are over 30 μg/ml, unusual drug intake, contamination, or technical difficulties in the laboratory should be suspected.

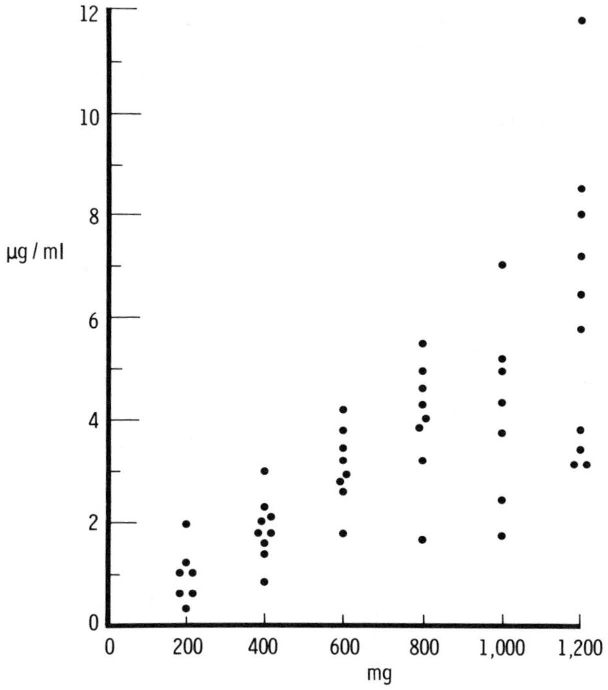

FIG. 2. Blood levels of carbamazepine on various dosages.

The saliva and CSF concentrations of carbamazepine constitute usually about 25% and those of 10,11-epoxide about 50% of their plasma levels, respectively.

EFFECTIVE PLASMA CARBAMAZEPINE LEVELS

Much still remains to be learned about the clinically effective plasma carbamazepine concentrations. The evaluation of this aspect is complicated by the presence of one known pharmacologically active metabolite, the 10,11-epoxide, and there may be others. Furthermore, more often than not, carbamazepine is used in combination with other antiepileptic drugs. Nevertheless, it appears that in studies where an attempt was made to evaluate the plasma level and efficacy relations, the value of 4 μg/ml is cited as the low end of the effective range (6,16). It is obvious that this is a compromise figure. There are patients who seem to benefit from levels lower than 4 μg/ml, and there are others who do not improve with levels double that. This, of course, reflects the differences in the nature and severity of the epileptic process among individual patients. In the evaluation of the contribution of antiepileptic effects from the 10,11-epoxide, one has to consider that although its levels are low, being only 50% bound, the concentration of epoxide reaching the site of action may be significant. More data need to be accumulated to evaluate the role of the epoxide. Currently, however, it appears fair to recommend achieving plasma carbamazepine levels over 4 μg/ml if seizure control is inadequate in a given patient. Alleviation of symptoms of trigeminal neuralgia has been seen in patients whose plasma carbamazepine levels ranged from 3 to 12 μg/ml.

TOXIC PLASMA CARBAMAZEPINE LEVELS

The dose- and plasma level-related toxic effects of carbamazepine are somewhat similar to those of phenytoin and include eye muscle imbalance resulting in nystagmus and blurred vision, unsteadiness, drowsiness, dizziness, and also nausea, vomiting, and headache. Some adaptation to those effects takes place over a period of time even without reduction of dosage, and there are marked interindividual variations in the severity of these manifestations among patients having similar carbamazepine plasma levels. Generally, some transient nystagmus may be seen with levels 6 μg/ml or less, but this rarely necessitates reduction of the dose. Levels over 9 to 12 μg/ml, however, may cause incapacitating unsteadiness, dizziness, and generally poor performance in the majority of patients and may thus be considered to be in the toxic range (3,7,16,18). However, if the high level is needed to achieve seizure control and the patient has adapted to that and has no side effects, there is no need to reduce the dose just because the level is over 10 μg/ml.

Since several carbamazepine side effects (nystagmus, ataxia) are similar to those of phenytoin, they seem to add up in some patients who are on combined medication and have high plasma phenytoin levels (16). Figure 3 illustrates one such patient whose plasma phenytoin level was in the range of 30 μg/ml and who had some nystagmus and was slightly unsteady from that. After carbamazepine was added to his medication and the plasma level reached 3.5 μg/ml, the patient became quite unsteady, the nystagmus increased markedly, and the patient complained of blurred vision. After the end of the controlled study protocol period, phenytoin dose was reduced, carbamazepine dose was increased to reach levels of 6 to 8 μg/ml, and the patient did well without excessive toxicity. Thus in patients on several antiepileptic drugs, including phenytoin, it is advisable to determine all drug levels when evaluating the toxic symptomatology, and one may find that relatively low carbamazepine levels may be incapacitating.

Other rare toxic effects of carbamazepine, such as depression of the hematopoietic system and skin rashes, do not seem to be related to the dose and blood level, although data in this respect are scarce. Hematological monitoring in patients taking carbamazepine, however, is mandatory.

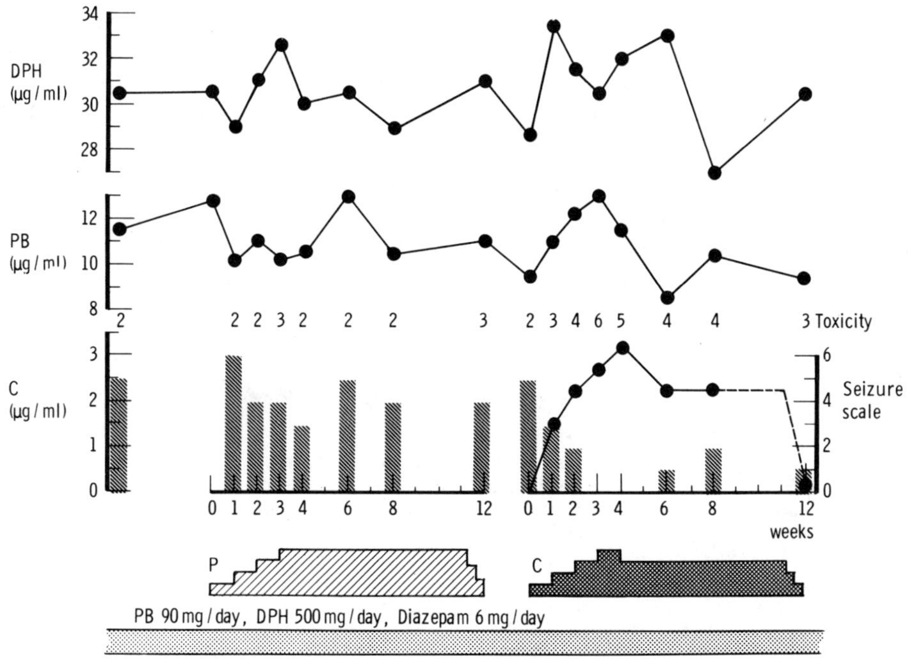

FIG. 3. **Blood levels of phenytoin (DPH), phenobarbital (PB), and carbamazepine (C) in a 19-year-old patient. Note marked increase of the toxicity score with relatively low blood levels of carbamazepine. The bars indicate the number of seizures per week during the preceding observation period (scale on the right).**

INTERACTIONS WITH OTHER DRUGS

Carbamazepine has been observed to cause a decline in plasma phenytoin and warfarin levels in some patients (11). It has also increased the phenobarbital to primidone ratio in the plasma (Chapter 24). All these effects are thought to be caused by the induction of microsomal enzyme activity by carbamazepine.

SUMMARY

Carbamazepine is a tricyclic compound that is effective against psychomotor and grand mal seizures and also alleviates symptoms of trigeminal neuralgia. It is slowly and incompletely absorbed and biotransformed extensively, yielding an active metabolite, 10,11-epoxide, which also circulates. The major urinary elimination product is 10,11-dihydroxide. The apparent plasma half-life is 15 to 30 hr for the parent compound and 5 to 15 hr for the epoxide metabolite; plasma protein binding is 75% for the parent compound and 50% for the epoxide metabolite. Time to reach steady-state plasma level is 2 to 4 days; up to 50% diurnal variation may occur in the plasma level. The effective plasma level of carbamazepine may be considered to be over 4 μg/ml; toxic effects are frequent with levels over 12 μg/ml, but may occur with lower values in patients with high phenytoin levels. Data are still incomplete with regard to the role of plasma 10,11-epoxide levels in the efficacy and toxicity in patients taking carbamazepine.

All numerical values and averages regarding carbamazepine cited in this chapter are based on relatively few patients studied so far (compared to phenytoin literature) and may change as the general reported experience increases.

REFERENCES

1. Baker, K. M., Csentenyi, J., Frigerio, A., Morselli, P. L., Parravicini, F., and Pifferi, G. (1973): 10,11-dihydro-10,11-dihydroxy-5H-dibenz/b,f/azepine 5-carboxamide, a metabolite of carbamazepine isolated from human and rat urine. *J. Med. Chem.,* 16:703–705.
2. Blom, S. (1963): Tic doloreux treated with a new anticonvulsant. *Arch. Neurol.,* 9:285–290.
3. Cereghino, J. J. (1975): Serum carbamazepine concentration and clinical control. In: *Complex Partial Seizures and Their Treatment,* Advances in Neurology, Vol. 11, edited by J. K. Penry and D. D. Daly, pp. 309–330. Raven Press, New York.
4. Cereghino, J. J., Brock, J. T., Van Meter, J. C., Penry, J. K., Smith, L. D., and White, B. G. (1974): Carbamazepine for epilepsy. A controlled prospective evaluation. *Neurology* (Minneap.), 24:401–410.
5. Christiansen, J., and Dam, M. (1973): Influence of phenobarbital and diphenylhydantoin on plasma carbamazepine levels in patients with epilepsy. *Acta Neurol. Scand.,* 49:543–546.
6. Dam, M., Jensen, A., and Christiansen, J. (1975): Plasma level and effect of carbamazepine in grand mal and psychomotor epilepsy. *Acta Neurol. Scand. Suppl.,* 60:33–38.
7. Eichelbaum, M., Bertilsson, L., Lund, L., Palmer, L., and Sjöqvist, F. (1976): Plasma levels of carbamazepine and carbamazepine-10,11-epoxide during treatment of epilepsy. *Eur. J. Clin. Pharmacol.,* 9:417–421.
8. Eichelbaum, M., Ekbom, K., Bertilsson, L., Ringberger, V. A., and Rane A. (1975): Plasma kinetics of carbamazepine and its epoxide metabolite in man after single and multiple doses. *Eur. J. Clin. Pharmacol.,* 8:337–341.
9. Faigle, J. W., and Feldman, K. F. (1974): Pharmacokinetic data of carbamazepine and its major metabolites in man. In: *Clinical Pharmacology of Antiepileptic Drugs,* edited by H. Schneider, D. Janz, C. Gardner-Thorpe, H. Meinardi, and A. L. Sherwin. Springer Verlag, Berlin.
10. Frigerio, A., and Morselli, P. L. (1975): Carbamazepine: Biotransformation. In: *Complex Partial Seizures and Their Treatment,* Advances in Neurology, Vol. 11, edited by J. K. Penry and D. D. Daly, pp. 295–308. Raven Press, New York.
11. Hansen, J. M., Siersboek-Nielsen, K., and Skovsted, L. (1971): Carbamazepine induced acceleration of diphenylhydantoin and warfarin metabolism in man. *Clin. Pharmacol. Ther.,* 12:539–543.
12. Hooper, W. D., Dubetz, D. K., Bochner, F., Cotter, L. M., Smith, G. A., Eadie, M. J., and Tyrer, J. H. (1975): Plasma protein binding of carbamazepine. *Clin. Pharmacol. Ther.,* 17:433–440.
13. Julien, R. M., and Hollister, R. P. (1975): Carbamazepine: Mechanism of action. In: *Complex Partial Seizures and Their Treatment,* Advances in Neurology, Vol. 11, edited by J. K. Penry and D. D. Daly, pp. 263–277. Raven Press, New York.

14. Krupp, P. (1969): The effect of Tegretol on some elementary neuronal mechanisms. *Headache,* 9:42–46.
15. Kutt, H. (1975): Carbamazepine: Chemistry and methods of determination. In: *Complex Partial Seizures and Their Treatment,* Advances in Neurology, Vol. 11, edited by J. K. Penry and D. D. Daly, pp. 249–261. Raven Press, New York.
16. Kutt, H., Solomon, G., Wasterlain, C., Peterson, H., Louis, S., and Carruthers, R. (1975): Carbamazepine in difficult to control epileptic out-patients. *Acta Neurol. Scand. Suppl.,* 60:27–32.
17. Levy, R. H., Pitlick, W. H., Troupin, A. S., Green, J. R., and Neal, J. M. (1975): Pharmacokinetics of carbamazepine in normal man. *Clin. Pharmacol. Ther.,* 17:657–668.
18. Meinardi, H. (1972): Carbamazepine. In: *Antiepileptic Drugs,* edited by D. M. Woodbury, J. K. Penry, and R. P. Schmidt, pp. 487–496. Raven Press, New York.
19. Morselli, P. L. (1975): Carbamazepine: Absorption, distribution and excretion. In: *Complex Partial Seizures and Their Treatment,* Advances in Neurology, Vol. 11, edited by J. K. Penry and D. D. Daly, pp. 279–293. Raven Press, New York.
20. Parsonage, M. (1975): Treatment with carbamazepine: Adults. In: *Complex Partial Seizures and Their Treatment.* Advances in Neurology, Vol. 11, edited by J. K. Penry and D. D. Daly, pp. 221–236. Raven Press, New York.
21. Rane, A., Bertilsson, L., and Palmer, I. (1975): Disposition of placentally transferred carbamazepine (Tegretol®) in the newborn. *Eur. J. Clin. Pharmacol.,* 8:283–284.
22. Rane, A., Höjer, B., and Wilson, J. T. (1976); Kinetics of carbamazepine and its 10,11-epoxide metabolite in children. *Clin. Pharmacol. Ther.,* 19:276–283.
23. Rawlins, M. D., Collste, P., Bertilsson, L., and Palmer, L. (1975): Distribution and elimination kinetics of carbamazepine. *Eur. J. Clin. Pharmacol.,* 8:91–96.
24. Theobald, W., and Kunz, H. A. (1963): Zur Pharmakologie des Antiepilepticums 5-carbamul-5H-dibenzo(b,f)azepin. *Arzneim. Forsch.,* 13:122–125.
25. Troupin, A. S., Green, J. R., and Halpern, L. M. (1975): Carbamazepine (Tegretol) as an anticonvulsant. A controlled double-blind comparison with diphenylhydantoin (Dilantin). *Acta Neurol. Scand. Suppl.,* 60:13–26.

Antiepileptic Drugs: Quantitative Analysis and Interpretation, edited by C. E. Pippenger, J. K. Penry, and H. Kutt, Raven Press, New York, © 1978.

Chapter 27

Evaluation of Unusual Antiepileptic Drug Concentrations

Henn Kutt

Nonroutine assays are used mostly to evaluate further those patients whose observed blood concentrations of antiepileptic drugs are considered unusual or unexpected. The unusual or unexpected values may occur in two respects: unexpectedly high or low levels relative to the dose, and unexpected levels relative to the clinical response. The patient whose blood drug level is unexpected relative to the dose can be evaluated further by studies of urinary output of the drug and its metabolites. The patient whose blood drug level is unusual relative to the clinical response can be evaluated further by plasma drug protein-binding studies.

EXPECTED RANGE OF BLOOD LEVELS RELATIVE TO DOSE

In order to recognize or define an observed blood drug level unexpectedly high or low relative to the dose, one needs to know what the expected level is. Based on the general experience reported by various laboratories (4,5,17), it is apparent that lower doses usually produce lower levels and higher doses produce higher levels. However, there can be considerable variations of levels among individuals receiving the same dose, as evidenced by the wide scatter of values in various published diagrams. The reasons for variations in the steady-state levels among patients receiving equivalent doses include differences in the rate and completeness of drug absorption, biotransformation, and elimination, aspects that can be influenced by genetic and environmental factors (15). Furthermore, the scatter of values is usually greater in diagrams that include outpatients, where the ingested dose is less likely to equal the prescribed dose; it is less in studies reporting hospitalized patients studied under controlled conditions.

Allowing the average variations caused by factors mentioned above, it is possible to define empirically the expected ranges of blood levels into which the majority of patients would fall when receiving the common doses (17). When the observed blood level is considerably below or above the expected range values, there is usually something wrong technically or the factors mentioned above are operational in the extreme. Table 1 gives the common doses and the corresponding expected blood-level ranges for the major antiepileptic drugs, compiled and interpolated from the literature.

TABLE 1. *Dose and blood-level relations*

Drug	Average dose (mg/day)	Expected level (μg/ml) Range	Average
Phenytoin	300	5–20	10
Phenobarbital	120	10–30	20
Primidone	750	5–15	8
Carbamazepine	1,200	3–12	6
Ethosuximide	750	20–70	50
Trimethadione	900	300–800(as DMO)	
Diazepam	15	0.1–0.3	
Clonazepam	4	0.015–0.050	
Valproate	1,000	50–90	

Accepting that an observed blood-level value is unexpectedly high or low would lead to further evaluation of the patient. The first step is an in-depth interview which may reveal (as a confession by the patient) that the ingested dose was not equal to the prescribed dose, that is, noncompliance by the patient. A chart review may reveal intake of other drugs causing drug-drug interactions. Further causes for unexpected blood levels include low drug absorption or unusually slow or fast drug metabolism.

In order to ascertain if the unexpected blood drug level with a given dose is caused by poor absorption from the intestinal tract or by an unusual rate of drug metabolism or by noncompliance not admitted to by the patient, determination of the urinary output of the drug and its metabolites is of value.

Utilization of studies of urinary output of the drug and its metabolites is based on the assumption or realization that there is an expected range of amounts of drug products found in the urine with a given dosage. Reasonably good and reliable data in this respect are available for phenytoin and its major metabolite *p*-hydroxy diphenylhydantoin (HPPH), and to some extent for phenobarbital and *p*-hydroxy phenobarbital (13); less firm data are on hand for the other antiepileptic drugs. The available data in the literature are compiled in Table 2.

Determination of the urinary output of HPPH and *p*-hydroxy phenobarbital are the two assays that most laboratories may consider to perform. The original procedures were published by Butler (6,7) and consisted of liberation of conjugated metabolites by hydrolysis followed by solvent extraction and then quantitation by spectrophotometry. In later reports, quantification has been attempted by paper chromatography (19) and thin-layer chromatography (12,21) in combination with colorimetry. More recently, gas chromatography has been used for quantitation of HPPH and *p*-hydroxy phenobarbital. Chang and Glazko (8) have recommended silylation before injection into the gas chromatograph, whereas others have utilized on-column methylation (10,13,14).

The procedure used for quantification of HPPH and *p*-hydroxy phenobar-

TABLE 2. *Urinary recoveries as percent of dose*

Drug	Range	Average	Total equivalent
Phenytoin	0.1–3	1.0	
p-HPPH	50–75	65	65
Phenobarbital	10–40	30	
p-OH-Pb	10–40	30	60
Primidone	30–60		
PEMA	10–30		
Pb + p-OH-Pb	5–10		75
Carbamazepine	< 1		
Epoxy + Dihydro Met's	30		
Ethosuximide	10–20		
Met's	?		

bital in the author's laboratory is described in detail in Appendix II of this volume. It should be emphasized first that of great importance is the accuracy of the 24-hr urine collection, because meaningful results are usually obtained from the recovery of compounds as percent of dose per 24 hr. When evaluating steady state, we prefer three consecutive 24-hr collections. An aliquot, usually 0.5 to 2.0 ml, is then added to an equal volume of concentrated hydrochloric acid and the appropriate internal standards, *p*-methylphenylphenyl hydantoin (MPPH) or *p*-methyl phenobarbital (MPB). The mixture is heated to boil for 30 min, let cool, and set with NaOH to bring the pH to around 5. Instead of acid hydrolysis, glusulase may be used to liberate the conjugate, but this takes longer. Calibration samples consisting of control urine with added known amounts of HPPH and *p*-hydroxy phenobarbital, and their internal standards are prepared in a similar manner.

Extraction of drug components is carried out with ethyl acetate. The extract may be purified by passing through a Celite column, particularly when *p*-hydroxy phenobarbital is the substance of interest, as some impurities may "crowd" that peak in the gas chromatogram. The solvent is then evaporated to dryness and the residue reconstituted with trimethylphenylammonium hydroxide (TMPAH). It is important to use TMPAH of sufficient molar strength, such as 0.3 to 0.5, to assure complete methylation.

Gas chromatography is carried out with 5% OV-17 columns. Our instruments are HP 402, 7610 and 5830. The *p*-hydroxy phenobarbital appears between MPB and MPPH, whereas HPPH appears after MPPH (see Fig. 1). Suitable isothermal oven temperatures for *p*-hydroxy phenobarbital are around 200°C, whereas 260°C may be used for HPPH to save time. The concentration of unknowns are computed from the calibration curve and calculated to express total 24-hr output.

Using acid hydrolysis in HPPH determination has been criticized (14) for the following reasons. There is usually a small amount of dihydrodiol metabolite also present in the urine of patients taking phenytoin. This com-

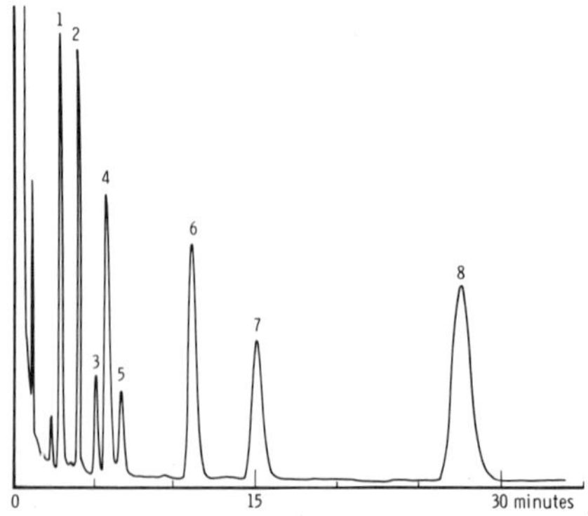

FIG. 1. GLC tracing indicating the position of major antiepileptic drugs and their metabolites. The peaks are (1) phenobarbital; (2) *p*-methyl phenobarbital (MPB); (3) iminostilbene; (4) primidone; (5) *p*-OH-phenobarbital; (6) phenytoin; (7) *p*-methylphenylphenylhydantoin (MPPH); (8) HPPH. Instrument: HP 402; column 5% OV-17; column temperature 220°C isothermal.

pound converts in acid hydrolysis to *p*-HPPH and *m*-HPPH, adding slightly to the quantity of the *p*-HPPH value, but probably no more than 10% of the total. This problem can be circumvented by extracting the urine with isoamyl alcohol prior to hydrolysis. On the other hand, having the dihydrodiol metabolite included in the total may even be an advantage, particularly if the question is what portion of the dose can be accounted for.

The results of *p*-HPPH determination can then be applied to evaluate patients with unexpected blood levels in the following manner (15).

1. *Patients with unexpectedly low blood levels:* Malabsorption of phenytoin is indicated by low blood level and low HPPH (less than 30% of the dose) output even under supervised drug intake. No significant increase occurs upon increase of the dose.

Rapid metabolism of phenytoin is indicated by low blood level but adequate (over 60% of the dose) output of urinary p-HPPH. Upon increase of dosage, both blood level and *p*-HPPH output will increase.

Nonconfessed noncompliance is indicated by low blood level and low *p*-HPPH output initially but an increase of both takes place when drug intake is supervised.

2. *Patients with unexpectedly high blood levels:* Slow metabolism of phenytoin is indicated by high blood level in patients receiving average or low doses. The *p*-HPPH output is on the low side and does not increase while the blood level is rising.

Nonconfessed noncompliance is indicated by high blood level and higher than expected *p*-HPPH output (over 90% of the "dose"). There are patients who like to take extra doses for fear of having another seizure or simply forgetting that they have already taken their daily doses.

DRUG-DRUG INTERACTIONS

Drug-drug interactions may cause unexpectedly low or high plasma levels relative to the dose. Most instances of reported interactions involve pheny-

TABLE 3. *Drugs found to cause changes of blood phenytoin level*

	Increase	
Decrease	Predictable	Sporadic
Phenobarbital	Disulfiram	Methylphenidate
Carbamazepine	Sulthiame	Dicoumarol
Tolbutamide	Isoniazid (slow inactivators)	Phenylbutazole
Ethanol		Sulfa
DDT		Chloramphenicol
		Phenothiazines
		Benzodiazepines
		Phenobarbital

toin and include both interactions where the other drug caused a decline (usually enzyme induction) of plasma phenytoin level or a rise (usually enzyme inhibition) (16). Table 3 lists the drugs thus implicated. It is to be emphasized that with the majority of these agents clinically significant plasma phenytoin level changes do not take place in all patients taking these drugs in combination. There seems to be marked variability in the individual susceptibility, and many patients can take these drug combinations, without difficulties, when needed. The only exceptions are disulfiram and sulthiame, as well as isoniazid (in slow isoniazid inactivators only), which predictably cause plasma phenytoin level elevations.

Lowering of plasma phenytoin levels is caused in some patients by phenobarbital, carbamazepine, and tolbutamide, among others. Again, marked changes are seen only in patients with unusualy marked (so far unexplained) susceptibility, and these are not frequent.

Studies of urinary output of *p*-HPPH can sometimes be helpful in confirming the drug-drug interactions taking place, particularly if carried out during the phase when the plasma level is changing. This, however, is rarely possible in most clinical cases, and the *p*-HPPH determinations from the later urine collections during new steady states are not particularly helpful.

BINDING STUDIES

Studies of plasma protein binding of antiepileptic drugs are usually carried out to evaluate patients whose clinical response is unusual relative to the observed plasma level (2). The rationale of this is based on the assumption that if less than average of the drug is bound, more free drug is on hand to arrive at the sites of action in the tissue, and effectiveness and/or intoxication may occur at lower than average total plasma concentrations. This assumption may not always hold true because it is conceivable that the free drug reaching the liver is simply metabolized and then eliminated without leading to higher than average concentrations in the nervous tissue. No concrete evidence is available to prove one or the other possibility, but empirically it has been observed that in some patients with low plasma protein binding, relatively low total plasma levels are effective or levels of moderate height may be causing signs of intoxication. Thus carrying out the protein-binding studies may enhance the understanding of unexpected clinical response in some patients.

Lower than average plasma protein binding of phenytoin has been observed frequently in patients with chronic uremia (20,23) or liver disease (11). It may also occur when other drugs such as salicylates (20) have occupied some of the binding sites; or in babies (9); or for reasons so far unknown.

The methods for studying the plasma protein binding of antiepileptic drugs and for determining the unbound fraction of the drug include equilibrium dialysis, ultrafiltration, red blood cell content, and saliva or CSF content.

EQUILIBRIUM DIALYSIS

In equilibrium dialysis, 1 to 2 ml of plasma secured in a cellophane bag is placed in a large volume of buffered dialysis fluid with low drug concentration ("tank dialysis"). The final ratio of the concentration of dialysate over that of plasma in the bag gives the percent unbound. This technique is sensitive to temperature, and day-to-day reproducibility is not perfect. Furthermore, it is not suitable for studies of binding alterations caused by other drugs occupying the binding sites in a native clinical sample, because the interfering drugs would disappear into the dialysis fluid. Equilibrium dialysis can be used, however, for general evaluation of displacement capacity of another drug when this agent is placed into the dialysis fluid. An alternative to "tank dialysis" is a dialysis cell in which the plasma and the buffer are separated by a membrane. Results of studies applying this technique have been published by Ehrnebo et al. (9), Odar-Cederlöf and Borga (20), and Troupin and Friel (25), among others.

ULTRAFILTRATION

Theoretically, ultrafiltration could be the best method for the binding studies, as the concentration of drug in the ultrafiltrate is a true representative of the unbound fraction. The binding sites occupied by other drugs or substances in the original plasma sample remain unaffected during ultrafiltration (unlike the situation in equilibrium dialysis). The available membranes, however, are not perfect as yet. The membranes may leak protein or clog up or bind some of the drug. It is important to pay careful attention to these possible pitfalls when using ultrafiltration for the binding studies. Results obtained by ultrafiltration have been published by Booker and Darcey (2), Bochner et al. (1), Hooper et al. (11), Lund et al. (18), Porter and

Layzer (22), and Reidenberg et al. (23), among others. With the expected improvements in technology regarding membrane structure and apparatus design, ultrafiltration may well become the procedure of choice for binding studies.

RED CELL- OR BLOOD-TO-PLASMA RATIO AS INDICATOR OF UNBOUND DRUG FRACTION

Determinations of red cell- or blood-to-plasma ratio have given values that are within the same range as free drug fractions determined by equilibrium dialysis or ultrafiltration. The procedures are time consuming and may involve addition of radioactive drugs. Results of these studies have been published by Borondy et al. (3) and by Wilkinson and Kurata (26), among others.

SALIVA AND CSF CONTENT AS INDICATOR OF UNBOUND DRUG FRACTION

Saliva and CSF may be viewed as naturally occurring ultrafiltrates. Their concentration of phenytoin and carbamazepine corresponds quite closely with the free drug fraction determined by other techniques. Since obtaining saliva samples is an innocuous procedure, the study material is easily available. Results comparing saliva or cerebrospinal fluid concentrations of drug with plasma free drug fraction determined by other techniques have been published by Bochner et al. (1), Schmidt and Kupferberg (24), Troupin and Friel (25), and Lund et al. (18), among others.

Quantitation of the drug concentration in the study material, whether ultrafiltrate, dialysis fluid, saliva, or CSF, requires extra care. The drug concentration representing the unbound fraction is usually low, 10 to 30% of that of the total plasma concentration. To ascertain accuracy, larger than average sample size may be used, if available, such as when dealing with dialysis fluid. Best results are obtained with quantitation techniques that have proved to be most reliable in a given operator's hands.

REFERENCES

1. Bochner, F., Hooper, W. D., Sutherland, J. M., Eadie, M. J., and Tyrer, J. H. (1974): Diphenylhydantoin concentration in saliva. *Arch. Neurol.* 31:57–59.
2. Booker, H. E., and Darcey, B. (1973): Serum concentrations of free diphenylhydantoin and their relationships to clinical intoxication. *Epilepsia,* 14:171–184.
3. Borondy, P., Dill, W. A., Chang, T., Buchanan, R. A., and Glazko, A. J. (1973): Effects of protein binding on the distribution of 5,5-diphenylhydantoin between plasma and red cells. *Ann. N.Y. Acad. Sci.,* 226:82–87.
4. Buchthal, F., and Lennox-Buchthal, M. A. (1972): Diphenylhydantoin. Relation of anticonvulsant effect to concentration in serum. In: *Antiepileptic Drugs,* edited by D. M. Woodbury, J. K. Penry, and R. P. Schmidt, pp. 193–209. Raven Press, New York.

5. Buchthal, F., and Svensmark, O. (1971): Serum concentration of diphenylhydantoin (phenytoin) and phenobarbital and their relation to therapeutic and toxic effects. *Psychiatr. Neurol. Neurochir.,* 74:7–36.
6. Butler, T. C. (1956): The metabolic hydroxylation of phenobarbital. *J. Pharmacol. Exp. Ther.,* 116:326–336.
7. Butler, T. C. (1957): The metabolic conversion of 5,5-diphenylhydantoin to 5-(*p*-hydroxyphenyl)-5-phenyl hydantoin. *J. Pharmacol. Exp. Ther.,* 119:1–11.
8. Chang, T., and Glazko, A. J. (1970): Quantitative assay of 5,5-diphenylhydantoin Dilantin®) and 5-(*p*-hydroxyphenyl)-5-phenyl hydantoin by gas-liquid chromatography. *J. Lab. Clin. Med.,* 75:145–155.
9. Ehrnebo, M., Agurell, S., Jalling, B., and Boreus, L. O. (1971): Age differences in drug binding by plasma proteins: Studies on human fetuses, neonates and adults. *Eur. J. Clin. Pharmacol.,* 3:189–193.
10. Hammer, R. H., Wilder, B. J., Streiff, R. R., and Mayersdorf, A. (1971): Flash methylation and GLC of diphenylhydantoin and 5-(*p*-hydroxyphenyl)-5-phenylhydantoin. *J. Pharm. Sci.,* 60:327–329.
11. Hooper, W. D., Bochner, F., Eadie, M. J., and Tyrer, J. H. (1974): Plasma protein binding of diphenylhydantoin. *Clin. Pharmacol. Ther.,* 15:276–282.
12. Huisman, J. W. (1966): The estimation of some important anticonvulsant drugs in serum. *Clin. Chim. Acta,* 13:323–328.
13. Kallberg, N., Agurell, S., Ericsson, O., Bucht, E., Jalling, B., and Boreus, L. O. (1975): Quantitation of phenobarbital and its main metabolites in human urine. *Eur. J. Clin. Pharmacol.,* 9:161–168.
14. Karlen, B., Garle, M., Rane, A., Gutova, M., and Lindborg, B. (1975): Assay of the major (4-hydroxylated) metabolites of diphenylhydantoin in human urine. *Eur. J. Clin. Pharmacol.,* 8:359–363.
15. Kutt, H. (1971): Biochemical and genetic factors regulating Dilantin metabolism in man. *Ann. N.Y. Acad. Sci.,* 179:704–722.
16. Kutt, H. (1975): Interactions of antiepileptic drugs. *Epilepsia,* 16:393–402.
17. Kutt, H., and Penry, J. K. (1974): Usefulness of blood levels of antiepileptic drugs. *Arch. Neurol.,* 31:283–288.
18. Lund, L., Berlin, A., and Lunde, P. K. M. (1970): Plasma protein binding of diphenylhydantoin in patients with epilepsy. Agreement between the unbound fractions in plasma and the concentration in the cerebrospinal fluid. *Clin. Pharmacol. Ther.,* 11:846–855.
19. Maynert, E. W. (1960): The metabolic fate of diphenylhydantoin in the dog, rat and man. *J. Pharmacol. Exp. Ther.,* 130:275–284.
20. Odar-Cederlöf, I., and Borga, O. (1976): Impaired plasma protein binding of phenytoin in uremia and displacement effect of salicylic acid. *Clin. Pharmacol. Ther.,* 20:36–47.
21. Olesen, O. V. (1968): Determination of 5-(*p*-hydroxyphenyl)-5-phenylhydantoin (HPPH) in urine by thin-layer chromatography. *Acta Pharmacol. Toxicol.* (Kbh.), 26:222–228.
22. Porter, R. J., and Layzer, R. B. (1975): Plasma albumin concentration and diphenylhydantoin binding in man. *Arch. Neurol.,* 32:298–303.
23. Reidenberg, M. M., Odar-Cederlöf, I., von Bahr, C., Borga, O., and Sjöqvist, F. (1971): Protein binding of diphenylhydantoin and desmethylimipramine in plasma from patients with poor renal function. *N. Engl. J. Med.,* 285:264–267.
24. Schmidt, D., and Kupferberg, H. J. (1975): Diphenylhydantoin, phenobarbital and primidone in saliva, plasma and cerebrospinal fluid. *Epilepsia,* 16:735–741.
25. Troupin, A. S., and Friel, P. (1975): Anticonvulsant level in saliva, serum and cerebrospinal fluid. *Epilepsia,* 16:223–227.
26. Wilkinson, G. R., and Kurata, D. (1974): The uptake of diphenylhydantoin by the human erythrocyte and its application to the estimation of plasma binding. In: *Drug Interactions,* edited by P. L. Morselli, S. Garattini, and S. N. Cohen, pp. 289–297. Raven Press, New York.

Antiepileptic Drugs: Quantitative Analysis and Interpretation, edited by C. E. Pippenger, J. K. Penry, and H. Kutt, Raven Press, New York, © 1978.

Chapter 28

Pediatric Clinical Pharmacology of Antiepileptic Drugs: A Special Consideration

C. E. Pippenger

The onset of seizures in childhood, particularly absence seizures, is a common occurrence. The successful control of seizures in children, however, is essential for their development into productive members of society. The management of seizure disorders in children has been extensively reviewed (6,7,10).

For several years, clinicians and investigators have recognized the existence of an age-related difference between children and adults in the utilization of antiepileptic drugs (2–5,12,17). Unfortunately, most of these investigations have been concerned with the effects of only one drug regardless of the number of agents the patient was receiving. We have described our experience with therapeutic monitoring of antiepileptic drugs in a pediatric population receiving multiple-drug therapy (14). This chapter summarizes these findings and alerts physicians and laboratories engaged in pediatric therapeutic drug monitoring to the remarkable differences between children and adults in the utilization of drugs.

Serum antiepileptic drug concentrations were analyzed by gas-liquid chromatography or homogeneous enzyme immunoassay (EMIT) (13) in 828 specimens from children and adolescents 1 to 20 years of age who were receiving multiple antiepileptic drugs. The results of this study are summarized in Table 1 as the anticipated steady-state plasma antiepileptic drug concentrations following a hypothetical 1-mg/kg dose in children of different ages receiving single- or multiple-drug therapy. An age-dependent relationship between plasma concentration and dose is clearly evident. Children below the age of 11 years rapidly utilize phenytoin, phenobarbital, and primidone. Recently, other investigators have reported rapid utilization of carbamazepine (11) and ethosuximide (16). Serum concentrations in a pediatric population tend to be significantly lower than those in an adult population on equivalent mg/kg dosages. Consequently, children should receive higher maintenance dosages of a given drug to achieve optimal antiepileptic drug concentration.

A marked decrease in antiepileptic drug utilization is observed as children enter the early stages of puberty. Pubescent children achieve serum concentrations that approximate more closely those expected in adults on the

TABLE 1. *Anticipated steady-state plasma antiepileptic drug concentrations in children after dose of 1 mg/kg*

Drugs	Plasma concentrations (μg/ml) by age (years) 1–5	6–10	11–15	16–20
Phenytoin (DPH)				
DPH alone	1.3	1.8	2.0	2.9
DPH + PB	1.1	1.7	1.9	2.4
DPH + PR	1.3	1.5	1.8	2.3
Phenobarbital (PB)				
PB alone	3.7	5.3	7.5	9.9
DPH + PB	5.5	7.5	9.3	12.2
Primidone (PR)				
PR alone	—	0.46	0.72	0.71
PR + DPH	0.41	0.34	0.86	0.57
Phenobarbital derived from primidone				
PR alone	—	1.2	1.4	1.9
PR + DPH	1.7	1.1	1.8	2.2

To determine the expected plasma concentration for a child of a given age receiving the indicated drug or drug combination, multiply the expected plasma concentration for a given age group by the total daily dosage (mg/kg).

same mg/kg dosage. By the time children reach late adolescence (16 to 20 years), their drug patterns are essentially identical to those of adults. Morselli and colleagues (12) reported, and we have confirmed, a marked decrease in serum phenytoin concentrations and an elevation of serum phenobarbital concentrations after phenobarbital was added to the regimens of children on phenytoin therapy. Children at every age level medicated with a combination of phenytoin and phenobarbital consistently exhibited lower serum phenytoin and higher phenobarbital concentrations than children receiving the same mg/kg dosage of these agents as single drug therapy. Children receiving primidone and phenytoin also exhibited decreased phenytoin and increased phenobarbital concentrations, suggesting that an interaction also occurs between phenytoin and the phenobarbital derived from primidone.

The disposition of phenobarbital derived from primidone follows the same pattern of utilization in children that is observed when phenobarbital is administered alone. Thus, the age-dependent phenobarbital utilization patterns will also be present after primidone administration. Unfortunately, the practice of prescribing primidone in conjunction with phenobarbital is widespread. In our patient population, 176 patients were receiving primidone in combination with another drug, and 57 were receiving phenobarbital with the primidone. The metabolic pathways for primidone and its conversion to phenobarbital and phenylethylmalonamide (PEMA) have been well documented by Gallagher et al. (8,9) and Baumel et al. (1).

Traditionally, the clinical "rule of thumb" for multiple-drug treatment of epilepsy has been to initiate therapy with either phenytoin or phenobarbital, or both, and increase dosages until control is achieved or clinical toxicity develops. If the seizures remain uncontrolled, primidone may be added to the regimen. Often, the drug toxicity that develops after the institution of primidone is attributed clinically to the primidone. However, patients receiving both phenobarbital and primidone will show a marked elevation of the serum phenobarbital concentration because of phenobarbital accumulation from both agents. In our experience, the clinical toxicity observed after the administration of primidone to patients on chronic antiepileptic drug therapy is attributable to toxic serum phenobarbital concentrations resulting from the simultaneous administration of primidone and phenobarbital rather than to toxic levels of primidone itself.

One of the major problems associated with the treatment of epilepsy in children is the deterioration that often occurs as they approach puberty. This may be characterized clinically by an exacerbation of seizures or increased lethargy and dullness. We suggest that many of the problems associated with seizure control in pubescent children may be directly related to the alteration of their drug-utilization patterns. The importance of this problem is demonstrated by two hypothetical examples based on our clinical experience.

First, consider the child who, at the age of 9, is placed on a standard pediatric dosage of phenobarbital (6 mg/kg) and achieves a serum phenobarbital concentration of 30 μg/ml. Drug levels are carefully monitored, seizures are well controlled, and he is seen by his pediatric neurologist once a year. Between his yearly visits, the parents and teachers become aware of a gradually increased lethargy in the child. On his yearly return visit, the serum phenobarbital concentrations are found to have increased from 30 to 60 μg/ml, reflecting the characteristic adult levels observed with a phenobarbital dosage of 6 mg/kg. This increased phenobarbital level is attributable directly to changes associated with puberty.

Chronic phenobarbital toxicity is subtle, often occurs without dramatic clinical changes, and may go undetected by the casual observer. Because a child's potential ability to learn is diminished by increasing lethargy, we urge that antiepileptic drug concentrations be monitored frequently (at least every 3 months) as a child approaches the age of early pubescence, regardless of whether or not the patient is seen by a physician. If serum drug concentrations increase, we recommend that appropriate dosage regulations be undertaken immediately. If such a procedure is followed, unnecessary phenobarbital toxicity could be virtually eliminated.

In the next example, consider the child who is 10 years old and receiving a phenytoin dosage of 8.6 mg/kg, with a therapeutic serum concentration of 17.2 μg/ml. At pubescence, there is a sudden exacerbation of seizures. If serum phenytoin concentrations are not measured, this exacerbation may be attributed to the increased seizure frequency that often accompanies the onset of puberty. Measurement of the serum concentration, however, demonstrates a level of 35.8 μg/ml, reflecting saturation of phenytoin metabolic pathways. This represents paradoxical phenytoin intoxication. In some individuals, extreme elevation of phenytoin concentrations may precipitate seizures (18).

We hope that progress in the relatively new field of pediatric clinical pharmacology will increase our now severely limited knowledge of drug utilization in children. Physicians should become increasingly aware that drug utilization patterns in children are different from those in adults, and that careful monitoring with appropriate medication adjustments to compensate for the process of maturation is essential for rational pediatric therapy. Failure to consider the unique drug utilization patterns in children will usually lead to severe drug interactions. The manifestations of such interactions may be increased lethargy or increased seizure frequency, both with consequent social sequelae in the child's development.

We urge any laboratory engaged in pediatric therapeutic drug monitoring to develop continuing education programs for pediatric neurologists and pediatricians, which will alert them to the potential problems of antiepileptic drug administration in children. Our goal is to achieve the knowledge that will assure children receiving antiepileptic medication of the best possible therapeutic regimen.

REFERENCES

1. Baumel, I. P., Gallagher, B. B., and Mattson, R. H. (1972): Phenylethylmalonamide (PEMA)—An important metabolite of primidone. *Arch. Neurol.,* 27:34–41.
2. Borofsky, L. G., Louis, S., and Kutt, H. (1973): Diphenylhydantoin in children—Pharmacology and efficacy. *Neurology* (Minneap.), 23:967–972.
3. Borofsky, L. G., Louis, S., Kutt, H., and Roginsky, M. (1972): Diphenylhydantoin: Efficacy, toxicity and dose-serum level relationships in children. *J. Pediatr.,* 81:995–1002.
4. Buchanan, R. A., and Allen, R. J. (1971): Diphenylhydantoin and phenobarbital levels in epileptic children. *Neurology* (Minneap.), 21:866–871.
5. Dawson, K. P. and Jamieson, A. (1971): Value of blood phenytoin estimation in management of childhood epilepsy *Arch. Dis. Child.,* 46:386–388.
6. Dodson, W. E., Prensky, A. L., DeVivo, D. C., Goldring, S., and Dodge, P. R. (1976): Management of seizure disorders: Selected aspects, Part I. *J. Pediatr.,* 89: 527–540.
7. Dodson, W. E., Prensky, A. L., DeVivo, D. C., Goldring, S., and Dodge, P. R. (1976): Management of seizure disorders: Selected aspects, Part II. *J. Pediatr.,* 89: 695–703.
8. Gallagher, B. B., Baumel, I. P., and Mattson, R. H. (1972): Metabolic disposition of primidone and its metabolites in epileptic subjects after single and repeated administration. *Neurology* (Minneap.), 22:1186–1192.
9. Gallagher, B. B., Smith, D. B., and Mattson, R. H. (1970): The relationship of the anticonvulsant properties of primidone to phenobarbital. *Epilepsia,* 11:293–301.
10. Low, N. L., and Pellock, J. M. (1976): Seizure disorders. In *Practice of Pediatrics,* Vol. IV, editor-in-chief, V. C. Kelley. Harper & Row, New York.
11. Monaco, F., Riccio, A., Benna, P., Covacich, A., Durelli, L., Fantini, M., Furlan, P., Gilli, M., Mutani, R., Troni, W., Gerna, M., Chim, P., and Morselli, P. L. (1976): Further observations on carbamazepine plasma levels in epileptic patients. *Neurology* (Minneap.), 26:936–943.

12. Morselli, P. L., Rizzo, M., and Garattini, S. (1971): Interaction between phenobarbital and diphenylhydantoin in animals and in epileptic patients. *Ann. N.Y. Acad. Sci.*, 179:88–107.
13. Pippenger, C. E., Bastiani, R. J., and Schneider, R. S. (1975): Evaluation of an experimental homogeneous enzyme immuno-assay for the quantification of phenytoin and phenobarbitone in serum or plasma. In *Clinical Pharmacology of Anti-Epileptic Drugs,* edited by H. Schneider, D. Janz, C. Gardner-Thorpe, H. Meinardi, and A. L. Sherwin, pp. 331–336. Springer-Verlag, Berlin.
14. Pippenger, C. E., Pellock, J. M., and Gold, A. P. (1977): Antiepileptic drug concentrations in children on multiple therapy. In *Antiepileptic Drug Monitoring,* edited by C. Gardner-Thorpe, D. Janz, H. Meinardi, and C. E. Pippenger, pp. 282–286. Pitman Medical, Kent.
15. Rowan, A. J., Pippenger, C. E., McGregor, P. A., and French, J. H. (1975): Seizure activity and anticonvulsant drug concentration. *Arch. Neurol.,* 32:281–288.
16. Sherwin, A. L., and Robb, J. P. (1972): Ethosuximide: Relation of plasma levels to clinical control. In *Antiepileptic Drugs,* edited by D. M. Woodbury, J. K. Penry, and R. P. Schmidt, Raven Press, New York.
17. Svensmark, O., and Buchthal, F. (1964): Diphenylhydantoin and phenobarbital serum levels in children. *Am. J. Dis. Child.,* 108:82–88.
18. Troupin, A. S., and Ojemann, L. M. (1975): Paradoxical intoxication—A complication of anticonvulsant administration. *Epilepsia,* 16:753–758.

Appendix I
Physicochemical and Pharmacological Properties of Antiepileptic Drugs

This Appendix is intended to serve as a concise summary of the relevant chemical and pharmacological properties of the most commonly used antiepileptic drugs. The information was compiled from a wide variety of sources, and the clinical data are based on reported studies in man. The pharmacological properties of many drugs, even though the drugs have been marketed for a number of years, have not been fully established in man. Thus, the data presented for certain drugs are incomplete. To conserve space, we have omitted categories for which the information is unknown. If, for example, the partition coefficient of a particular drug is not known, then that category will not appear for that drug.

The reader must bear in mind the fundamental principles related to the clinical pharmacology of antiepileptic drugs, particularly the wide variability among patients in drug utilization, therapeutic response at a given serum drug concentration, effects of multiple-drug therapy on drug utilization, and potential drug interactions. For more detailed information on specific drugs, the reader is referred to the numerous monographs and reviews that have been published on the antiepileptic drugs.

Generic name: **Carbamazepine**
Chemical name: 5H-Dibenz[b,f]azepine-5-carboxamide
Trade name: Tegretol
Molecular weight: 236.26
Melting point: 190–193°C
Conversion factor (μg/ml to μM): 4.232
Solubility in water: Insoluble
Partition Coefficient: 94 (chloroform/water at pH 3.4)

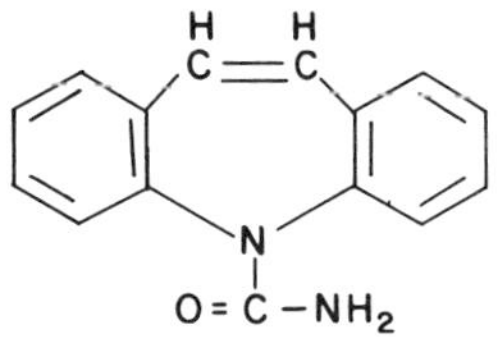

Absorption
  Time to peak: 6–18 hr
  Percentage absorbed: 70%
Protein binding
  Percentage bound: 60–73%
  Percentage unbound: 27–40%
Tissue distribution
  V_d: 0.8–1.4 liters/kg
  CSF/plasma: 0.2
  Brain/plasma: 1.0–2.3

Metabolism and excretion

Parent drug and major metabolites[a]	Active	Blood	Percent daily dose excreted in urine	
			Free	Conjugated
Carbamazepine	+	+	0.5–1.0	--
10,11-Epoxycarbamazepine	+	+	1–2	--
2-Hydroxycarbamazepine	—	--	—	2–10
3-Hydroxycarbamazepine	—	--	—	2–10
1-Hydroxycarbamazepine	—	--	—	2–10
trans-10,11-Dihydroxy-10,11-di-H-carbamazepine	—	--	—	10–30
9-Hydroxymethyl-10-carbamoylacridan	—	--	—	2–10

[a] Major metabolites of the 13 reported in the urine.
—, negative; --, unknown.

Clinical pharmacology

	Adults	Children
Recommended therapeutic dose (mg/kg)	20	20
Half-life (hr)	10–25	8.5–19
Time to reach steady state (days)	4–6	4–6
Effective levels (μg/ml)	6–10	6–10
Toxic levels (μg/ml)	>15	>15
Steady-state level expected from 1 mg/kg/day (μg/ml)	0.1–0.5	0.1–0.5

Generic name: **Clonazepam**
Chemical name: 5-(*o*-Chlorophenyl)-1,3-dihydro-7-nitro-2H-1,4-benzodiazepin-2-one
Trade name: Clonopin
Molecular weight: 315.7
Conversion factor (μg/ml to μM): 3.168
Solubility in water: Insoluble
pK_a: 10.5

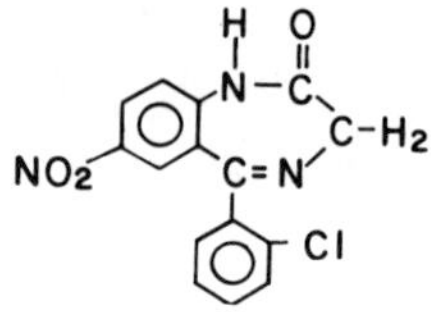

Absorption
Time to peak: 1–2 hr
Percentage absorbed: 90%
Protein binding
Percentage bound: 82%
Percentage unbound: 18%
Tissue distribution
V_d: 2.5 liters/kg

Metabolism and excretion

Parent drug and major metabolites	Active	Blood	Percent daily dose excreted in urine	
			Free	Conjugated
Clonazepam	+	+	0.1–0.5	—
7-Aminoclonazepam	—	+	2.3–18	—
7-Acetamidoclonazepam	—	+	1.2–7.8	—
3-Hydroxyclonazepam	—	--	—	—
3-Hydroxy-7-aminoclonazepam	—	--	—	—
3-Hydroxy-7-acetamidoclonazepam	—	--	—	—

—, negative; --, unknown.

Clinical pharmacology

	Adults	Children
Recommended therapeutic dose (mg/kg)	0.2	0.2
Half-life (hr)	19–46	13–33
Time to reach steady state (days)	4–6	4–5
Effective levels (μg/ml)	0.03–0.06	0.03–0.06
Toxic levels (μg/ml)	>0.08	>0.08
Steady-state level expected from 1 mg/kg/day (μg/ml)	0.03	0.03

Generic name: **Diazepam**
Chemical name: 7-Chloro-1,3-dihydro-1-methyl-5-phenyl-2H-1,4-benzodiazepin-2-one
Trade name: Valium

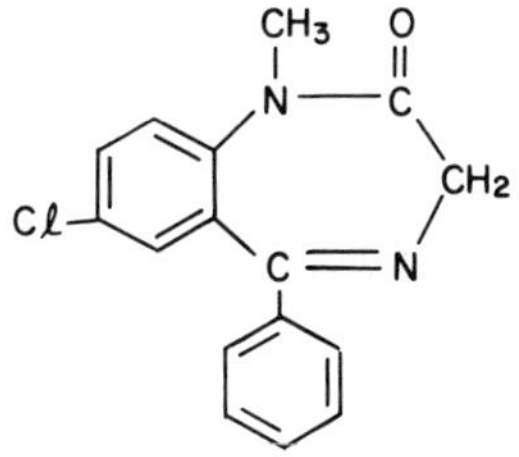

Molecular weight: 284.76
Melting point: 125–126°C
Conversion factor (μg/ml to μM): 3.511
Solubility in water: Insoluble
pK_a: 3.4
Absorption
  Time to peak: 1–2 hr
  Percentage absorbed: 90%
Protein binding
  Percentage bound: 96%
  Percentage unbound: 4%
Tissue distribution
  V_d: 1–2 liters/kg

Metabolism and excretion

Parent drug and major metabolites	Active	Blood	Percent daily dose excreted in urine	
			Free	Conjugated
Diazepam (DZP)	+	+	1–2	4
N-Desmethyldiazepam (DDZP)	+	+	—	10
N-Desmethyl-3-hydroxydiazepam	+	+	—	—
3-Hydroxydiazepam	—	—	—	—
Oxazepam	—	+	—	—
5-*p*-Hydroxyphenyldesmethyldiazepam	—	—	—	—
5-*p*-Hydroxyphenyloxazepam	—	—	—	—

Clinical pharmacology

		Adults	Children
Recommended therapeutic dose (mg/kg)		0.2–0.4	—
Half-life (hr)	DZP	20–40	18
	DDZP	60–95	—
Time to reach steady state (days)	DZP	4–6	3–5
	DDZP	15–21	15–21
Effective levels (μg/ml)	DZP	0.2–0.5	—
	DDZP	0.6–1.5	—
Toxic levels (μg/ml)	DZP	>1	>1
	DDZP	>2	—
Steady-state level expected from 1 mg/kg/day (μg/ml)	DZP	0.1	—
	DDZP	0.2	—

Generic name: **Ethosuximide**
Chemical name: 2-Ethyl-2-methylsuccinimide
Trade name: Zarontin
Molecular weight: 141.17
Melting point: 64–65°C
Conversion factor (μg/ml to μM): 7.083
Solubility in water: 190 mg/ml at 25°C, pH 3–7.9
Partition coefficient: 9 (chloroform/water at pH 4)

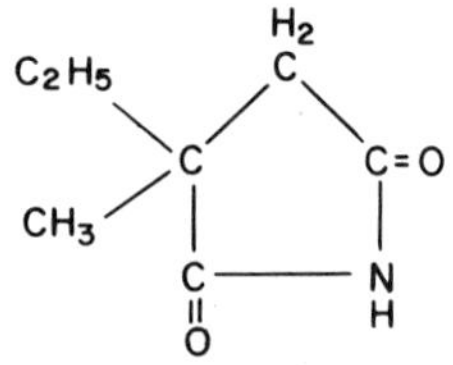

Absorption
  Time to peak: 1–2 hr
  Percentage absorbed: 100%
Protein binding
  Percentage bound: 0%
  Percentage unbound: 100%
Tissue distribution
  V_d: 0.7 liter/kg
  CSF/plasma: 1.0

Metabolism and excretion

Parent drug and major metabolites	Active	Blood	Percent daily dose excreted in urine	
			Free	Conjugated
Ethosuximide	+	+	20	—
2-Hydroxyethyl-2-methylsuccinimide	—	—	14	20

Clinical pharmacology

	Adults	Children
Recommended therapeutic dose (mg/kg)	15	20
Half-life (hr)	60	30
Time to reach steady state (days)	4–8	2–5
Effective levels (μg/ml)	40–100	40–100
Toxic levels (μg/ml)	>150	>150
Steady-state level expected from 1 mg/kg/day (μg/ml)	2–3	1–2

Generic name: **Ethotoin**
Chemical name: 3-Ethyl-5-phenylhydantoin
Trade name: Peganone
Molecular weight: 204.22
Melting point: 94°C
Conversion factor (μg/ml to μM): 4.896
Solubility in water: Slight

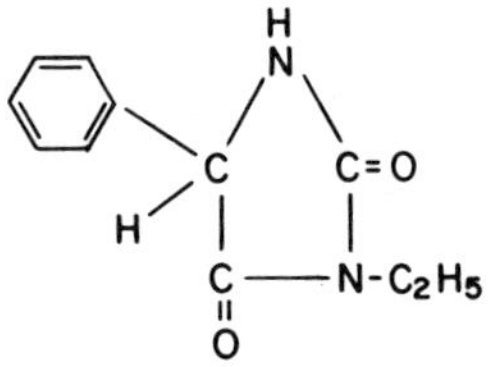

Metabolism and excretion

Parent drug and major metabolites	Active	Blood	Percent daily dose excreted in urine	
			Free	Conjugated
Ethotoin	+	+	—	—
2-Phenylhydantoic acid	—	—	—	—

Generic name: **Mephenytoin**
Chemical name: 5-Ethyl-3-methyl-5-phenylhydantoin
Trade name: Mesantoin
Molecular weight: 218.25
Melting point: 136–137°C
Conversion factor (μg/ml to μM): 4.581
Solubility in water: Insoluble
Absorption
  Time to peak: 2–4 hr
Protein Binding
  Percentage bound: 20–50%
  Percentage unbound: 50–80%
Tissue Distribution
  CSF/plasma: 0.5–0.8

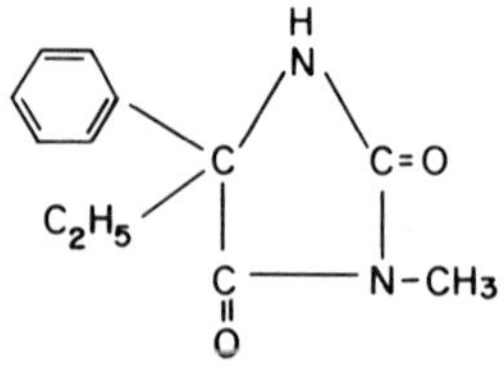

Metabolism and excretion

Parent drug and major metabolites	Active	Blood	Percent daily dose excreted in urine: Free	Conjugated
Mephenytoin (MHT)	+	+	—	—
5-Ethyl-5-phenylhydantoin (Nirvanol)	+	+	—	—
5-Ethyl-5-p-hydroxyphenylhydantoin	—	—	—	—

Clinical pharmacology

		Adults	Children
Recommended therapeutic dose (mg/kg)		5–10	3–10
Time to reach steady state (days)		5–7	—
Effective levels (μg/ml)	MHT	5–16	—
	Nirvanol	25–40	—
Toxic levels (μg/ml)	MHT	>20	—
	Nirvanol	>50	—

Generic name: **Metharbital**
Chemical name: 5,5-Diethyl-1-methyl-barbituric acid
Trade name: Gemonil
Molecular weight: 198.22
Melting point: 155°C
Conversion factor (μg/ml to μM): 5.044
Solubility in water: 1.2 mg/ml
pK_a: 8.45

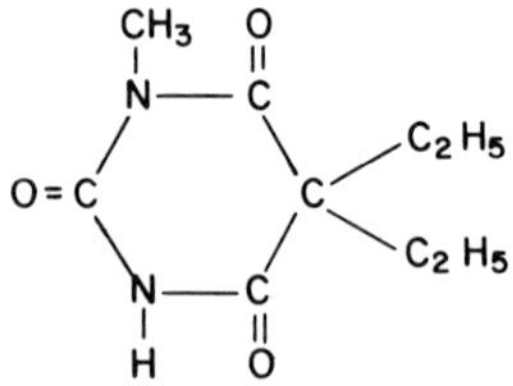

Metabolism and excretion

Parent drug and major metabolites	Active	Blood	Percent daily dose excreted in urine	
			Free	Conjugated
Metharbital	+	±	1–2	—
5,5-Diethylbarbituric acid (Barbital)	+	+	84–95	—

Generic name: **Methsuximide**
Chemical name: N,2-Dimethyl-2-phenylsuccinimide
Trade name: Celontin
Molecular weight: 203.23
Melting point: 52–53°C
Conversion factor (μg/ml to μM): 4.920
Solubility in water: 2.8 mg/ml at 25°C
Absorption
Time to peak: 1–4 hr

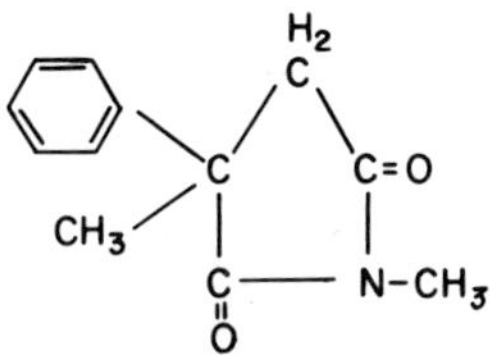

Metabolism and excretion

Parent drug and major metabolites	Active	Blood	Percent daily dose excreted in urine	
			Free	Conjugated
Methsuximide (MSM)	+	+	—	—
N-Desmethylmethsuximide (DMSM)	+	+	—	—

Clinical pharmacology

		Adults	Children
Recommended therapeutic dose (mg/kg)		20	20
Half-life (hr)	MSM	1.2–1.6	—
	DMSM	28–36	—
Time to reach steady state (days)		6–8	6–8
Effective levels (μg/ml)	MSM	0.1–1.4	0.1–1.4
	DMSM	10–40	10–40
Toxic levels (μg/ml)	MSM	—	—
	DMSM	>60	>60
Steady-state level expected from 1 mg/kg/day (μg/ml)	MSM	—	—
	DMSM	1.62	—

Generic name: **Methylphenobarbital**
Chemical name: 5-Ethyl-1-methyl-5-phenylbarbituric acid
Trade name: Mebaral
Molecular weight: 246.26
Melting point: 178°C
Conversion factor (μg/ml to μM): 4.060
pK_a: 7.8
Absorption
Time to peak: 5 hr
Percentage absorbed: 50–60%

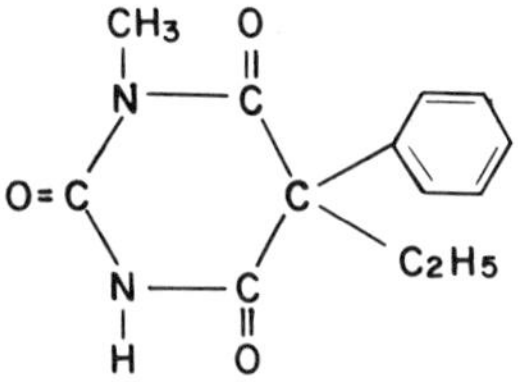

Metabolism and excretion

Parent drug and major metabolites	Active	Blood	Percent daily dose excreted in urine: Free	Percent daily dose excreted in urine: Conjugated
Methylphenobarbital (MPB)	+	+	0.8	—
Phenobarbital (PB)	+	+	50	—
p-Hydroxyphenobarbital	—	—	5–10	20–40

Clinical pharmacology

		Adults	Children
Recommended therapeutic dose (μg/ml)		10	10
Half-life (hr)	MPB	1–3	—
	PB	50–150	40–70
Time to reach steady state (days)	MPB	—	—
	PB	14–21	—
Effective levels (μg/ml)	MPB	—	—
	PB	20–40	15–40
Steady-state level expected from 1 mg/kg/day (μg/ml)	MPB	—	—
	PB	2	—

Generic name: **Paramethadione**
Chemical name: 5-Ethyl-3,5-dimethyl-oxazolidine-2,4-dione
Trade name: Paradione
Molecular weight: 157.17
Specific gravity: 1.118
Conversion factor (μg/ml to μM): 6.362
Solubility in water: Slight

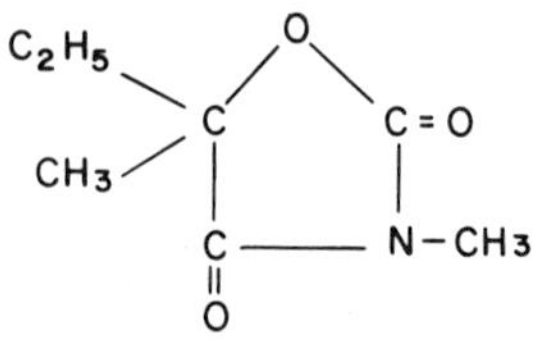

Metabolism and excretion

Parent drug and major metabolites	Active	Blood	Percent daily dose excreted in urine	
			Free	Conjugated
Paramethadione	+	+	—	—
5-Ethyl-5-methyloxazolidine-2,4-dione	+	+	—	—

Generic name: **Phenacemide**
Chemical name: 1-(2-Phenylacetyl)-urea
Trade name: Phenurone
Molecular weight: 178.19
Melting point: 212–216°C
Conversion factor (μg/ml to μM): 5.611
Solubility in water: Slight
Absorption
  Time to peak: 3–5 hr

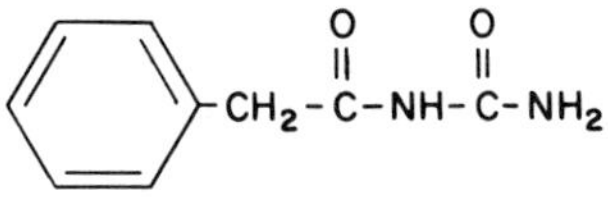

Metabolism and excretion

Parent drug and major metabolites	Active	Blood	Percent daily dose excreted in urine	
			Free	Conjugated
Phenacemide	+	+	—	—
p-Hydroxyphenacemide	—	—	100	—

Generic name: **Phenobarbital**
Chemical name: 5-Ethyl-5-phenylbarbituric acid
Trade name: Luminal
Molecular weight: 232.23
Melting point: 176°C
Conversion factor (μg/ml to μM): 4.306
Solubility in water: Phenobarbital sodium, freely soluble; free acid, sparingly
pK_a: 7.3
Partition coefficient: 4.2 (chloroform/water at pH 3.4)
Absorption
  Time to peak: 6–18 hr
  Percentage absorbed: 80%
Protein binding
  Percentage bound: 45–50%
  Percentage unbound: 50–55%
Tissue distribution
  V_d: 0.7 liter/kg
  CSF/plasma: 0.5
  Brain/plasma: 0.9–1.0

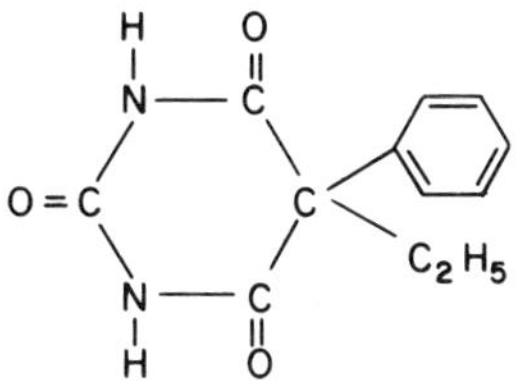

Metabolism and excretion

Parent drug and major metabolites	Active	Blood	Percent daily dose excreted in urine: Free	Conjugated
Phenobarbital	+	+	10–30	—
p-Hydroxyphenobarbital	—	—	5–10	20–40
N-Hydroxyphenobarbital	--	--	20–30	—

—, negative; --, unknown.

Clinical pharmacology

	Adults	Children
Recommended therapeutic dose (mg/kg)	2	4
Half-life (hr)	50–120	40–70
Time to reach steady state (days)	14–21	10–18
Effective levels (μg/ml)	20–40	15–40
Toxic levels (μg/ml)	>50	>50
Steady-state level expected from 1 mg/kg/day (μg/ml)	10	5

Generic name: **Phensuximide**
Chemical name: N-Methyl-2-phenylsuccinimide
Trade name: Milontin
Molecular weight: 189.21
Melting point: 71–73°C
Conversion factor (μg/ml to μM): 5.285
Solubility in water: 4.2 mg/ml at 25°C
Absorption
Time to peak: 1–4 hr

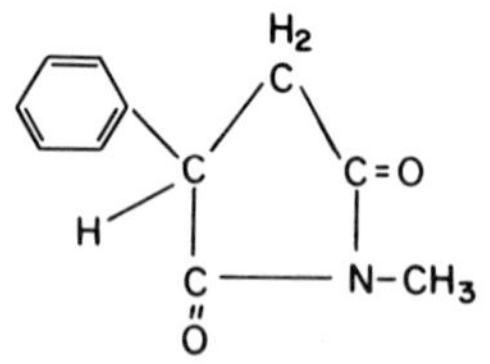

Metabolism and excretion

Parent drug and major metabolites	Active	Blood	Percent daily dose excreted in urine: Free	Conjugated
Phensuximide (PSM)	+	+	—	—
N-Desmethylphensuximide (DPSM)	+	+	—	—
2-Phenylsuccinamic acid	—	--	—	—

Clinical pharmacology

		Adults	Children
Recommended therapeutic dose (mg/kg)		20–40	—
Half-life (hr)	PSM	6–8.5	—
	DPSM	6–8.5	—
Time to reach steady state (days)		2–4	2–4

Generic name: **Phenytoin**
Chemical name: 5,5-Diphenylhydantoin
Trade name: Dilantin
Molecular weight: 252.26
Melting point: 295–298°C
Conversion factor (μg/ml to μM): 3.964
Solubility in water: 14 μg/ml at pH 1–7 (free acid, 165 μg/ml at pH 9.1; phenytoin sodium, highly soluble at alkaline pH)
pK_a: 8.3
Partition coefficient: 28.8 (chloroform/water at pH 3.4)

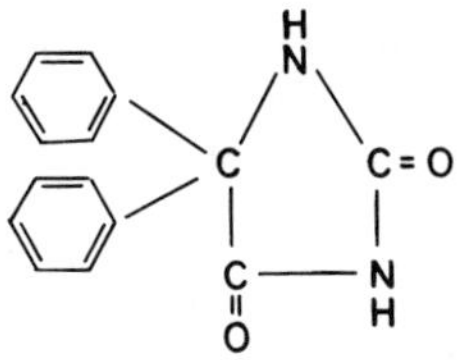

Absorption
Time to peak: 4–8 hr
Percentage absorbed: 90%
Protein binding
Percentage bound: 87–93%
Percentage unbound: 7–13%
Tissue distribution
V_d: 0.5–0.8 liter/kg
CSF/plasma: 0.1
Brain/plasma: 1.2–1.6

Metabolism and excretion

Parent drug and major metabolites	Active	Blood	Percent daily dose excreted in urine: Free	Percent daily dose excreted in urine: Conjugated
Phenytoin	+	+	1–5	—
5-(4-Hydroxyphenyl)-5-phenylhydantoin (HPPH)	−	+	10	50–70
5-(3,4-Dihydroxyphenyl)-5-phenylhydantoin	−	−	—	—
5-(3-o-Methyl-4-hydroxyphenyl)-5-phenylhydantoin	−	−	—	—

Clinical pharmacology

	Adults	Children
Recommended therapeutic dose (mg/kg)	5	5–8
Half-life (hr)	22	18–22
Time to reach steady state (days)	5–7	5–7
Effective levels (μg/ml)	10–20	5–20
Toxic levels (μg/ml)	>25	>25
Steady-state level expected from 1 mg/kg/day (μg/ml)	2–3	1–2

Generic name: **Primidone**
Chemical name: 5-Ethyldihydro-5-phenyl-4,6(1H,5H)-pyrimidinedione
Trade name: Mysoline
Molecular weight: 218.25
Melting point: 182°C
Conversion factor (μg/ml to μM): 4.581
Solubility in water: 600 μg/ml at 37°C
Partition coefficient: 0.7 (chloroform/water at pH 3.4)
Absorption
  Time to peak: 2–4 hr
Protein binding
  Percentage bound: 0–30%
  Percentage unbound: 70–100%
Tissue distribution
  V_d: 0.6 liter/kg
  CSF/plasma: 0.7–1.1
  Brain/plasma: 0.87

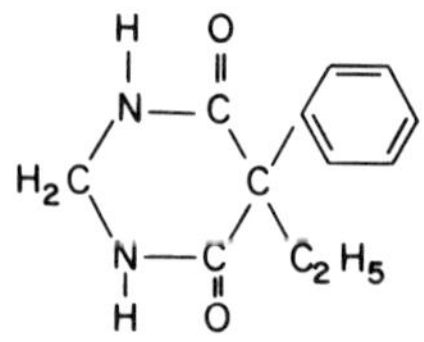

Metabolism and excretion

Parent drug and major metabolites	Active	Blood	Percent daily dose excreted in urine	
			Free	Conjugated
Primidone (PRM)	+	+	20–40	—
Phenobarbital (PB)	+	+	2–5	—
Phenylethylmalonamide (PEMA)	+	+	10–30	—
p-Hydroxyphenobarbital	—	—	2.5–5	2.5–5

Clinical pharmacology

		Adults	Children
Recommended therapeutic dose (mg/kg)		20	20
Half-life (hr)		6–8	—
Time to reach steady state (days)		2–3	2–3
Effective levels (μg/ml)		8–12	8–12
Toxic levels (μg/ml)		>15	>15
Steady-state level expected from 1 mg/kg/day (μg/ml)	PRM	0.5–0.7	0.5–0.7
	PB	1–4	0.5–2
	PEMA	1–2	—

Generic name: **Trimethadione**
Chemical name: 3,5,5-Trimethyl-oxazolidine-2,4-dione
Trade name: Tridione
Molecular weight: 143.15
Melting point: 46°C
Conversion factor (μg/ml to μM): 6.985 (DMO, 7.744)
Solubility in water: Sparingly
pK_a: (DMO, 6.15)
Absorption
  Time to peak: 0.5–1 hr
Protein binding
  Percentage bound: 0%
  Percentage unbound: 100%

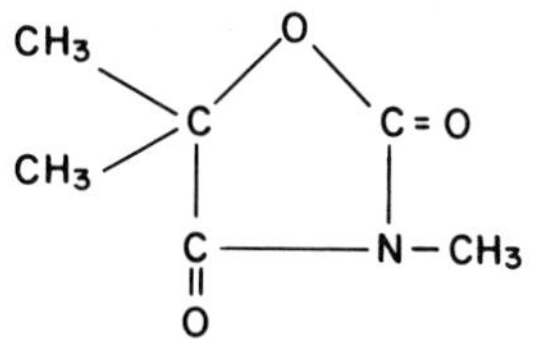

Metabolism and excretion

Parent drug and major metabolites	Active	Blood	Percent daily dose excreted in urine: Free	Percent daily dose excreted in urine: Conjugated
Trimethadione (TMO)	+	+	2–4	—
Dimethadione (DMO)	+	+	96	—

Clinical pharmacology

		Adults	Children
Recommended therapeutic dose (mg/kg)		30	30
Half-life (hr)	TMO	16–20	—
	DMO	240	—
Time to reach steady state (days)	TMO	4–7	4–7
	DMO	50–75	—
Effective levels (μg/ml)	TMO	20	20
	DMO	>700	>700
Toxic levels (μg/ml)	TMO	—	—
	DMO	>1,500	>1,500
Steady-state level expected from 1 mg/kg/day (μg/ml)	TMO	0.6	—
	DMO	12	—

Appendix II
Methodology and Sources

The first section of this Appendix contains detailed instructions for the performance of antiepileptic drug determinations by gas-liquid chromatography, using different methodologies. The publication of these techniques in a central source should provide easy and rapid access to procedures scattered throughout the literature, thereby helping laboratories to assess and compare the three most commonly used methodologies for antiepileptic drug analysis by gas-liquid chromatography.

Because of the many analytical pitfalls associated with the quantitation of carbamazepine by GLC on-column methylation procedures, we have included two different techniques for its determination. Also, the widespread use of mephenytoin (Mesantoin) in certain parts of the country has led to the inclusion of instructions for its determination by flash-heater ethylation. This section also includes a description of techniques that can be utilized in any laboratory for the preparation of appropriate internal standards.

In the next section, space prevents listing all commercial sources for the numerous items commonly used in antiepileptic drug assays. We have, however, included sources of commercially available antiepileptic drug controls in a biological matrix, sources for drug metabolites and internal standards, and instructions for obtaining commercially unavailable drugs and metabolites, which the laboratory may require for development of new assays.

A. Methodology

Phenobarbital, Carbamazepine, Primidone, and Phenytoin: Simultaneous Determination with On-Column Methylation (TMPAH)

Donald W. Sichler and C. E. Pippenger

PRINCIPLE

Phenobarbital, carbamazepine, primidone, and phenytoin are quantitated by an on-column methylation technique, using trimethylphenylammonium hydroxide (TMPAH). The drugs are extracted from plasma specimens into chloroform, and the extracts are washed with hexane to remove normal plasma constituents that could interfere with drug analysis.

PROCEDURE

1. To 1.0 ml of plasma (or standard) in a 13-ml centrifuge tube add 1.0 ml of 0.25 N HCl and mix by brief vortexing.

2. Add 6 ml of chloroform extracting solution, stopper with a Teflon stopper, and shake for 15 min on a Fisher Roto-Rack (speed setting on Roto-Rack = 9).
3. Filter through prewashed phase-separating filter paper (Whatman 1 PS 12.5 cm).
4. Discard the aqueous layer and evaporate the chloroform layer completely to dryness (Buchler Vortex Evaporatory Block Temp. 40°C).
5. To the dried $CHCl_3$ residue first add 2.0 ml of methanol followed by 1.0 ml of 0.25 N HCl and mix on Vortex mixer.
6. To the methanol-HCl mixture add 6 ml of hexane, stopper with a Teflon stopper, and shake for 10 min on Fisher Roto-Rack.
7. Aspirate the hexane layer (top layer) from the sample and discard.
8. To the remaining aqueous layer, add 6 ml of *pure* chloroform (no internal standards) and shake for 15 min on Fisher Roto-Rack.
9. Centrifuge the samples for 10 min at 2,500 rpm.
10. Completely remove the aqueous layer (top layer) and evaporate the remaining chloroform *completely* to dryness in the Vortex Evaporator.
11. To the dried residue add 0.1 ml of 0.2 M TMPAH and Vortex for at least 15 sec. The samples are now ready to be injected onto the gas chromatograph.

GAS CHROMATOGRAPH OPERATING PARAMETERS

Column: 6 ft × 2 mm i.d. glass
5% OV-17 on Gas Chrom Q, 80–100 mesh. Columns conditioned at 270°C for 48 hr prior to use with nitrogen flow.
Temperatures:
Injection port, 270°C
Column, 210°C
Detector, 290°C
Carrier gas: Nitrogen at a flow rate of 40 ml/min (secondary stage regulator at 35 psi).

REAGENTS

1. *0.25 N HCl:* 20.8 ml concentrated HCl diluted to 1,000 ml with distilled water.
2. *Chloroform:* Spectroanalyzed Fisher Scientific.
3. *Methanol:* Spectroanalyzed Fisher Scientific.
4. *Hexanes:* Spectroanalyzed Fisher Scientific.
5. *Internal standards:*
   (a) S_1-5-(*p*-Methylphenyl-5-phenylhydantoin, Aldrich Chemical Co.
   (b) S_2-5-Ethyl-5-*p*-Tolylbarbituric acid, Aldrich Chemical Co.
6. *Internal standard stock solution:* To a 500-ml volumetric flask add 50 mg of S_1 and 50 mg of S_2 q.s. to volume with chloroform. The final concentration of each internal standard is 100 μg/ml. The solution is transferred to and stored in a tightly capped amber glass bottle.
7. *Extracting solution:* Dilute 25 ml of internal standard stock solution to 500 ml with chloroform. The final concentration is 5 μg/ml of each internal standard. The total concentration of each internal standard in the plasma extracts is 30 μg/ml.
8. *Trimethylphenylammonium iodide,* obtained from Eastman Organic Chemicals, is recrystallized once from methanol prior to use.
9. *0.2 M Trimethylphenylammonium hydroxide (TMPAH):* Weigh 3.47 g of silver oxide (Fisher Scientific) and 5.26 g of trimethylphenylammonium iodide

into a 250-ml glass-stoppered Erlenmeyer flask. Add 100 ml of absolute methanol and a Teflon stirring bar. Place on a magnetic stirrer and stir for 2.5 hr.

(a) After mixing, the glass-stoppered Erlenmeyer flask containing TMPAH is stored in the refrigerator (4°C) over the silver oxide powder. This solution is stable for at least 1 month.

(b) If small quantities of TMPAH are used infrequently, it is advisable to make up smaller volumes of TMPAH at more frequent intervals.

(c) TMPAH supernatant (liquid above Ag_20) can be used directly or a small quantity can be filtered through Whatman no. 1 paper immediately prior to use.

(d) Water enhances the decomposition of various compounds in the presence of TMPAH; therefore, care should be taken to ensure that no moisture is present in the sample which is to be analyzed.

COMMENTS

1. The method described here is a modification of the Kupferberg method (*Clin. Chem. Acta,* 29:283–288, 1970) and is designed to process 20 to 40 patient samples per day. Although this method requires several extraction steps, it provides "clean" chromatograms. The hexane wash is essential to remove interfering lipids present in plasma. Attempts to eliminate certain steps in order to shorten the extraction time have resulted in chromatograms with interfering peaks.
2. It is imperative that both internal standards be utilized in the extraction. The erratic decomposition of phenobarbital in TMPAH has been well established. The only satisfactory method of correcting for this decomposition is to calculate phenobarbital concentrations with respect to *p*-tolylphenobarbital as the internal standard. As new internal standards become available for other drugs, such as primidone and carbamazepine, they should also be incorporated into this procedure.
3. Carbamazepine decomposes during flash methylation in TMPAH to iminostilbene (Rogers et al., *Clin. Chem.,* 19:590, 1973). We have found this decomposition to be related directly to the alkaline properties of TMPAH and to the method of injection of the specimen. With Hewlett-Packard automatic injection systems, the conversion of carbamazepine to iminostilbene is reproducible and can be utilized for quantitation. However, manual injection of carbamazepine in TMPAH *does not* result in reproducible conversion to iminostilbene. We *do not* recommend quantitation of carbamazepine following manual injection of the drug in TMPAH until an appropriate internal standard becomes available.
4. Teflon stoppers are recommended throughout the assay because glass-stoppered centrifuge tubes have a tendency to leak at the joint. *Do not* use stopcock grease on glass stoppers to prevent leaks. Stopcock grease is soluble in chloroform and will be carried through the extraction, giving numerous interfering peaks on the gas chromatograph.
5. Impurities that are present on the phase-separating filter paper are extracted by chloroform. These impurities can be removed by prewashing the phase-separating paper with chloroform and discarding the chloroform wash. Place 10 to 20 filters in a Buchler funnel connected to a suction flask. Pour 200 ml of chloroform over the filters. Remove the filters and dry at room temperature.
6. It is essential that the final chloroform layer be evaporated *completely* to dryness. The presence of water in any sample will cause an enhanced decomposition of phenobarbital in the presence of methylating agent.

7. Samples can be injected manually onto the gas chromatograph. Using a 10-μl Hamilton Syringe with Kel-F Guide, draw 1 or 2 μl of sample into syringe, wipe syringe needle with a Kimwipe, draw the plunger back so that all of the sample is visible in the barrel of the syringe, and then inject onto GLC column. After injection thoroughly rinse the syringe (at least 10 times) with solvent before proceeding to the next sample.

Phenytoin, Phenobarbital, Primidone, and Ethosuximide: Simultaneous Determination with On-Column Methylation (TMAH)

Elizabeth B. Solow

PRINCIPLE

Serum containing drugs is buffered with 0.3 M phosphate and is extracted with toluene containing internal standards. The anionic drugs and internal standards are extracted and concentrated from the solvent phase with a small quantity of a strong base, a methanolic solution of tetramethylammonium hydroxide (TMAH). A small aliquot of this final concentrated extract is injected into the gas chromatograph using the heated vaporizer of the instrument as a reaction chamber.

REAGENTS

1. *Phosphate buffer, 3 M:* Dissolve 414 g of sodium monobasic phosphate ($NaH_2PO_4 \cdot H_2O$) in 800 ml of deionized water contained in a liter volumetric flask. Dilute to volume with deionized water and mix well.
2. *Phosphate buffer, 0.3 M:* Dilute 100 ml of the 3 M buffer to a liter volume with deionized water.
3. *Tetramethylammonium hydroxide (TMAH):* 2 M in methanol (Cat. No. 705, Southwestern Analytical Chemicals, Austin, TX 78767). Refrigerate stock bottles of this reagent. Remove a small quantity each day and use this at normal room temperature.
4. *Toluene:* Analytical reagent grade.
5. *Reference compounds:* 5,5-Diphenylhydantoin (DPH), 5-(*p*-methylphenyl)-5-phenylhydantoin (MPPH), 5-ethyl-5-*p*-tolylbarbituric acid (MP), and α, α-dimethyl-β-succinimide (AA) (Aldrich Chemical Co., Inc., Milwaukee, WI 53233).

   5-Ethyl-5-phenylbarbituric acid (phenobarbital) (P) (Applied Science Laboratories, State College, PA 16801).

   5-Ethyl-5-phenylhexahydropyrimidine-4,6-dione, (primidone) (MY) (Ayerst Laboratories, New York, NY 10017).

   2-Ethyl-2-methylsuccinimide (ethosuximide) (Z) (Parke, Davis, and Co., Ann Arbor, MI 48106).

6. *Extraction reagents:*
   (a) Toluene containing internal standards MP and MPPH: To a liter volumetric flask add 5 mg of 5-ethyl-5-*p*-tolylbarbituric acid (MP) and 3 mg of 5-(*p*-methylphenyl)-5-phenylhydantoin (MPPH). Add toluene to the flask to dissolve the reference compounds and then dilute to volume with toluene. This solution now contains 25 μg of MP and 15 μg of MPPH per 5 ml of volume.
   (b) Toluene containing internal standards AA, MP, and MPPH: To a liter volumetric flask add 10 mg of α, α-dimethyl-β-methylsuccinimide (AA) and dilute to volume with toluene-MP-MPPH as prepared above. Mix well. This solution now contains 50 μg of AA, 25 μg of MP, and 15 μg of MPPH per 5 ml of volume.
7. *Stock solution of drugs:*
   (a) 5,5-Diphenylhydantoin (DPH) in ethanol, 10 mg/ml: Into a 10-ml volumetric flask weigh 100 mg of DPH, dissolve in ethanol and dilute to volume with the alcohol.
   (b) Phenobarbital (P), 10 mg/ml: Into a separate 10-ml volumetric flask weigh 100 mg of phenobarbital. Dissolve in ethanol and dilute to volume with alcohol.
   (c) Primidone (MY), 2 mg/ml: Into another 10-ml volumetric flask weigh 20 mg of primidone. Dissolve this in ethanol and dilute to volume with alcohol. *Store all the above stock ethanolic drugs at room temperature.*
   (d) Ethosuximide (Z), 10 mg/ml: Weigh 100 mg of ethosuximide into a 10-ml volumetric flask. Dissolve this drug in deionized water and dilute to volume with the water. Store this solution in the refrigerator.

INSTRUMENTATION

Column Specifications

Use a glass column, 180cm × 2 mm i.d., packed with 5% OV-17 w/w on Gas Chrom Q, 100/120 mesh (Applied Science Laboratories, State College, PA 16801).

Condition a new column by using a nitrogen flow of 40 ml/min and an oven temperature according to the following program: 1 hr at 250°C, 4 hr at 325°C, then overnight at 250°C.

Septa or disks used with the columns should be specifically designed for high-temperature conditions for minimal bleed characteristics (Applied Science Laboratories, State College, PA 16801).

Should columns require ferrule-swagelox connections, the graphite ferrules with an upper limit of 450°C should be used in order to decrease maintenance problems of the chromatograph (Supelco, Inc., Bellefonte, PA 16823).

OPERATING CONDITIONS

Injection port: Control the temperature at a constant setting. Depending on the design of the heated zone, this could be selected as low as 270°C or as high as 350°C.

Detector temperature: Depending on the physical design of the detector in relationship to the column, set the temperature at a constant setting 280 to 300°C.

Oven temperatures: for phenobarbital, primidone, and phenytoin, an isothermal mode of operation is preferable. Set the controls at an appropriate temperature for good separation of compounds, possibly 230 or 240°C. For ethosuximide an oven temperature of 100 or 110°C is suggested. A temperature-programmed mode is also acceptable for the above drugs being analyzed. Standardization must be carefully checked for each chromatographic system whether isothermal or programmed mode.

Flow rate of gases: Set flow valves controls as follows: nitrogen, 20 ml/min; air, 400 ml/min; and hydrogen 40 ml/min.

COLLECTION AND HANDLING OF SPECIMENS

Disposable vacuum containers or plastic tubes without anticoagulant are preferred for collection of blood samples. However, blood collected in tubes containing sodium fluoride, ethylenediaminetetraacetic acid, or heparin can be processed satisfactorily with this method.

Hemolysis should be avoided because red cells contribute to a minor increase in the quantity of DPH in serum. Red cells do not contribute to alteration of the phenobarbital results.

After centrifugation and separation of the serum from the clotted blood, the serum when stored in a refrigerator is stable for a week before processing. In a frozen state serum samples are stable for many months.

PROCEDURE

Preparation of Stock Plasma Standards

1. Phenytoin (DPH), 100 μg/ml: Deliver blood bank plasma to approximately half-full level of a 100-ml volumetric flask. Pipette 1.0 ml of the stock DPH solution to the plasma, slowly adding this alcoholic solution to the plasma, taking great care to prevent entrapment of the drug in denatured protein particles. Add more plasma to final volume and mix well. Add a minute drop of caprylic acid to the flask to eliminate the protein foam.
2. Phenobarbital (P), 100 μg/ml: Deliver plasma to another 100-ml volumetric flask, and add 1 ml of stock phenobarbital solution to this flask. Use the same delivery of alcoholic standard as described above for DPH standard. Also add a drop of caprylic alcohol. Add more plasma to the volumetric mark and mix thoroughly.
3. Plasma standard A, 10 μg of DPH and 30 μg of P/ml: Combine 10 ml of DPH standard 1 and 30 ml of P standard 2 in a 100-ml volumetric flask. Dilute to the volume mark with plasma and mix well.
4. Plasma standard B, μg of DPH and 30 μg of P/ml: Combine 20 ml of DPH standard 1 and 30 ml of standard 2 in a 100-ml volumetric flask. Dilute to volume and mix well.
5. Plasma standard C, 100 μg of ethosuximide (Z)/ml. Deliver 1 ml of stock solution of ethosuximide to a 100-ml volumetric flask. Dilute to volume with plasma and mix well.
6. Separately pipet 2 ml aliquots of plasma standards A, B, and C into stoppered tubes and place them in an upright position in a freezer (−20°C).

PROCEDURE FOR SERUM OR PLASMA EXTRACTIONS

Procedure A: Patient Sample

1. Add 1 ml of each serum or reference plasma standard to labeled 10-ml glass-stoppered conical centrifuge tubes.
2. Add 0.5 ml of phosphate buffer, 0.3 M, from an automatic dispensing pipette.

3. Add 5 ml of toluene containing appropriate internal standards from an automatic Machlett pipette equipped with a Teflon plug (Cat. No. 13,690-2a, Fisher Scientific Co., Pittsburgh, PA 15238). Stopper and shake thoroughly. Complete the extraction with a vortex-type mixer.
4. Centrifuge the tubes in a clinical model centrifuge (DYNAC, No. 0101, Clay-Adams, Div. of Becton, Dickinson and Co., Parsippany, NJ 07054), to separate the aqueous from the toluene extract phase.
5. Transfer the supernatant solvent phase to a Concentratube® (Laboratory Research Co., P.O. Box 36509, Los Angeles, CA 90863).
6. Add 25 μl of TMAH from an automatic pipette with a disposable polyethylene tip (Medical Laboratory Automation, Inc., Mt. Vernon, NY 10550). Tilt the tube and add this reagent close to the surface of the solvent. Stopper immediately and shake vigorously with a vortex-type mixer.
7. Centrifuge the mixture for 5 min in a clinical model centrifuge at maximum speed. The nippled tip on the tube is protected from breakage with a single-hole rubber stopper inserted to the bottom of a completely rubber-lined cushion for a 50-ml centrifuge shield.
8. Inject 1 or 2 μl of the TMAH phase from the bottom of the Concentratube® into the chromatograph. Inject less than 1 μl if unusually high drug values are obtained and a repeat injection is required.

Procedure B: Microadaptation

1. For a small serum sample, pipette 200 μl of *unknown* sample, 100 μl of phosphate buffer, and 1 ml of toluene containing internal standards into a glass-stoppered 2-ml volumetric flask. Follow the procedures as described above except for the addition of TMAH. Pipette 10 μl of TMAH to the surface of the toluene extraction mixture, and then mix well as described previously. Inject 2 to 3 μl of the TMAH phase into the chromatograph using the same attenuation on the electrometer.

   AA-internal standard elutes before ethosuximide. Phenobarbital, MP-internal standard, primidone, phenytoin, and MPPH-internal standard elute from the column in this order.

CALCULATIONS

1. Determine the peak height of each compound with the aid of a triangulator (Chemical Research Services, Inc., Addison, Ill. 60101). Read the peak height (mm) scale.
2. Calculate peak height ratio of P/MP, MY/MPPH, DPH/MPPH, and Z/AA.
3. For the graph identify the ordinate as peak height ratio and the abscissa as known amount of drug in micrograms per milliliter of serum. Plot the ratio for each point of DPH, P, and MY for both standard A and standard B, and standard C. Draw an appropriate line through zero for each drug. For the unknown results refer to the calibration curve for the individual peak height ratio. It is advisable that for each gas chromatographic system, linearity of the calibration curve be checked from 0 to 150 μg/ml for ethosuximide, 0 to 100 μg/ml for phenobarbital, 0 to 60 μg/ml for phenytoin, and 0 to 40 μg/ml for primidone.

PRECISION

At the level of 15 μg/ml for phenytoin the coefficient of variation (CV) of the assay is 3.1% between runs. For the 25-μg/ml level for phenobarbital the CV is 1.8%, and for primidone at the level of 10 μg/ml the CV is 6.1%.

INTERFERING SUBSTANCES

With isothermal mode for column temperature, glutethimide cannot be separated from phenobarbital by this method. The metabolite of mephobarbital is extracted and calculated as phenobarbital. Mephenytoin extracts with its method as the metabolite and when methylated it is the same as the parent compound and may interfere with the accuracy of phenobarbital calculations. However, at lower oven temperatures mephenytoin can be resolved from phenobarbital.

Phenobarbital, Primidone, and Phenytoin: Simultaneous Determination Without Derivatization

Harold E. Booker and Barbara A. Darcey

PRINCIPLE

The drugs are extracted from serum under acidic conditions and back-extracted into base to separate from neutral drugs. After reextraction into chloroform, the extracts are evaporated to dryness to concentrate the drugs. The extract residue is reconstituted using a suitable solvent and an aliquot is used for gas chromatography.

REAGENTS

1. *Hydrochloric acid:* 0.5 M and 6 M.
2. *Sodium hydroxide:* 0.5 M.
3. *Chloroform:* high purity (i.e., Nanograde, Mallinckrodt, St. Louis, MO 63147 or distilled in glass, Burdick & Jackson, Muskegon, MI 49442).
4. *Internal standards:* 5 ethyl-5-*p*-tolylbarbituric acid and 5-*p*-methylphenyl-5-phenylhydantoin (MPPH) (Aldrich Chemical, Milwaukee, WI 53233).
   a. Stock solutions of internal standard: Dissolve 25 mg of MPPH in methanol and dilute to 10 ml. Store in refrigerator. Dissolve 50 mg of 5-ethyl-5-*p*-tolylbarbituric acid in methanol and dilute to 10 ml. Store in refrigerator.
   b. Working internal standard solution: Transfer 1 ml of stock MPPH and 1 ml of stock 5-ethyl-5-*p*-tolylbarbituric acid solution to a 100-ml volumetric flask and dilute to 100 ml with water. Be sure that compounds are in solution. Solution should be clear. It is stable at room temperature for at least 4 weeks.
5. *Standards:* Compounds must be pure and anhydrous. Store dried compounds in a dessicator. Carefully weigh 100 mg of phenobarbital, 100 mg of phenytoin, and 50 mg of primidone. Dissolve in methanol and dilute to 100 ml. This solution is stable for several weeks if refrigerated tightly stoppered to prevent evaporation of the alcohol. Warm to room temperature before preparing working standards.

   Prepare serum standards with pooled negative serum.

Stock standard	Serum (ml)	Concentration (mg/liter)		
		Phenobarbital	DPH	Primidone
1	24	40	40	20
1	49	20	20	10
1	99	10	10	5

These standards are stable for at least a week. Store in refrigerator. Do not freeze as the drugs do not stay in solution.

Alternative preparation of aqueous standard:

32.6 mg of sodium phenytoin = 30 mg of DPH
54.7 mg of sodium phenobarbital = 50 mg of Pbt.
20 mg of primidone

Transfer to a 1-liter volumetric flask and add about 800 ml of water. Mix on a magnetic stirrer for several hours. Dilute to 1 liter. Store in refrigerator in amber glass. Prepare fresh once a month.

To prepare the standard curve:

ml of stock standard	Concentration (mg/liter)		
	Phenobarbital	DPH	Primidone
0.5	50	30	20
0.3	30	18	12
0.1	10	6	4

Transfer the 0.5, 0.3, and 0.1 ml of stock standard to 15-ml glass-stoppered centrifuge tubes. Add 0.5 ml of pooled negative serum and proceed as for unknowns.

Alternatively, use commercially available antiepileptic drug standards (Syva Corp. Palo Alto, CA 94309).

PROCEDURE

Prepare standards with every run of unknowns.

Transfer 0.5 ml of serum, 0.5 ml of HCl (0.5 M), and 0.5 ml of internal standard working solution to 15-ml glass-stoppered centrifuge tubes. Add 10 ml of chloroform and shake vigorously for 1 to 2 min. Centrifuge the tubes for 5 min at 1,500 rpm. Aspirate the top aqueous phase and carefully decant the chloroform to a clean 15-ml glass-stoppered tube.

Add 2.5 ml of sodium hydroxide (0.5 M) and shake for 1 to 2 min. Centrifuge for 5 min. Transfer the aqueous alkaline phase to a clean 15-ml glass-stoppered tube using a Pasteur pipette. Do not disturb the chloroform layer.

Add 0.3 ml of HCl (6 M). The aqueous phase must be acidic at this point. The concentrations of the acid and base are critical only to assure that the amount of acid added is sufficient to accomplish this.

Add 5 ml of chloroform. Shake for 1 to 2 min and centrifuge for 5 min. Aspirate the aqueous phase. Decant the chloroform to a plain 15-ml centrifuge tube. Evaporate to dryness under a gentle stream of clean, dry air or nitrogen in a water bath or Temp-Blok Heater at 50 to 60°C. Wash down the sides of the tubes with 50 μl of chloroform to concentrate the extract in the tip. Dry. Dissolve the dried residue in solvent (chloroform, carbon disulfide, methanol, or ethyl acetate) 50 μl. Use 2 to 3 μl for gas chromatography (if greater sensitivity is needed, dissolve the extract in 20 μl of solvent).

GAS CHROMATOGRAPHIC CONDITIONS

Column: 180 cm × 2 mm i.d. glass column packed with 3% OV-17 on Chromosorb W. H.P. 80 to 100 mesh. Columns are conditioned at least 3 hr at 290°C.

Column temperature, 260°C
Flash heater temperature, 290°C
Detector temperature, 290°C

Approximate retention times: Phenobarbital, 2.5 min; 5-ethyl-*p*-tolylbarbituric acid, 3.5; primidone, 7.5; DPH, 8.5; MPPH, 10.

Carrier gas flow is 40 ml/min.

Calibration Curves

Phenobarbital standards: Plot peak height of phenobarbital/peak height of 5-ethyl-5-*p*-tolylbarbituric acid versus concentration of phenobarbital for each standard.

Primidone standards: Plot peak height of primidone/peak height of MPPH versus concentration of primidone.

Phenytoin standards: Plot peak height of DPH/peak height of MPPH versus concentration of DPH.

For unknowns: Calculate peak height of unknown/peak height of internal standard.

Read concentrations from respective calibration curve.

COMMENTS

The addition of methanol to serum in the preparation of the working standards causes some precipitation of proteins. Mix thoroughly to ensure complete solution of the proteins.

Standards must be done with every run of unknowns. Inject the standards before the unknowns. Inject at least one standard after the last unknown. If more than 8 to 10 unknowns are done in one run, inject a standard midway through the run. If the solvent used to redissolve the standard extract has evaporated, add another drop.

If the column has been used for succinimides or other drugs that elute at a lower temperature, condition the column at 260°C for at least 1 hr before attempting to do phenobarbital, primidone, or phenytoin.

If a patient is on mephenytoin, its metabolite 5,5-phenylethylhydantoin (Nirvanol) will elute from the column very close to phenobarbital. It is advisable to keep an alcohol solution of Nirvanol on hand to inject into the column in order to determine if it would interfere with the quantitation of phenobarbital.

Phenylbutazone elutes from most columns very close to phenytoin and primidone. This is the only drug we have encountered that could be mistakenly identified as primidone or phenytoin when we use the double extraction technique.

Keep an alcoholic solution of the drugs and internal standards on hand (5 mg/ml of each in methanol). Inject 1 to 2 μl of this solution onto the gas chromatograph column to check column performance. The peaks should be sharp, with baseline separation of all five peaks. On a good column the equal concentration of primidone and phenytoin will produce equal peak heights. On an unsatisfactory column the phenytoin peak will be low and tailing will be significant. The phenobarbital peak will also be distorted. Sometimes several injections of this alcohol solution will "reconstitute" the column.

If peak height ratios are used for calibration, strive for operating parameters that will produce near full-scale recorder response with a phenobarbital concentration of 50 mg/liter. After phenobarbital and 5-ethyl-*p*-tolylbarbituric acid peaks come off, the attenuator may have to be reset to obtain near full-scale deflection with 30 mg/liter phenytoin concentration. This will allow accurately measurable peak heights over the range of concentrations most likely to be encountered.

Carbamazepine: Determination Without Derivatization

Harold E. Booker and Barbara A. Darcey

PRINCIPLE

Carbamazepine is extracted under alkaline conditions using chloroform containing *n*-tetracosane. After evaporation, the extract is dissolved in solvent and an aliquot is used for gas chromatography.

REAGENTS

1. *Chloroform:* high purity (i.e., Nanograde, Mallinckrodt, Inc., St. Louis, MO 63147 or distilled in glass from Burdick & Jackson, Muskegon, MI 49442).
2. *Hydrochloric acid:* 0.5 M.
3. *Sodium hydroxide:* 0.5 M.
4. *Carbon disulfide:* spectroanalyzed, Fisher Scientific, Fairlawn, NJ 07410.
5. *n*-Tetracosane, 1 mg/liter in chloroform (Applied Science Laboratories, State College, PA 16801).
6. *Carbamazepine:* (Ciba Pharmaceutical Co., Summit, NJ 07901).
7. *Stock standard:* 1 mg/ml in methanol. Store in refrigerator and prepare fresh monthly.
8. *Working standards:* dilute stock standard with serum known to be free of carbamazepine.

   100 μl diluted to 10 ml = 10 mg/liter
   50 μl diluted to 10 ml = 5 mg/liter
   20 μl diluted to 10 ml = 2 mg/liter

   Alternatively, use commercially available antiepileptic drug calibrators, Syva Corp., Palo Alto, CA 94304.

CHROMATOGRAPHIC CONDITIONS

1. The column used is a 180 cm × 2mm (i.d.) glass column packed with 3% OV-1 on Gas Chrom Q, 100 to 120 mesh (Applied Science Laboratories, State College, PA 16801).

2. Columns are conditioned as follows:
   (a) Turn on the carrier gas for 5 min and then turn it off.
   (b) Heat the column to 325°C without carrier gas flow for 1 hr.
   (c) Cool the column to room temperature.
   (d) Heat the column to 300°C with carrier gas flow for 3 hr.
3. The carrier gas (helium) flow is 40 ml/min.
4. The column, injector, and detector are maintained at 230°C. Because carbamazepine is unstable at high temperatures, it is extremely important to keep the injector and detector at this temperature.
5. The approximate retention times are carbamazepine, 3 min; *n*-tetracosane, 5 min.

These are typical conditions and may vary depending on the instrumentation, carrier gas, column, and other factors.

PROCEDURE

1. Transfer 0.5 ml of each standard, unknown, and a blank serum to 15-ml glass-stoppered centrifuge tubes. Add 0.5 ml of NaOH (0.5 M) and 5 ml of chloroform containing *n*-tetracosane (1 mg/liter).
2. Stopper and shake vigorously for 1 min. Centrifuge for 5 min at 1,500 rpm.
3. Aspirate the top aqueous phase and decant the chloroform extract to a clean, dry, 15-ml centrifuge tube. Backwash the extract with 2 ml of HCl (0.5 M). Centrifuge for 5 min.
4. Aspirate the top aqueous phase and decant the chloroform to a clean, dry tube. Evaporate the extract to dryness in a water bath or heating block at 50°C under a gentle stream of clean, dry air.
5. Wash down the sides of the tube with 50 μl of chloroform to concentrate the extract in the tip of the tube and evaporate to dryness again.
6. Dissolve the residue in 20 μl of carbon disulfide:chloroform (2:1) and inject 3 μl into the gas chromatograph. The extract may be dissolved in chloroform only.

CALIBRATION CURVE

Plot peak height ratio of carbamazepine:internal standard versus concentration of carbamazepine for each standard. For unknowns, calculate the peak height ratio of unknown to internal standard and read the concentration from the standard curve.

COMMENTS

The addition of the methanol to serum will cause some precipitation of protein. Be sure to mix the working standard thoroughly to ensure that these proteins are redissolved. Do not store the standards in silicone coated rubber stoppered tubes.

When blood specimens are drawn in tubes with silicone-coated rubber stoppers, the tube should be placed in an upright position as soon as possible to avoid contact of the blood with the stopper. A peak in the chromatogram between the carbamazepine and internal standard that is sometimes much higher than the other two peaks is caused by the stopper. If specimens are to be transported to another location for analysis, it would be advisable to ship the serum in a screw-top vial.

The best column sensitivity and column life is obtained with limited use of the column for other analyses.

If the carbamazepine peak starts to tail, remove the column and clean the injection end. Sometimes replacing 5 to 6 cm of packing at the injection end will improve column performance.

When the carbamazepine determinations are completed, increase the injector and detector temperatures approximately 50°C to burn off residual compounds that may be retained due to the low operating temperatures used for this analysis.

Strive for operating parameters that will produce about 75% of full-scale recorder deflection with the 10-mg/liter standard. This will allow accurately measurable peak heights over the range of concentration most likely to be encountered.

Carbamazepine: Determination by Silylation

Daniel L. Bius, Harvey J. Kupferberg, and Kenneth H. Dudley

PRINCIPLE

A method is described for the determination of carbamazepine levels in plasma by gas-liquid chromatography. The extraction procedure was designed to allow determination of five antiepileptic drugs (phenytoin, phenobarbital, primidone, ethosuximide, and carbamazepine) with 1 ml of plasma. Carbamazepine is determined as a silyl derivative, and the other drugs are determined by an on-column methylation technique. The procedure used for the extraction and silylation of carbamazepine is described below.

MATERIALS

USP-NF Reference Standard of carbamazepine (CBZ) was obtained from the U.S. Pharmacopeia (Rockville, MD). Cyheptamide, CYH (Ayerst Chemical Co., New York, NY) was provided by J. C. Van Meter (New Castle State Hospital, New Castle, IN). Anhydrous reagent-grade methanol, chloroform, and diethyl ether were used. Absolute ethanol was U.S.P. Reagent Quality and was obtained from U.S. Industrial Chemicals Company (New York, NY). Regisil® (BSTFA + 1% TMCS) was used as the silylating agent, and was obtained from Regis Chemical Company (Morton Grove, IL). Concentratubes® were obtained from Laboratory Research Company (Los Angeles, CA).

Drug-plasma Stock Solution (Spiked Plasma) for Calibration of CBZ

A solution was prepared by dissolving 10 mg of CBZ in 20 ml of absolute ethanol. This solution was stored in a tube with a Teflon-lined cap at 4°C indefinitely. Spiked plasma was prepared by diluting 1 ml of the ethanolic stock solution to 25 ml with blank plasma. The spiked plasma was stored at 4°C and was not used after five consecutive days.

Internal Standard Stock Solution (Spiked Buffer) for the Calibration and Determination of CBZ

A solution was prepared by dissolving 8.0 mg of cyheptamide (CYH) in 40 ml of absolute ethanol (other internal standards may be included in this solution).

This stock solution was stored in a tube with a Teflon-lined cap at 4°C indefinitely. Spiked buffer was prepared by diluting 1.0 ml of the ethanolic stock solution to 50 ml with 0.25 M sodium phosphate buffer (pH 7.6). Spiked buffer was stored at room temperature and was not used after 3 consecutive days.

METHODS

Preparation of Plasma Samples for Calibration of CBZ

Different volumes of spiked plasma and blank plasma were added to a series of tubes, the final volume of the blended mixture in each tube being 1.0 ml. These calibration samples provide a range of CBZ concentration of 2 to 20 μg/ml of plasma. A spiked plasma sample (1 ml) and spiked buffer (1 ml), the latter containing the internal standard, were mixed, and calibration was performed as described below.

Determination of CBZ: Gas Chromatography

Determinations of CBZ as its silylated derivative were carried out on a Hewlett-Packard model 5711 gas chromatograph equipped with hydrogen flame detectors. Columns were 1.2 m × 6 mm silanized glass with an inner diameter of 2 mm. The column packing was 3% SP-2401 on 100/120 mesh Supelcoport (Supelco, Inc., Bellefonte, PA). The carrier gas was nitrogen. Gas flow rates were as follows: nitrogen, 25 ml/min; hydrogen, 40 ml/min; and air, 250 ml/min. Other temperatures were injection port, 250°C; detector, 300°C; and oven (isothermal analysis), 200°C. Prior to use, columns were conditioned at 100°C for 1 hr, and the temperature was raised to 220°C at 1°C/min and maintained at 220°C for about 48 hr. The flow of the carrier gas was maintained at 25 ml/min at all times.

Determination of CBZ: Extraction Method and Preparation of Silylated Derivative

A spiked plasma sample or patient plasma sample (1 ml) and spiked buffer (1 ml) were mixed, and 8 ml of ether (previously saturated with 0.25 M sodium phosphate buffer of pH 7.6) was added. The tubes were capped and placed on a reciprocating shaker for 5 min, and were centrifuged (2,000 rpm) for 5 min. The ether phase was transferred to a concentratube and extracted with 100 μl of 0.3 M trimethylphenylammonium hydroxide (TMPAH). The extraction with TMPAH may be omitted if other antiepileptic drugs are not present in the sample. After centrifugation, the ether phase was transferred to a clean tube and was washed successively with 2 ml of 1 N NaOH and 2 ml of 1 N HCl. The ether phase was transferred to a 10-ml centrifuge tube and was evaporated to dryness. The residue was taken up in 0.5 ml of methanol, one drop of water was added, and then 6 ml of hexane was added. The tubes were placed on a reciprocating shaker for 5 min and were centrifuged for 5 min. The hexane was carefully removed and discarded. To each tube was added 1 ml of chloroform (to aid evaporation), and the solvent was evaporated. The tubes were dried *in vacuo* (40°C) over a drying agent for at least 45 min. To the dry tubes was added 30 μl of Regisil (BSTFA + 1% TMCS), and the tubes were rotated to ensure silylation of residue on the walls of the tubes. After standing at room temperature for at least 20 min, a sample (1.5 μl) was injected into the gas chromatograph. Calibration curves were constructed by plotting the ratio of the peak height of the drug to the peak height of its internal standard against the concentration of the drug (μg/ml).

Ethosuximide: Determination Without Derivatization

Harold E. Booker and Barbara A. Darcey

PRINCIPLE

Ethosuximide is extracted from serum under acidic conditions with chloroform. The chloroform is concentrated and an aliquot is used for gas chromatography. α,α-dimethyl-β-methylsuccinimide is used for the internal standard.

Adapted from W. A. Dill, L. Peterson, T. Chang, and A. J. Glazko, Physiologic disposition of 2-methyl-2-ethyl succinimide (ethosuximide: Zarontin) in animals and man. American Chemical Society 149th National Meeting, Detroit, Michigan, April 5–9, 1965, Abstracts page 30N.

REAGENTS

1. *Chloroform:* high purity (i.e., Nanograde, Mallinckrodt, St. Louis, MO 63147, or distilled in glass from Burdick and Jackson Labs, Muskegon, MI 49442).
2. *Hydrochloric acid:* 0.5 M.
3. α,α-dimethyl-β-methylsuccinimide for internal standard, 50 mg/liter in water (available from Aldrich Chemical, Milwaukee, WI 53233).
4. *Ethosuximide:* (available from Aldrich Chemical, Milwaukee, WI 53233).
   a. Stock standard: 500 mg/liter in distilled water. Store in refrigerator. Prepare fresh monthly.
   b. Working standards: Dilute the stock standard with serum known to be free of ethosuximide. Prepare fresh weekly.

1:20 dilution = 25 mg/liter
1:10 dilution = 50 mg/liter
1:5 dilution = 100 mg/liter

Alternatively, use commercially available antiepileptic drug calibrators (Syva Corp., Palo Alto, CA 94304.

PROCEDURE

1. Transfer 200 μl of each standard and unknown to a 15-ml glass-stoppered centrifuge tube. Add 0.5 ml of HCl (0.5 M) and 200 μl of the internal standard.
2. Add 5 ml of chloroform, stopper and shake vigorously for 1 min.
3. Centrifuge for 5 min at 1,500 rpm.
4. Aspirate the top aqueous layer and decant the chloroform to a clean, dry 15-ml centrifuge tube.
5. Evaporate all extracts to approximately 0.5 ml under a gentle stream of clean, dry air. *Do not evaporate to dryness.*
6. When ready to make each injection, spin the individual tube on a vortex while introducing a gentle stream of air into the tube. The extract can be concentrated to about 50 μl in less than 30 sec. Inject 3 μl of the concentrated extract into the gas chromatograph.

CALIBRATION CURVE

Plot the peak height ratio of the ethosuximide:internal standard versus the concentration of ethosuximide for each standard. For unknowns, calculate peak height ratios of unknown:internal standard and read concentrations from the standard curve.

CHROMATOGRAPHIC CONDITIONS

Columns are 180 cm × 2 mm (i.d.) glass columns packed with 3% OV-17 on Chromosorb WHP, 80 to 100 mesh (Hewlett-Packard).

Columns are conditioned at 300°C for at least 3 hr.

Carrier gas (helium) is 40 ml/min.

Column temperature is 125°C and the flash heater and detector at 160°C.

Approximate retention times: ethosuximide, 6 min; internal standard, 5 min.

COMMENTS

1. Trimethadione (TMO), paramethadione (PMO), and their *n*-demethylated metabolites will elute from this column at this temperature. The order of elution is TMO, PMO, *n*-demethylated TMO (DMO), internal standard, ethosuximide, *n*-demethylated PMO.
2. TMO and PMO can be quantitated successfully by this procedure. The recovery of DMO is low, and concentration of the extract to less than 0.5 ml results in distorted DMO peaks.
3. We have no experience with quantitation of *n*-demethylated PMO. In patients receiving PMO, the quantity of demethlyated PMO present is sufficient to swamp the ethosuximide peak. Quantitation of ethosuximide in the presence of high concentrations of demethylated PMO would be difficult.
4. Other drugs that are administered in conjunction with ethosuximide (i.e., phenobarbital, primidone, phenytoin, and carbamazepine) will be present in the extracts but will not elute from the column at this low temperature. After all of the ethosuximide determinations are completed, turn the column temperature to 300°C for about an hour to elute these compounds before using the column for other drug determinations.
5. Strive for operating parameters that will produce near full-scale recorder response with the 100-mg/liter standard. This will allow accurately measurable peak heights over the range of concentration most likely to be encountered.

Ethosuximide: Determination Without Derivatization

Christine D. Harvey and Allan L. Sherwin

PRINCIPLE

Ethosuximide is extracted from serum or plasma into chloroform. The extract is evaporated to dryness and injected directly into 3% XE 60 for analysis.

REAGENTS AND MATERIALS

1. Standard solution of ethosuximide in distilled water (Aldrich Chemical Co., Inc., Milwaukee, Wisc.), 100 μg/ml
2. Internal standard, α,α-dimethyl-β-methylsuccinimide in distilled water (Aldrich Chemical Co.), 200 μg/ml
3. 1.0 N hydrochloric acid.
4. Redistilled chloroform (Fisher Scientific Co., Montreal, Que.)
5. Isoamyl acetate (Aldrich Chemical Co.)
6. Whatman phase-separating filter paper IPS (Fisher Scientific Co.)
7. Glass-stoppered test tubes, 14 × 100 mm (Canadian Laboratory Supplies, Toronto, Ont.)
8. Polypropylene funnels, 66 mm i.d. (Canadian Laboratory Supplies)
9. 15-ml conical test tubes (Fisher Scientific Co.)
10. Eppendorf automatic pipette, 0.1 ml, 0.5 ml (Fisher Scientific Co.)

PROCEDURE

To prepare samples for the standard curve the volume of the indicated reagent is added in order:

Internal standard (200 μg/ml)	0.1	0.1	0.1	0.1	0.1	0.1
Blank plasma	0.5	0.5	0.5	0.5	0.5	0.5
Ethosuximide (100 μg/ml)	0.05	0.1	0.2	0.3	0.4	0.5
Distilled H_2O	0.45	0.4	0.3	0.2	0.1	—
1.0 N HCl	0.1	0.1	0.1	0.1	0.1	0.1
Total volume	1.2 ml	1.2 ml	1.2 ml	1.2 ml	1.2 ml	1.2 ml

Samples of unknown drug concentration:

Internal Standard	0.1 ml
Plasma	0.5 ml
Distilled H_2O	0.5 ml
1.0 N HCl	0.1 ml
Total volume	1.2 ml

1. To each tube is added, in order, 0.1 ml of internal standard; 0.5 ml of plasma; 0.5 ml of distilled water; 0.1 ml of 1.0 N HCl; 5 ml of redistilled chloroform.
2. The glass-stoppered test tube is then shaken for 10 min in an upright position.
3. During the extraction period, the Whatman IPS filter paper is folded and placed in a funnel. It is rinsed with 2 ml of chloroform, which is then discarded.
4. The sample is filtered through the Whatman IPS phase-separating paper that has been previously rinsed with chloroform into a 15-ml conical tube.
5. When filtration has *almost* ceased, the aqueous phase held back is returned to the original tube by pouring it from the filter cone, which is then rinsed with 2 ml of fresh chloroform and also added to the original tube. The aqueous phase is reextracted with the chloroform rinse plus an additional 2 ml of chloroform by hand shaking for 10 sec. The two phases are then emptied into the same filter cone. Finally, before filtration has ceased, the filter cone is discarded.

6. Three drops of isoamyl acetate are added to each tube, along with a carborundum chip.
7. The tubes are placed in a water bath, maintained at 65°C, in a fume hood.
8. The sample is allowed to evaporate to approximately 20 μl.
9. It is reconstituted with 30 μl of chloroform, the tube buzzed on a vortex, and 1 μl injected into a gas-liquid chromatograph.

Mephenytoin: Determination by Flash-Heater Ethylation

Patrick N. Friel and Allan S. Troupin

PRINCIPLE

The antiepileptic drugs measured in this procedure are weak organic acids, which when buffered to pH 6 exist mainly in their undissociated (acid) forms. They are extracted into ether/toluene, which is then mixed with a small volume of triethylphenylammonium hydroxide (TEPAH) in ethanol. Salts are formed between the alkaline TEPAH and the acidic antiepileptic drugs. Following centrifugation, the (lower) TEPAH layer containing the drugs of interest is sampled with a microsyringe and injected into a gas-liquid chromatograph (GLC). The high temperature of the injection port causes the salts to undergo a Hofmann degradation, yielding the ethyl derivatives of the antiepileptic drugs plus diethylaniline. The ethyl derivatives are separated by the GLC and quantitated using internal standards.

MATERIALS

1. *Phosphate buffer:* (0.25 M, pH 6.0): Dissolve 34 g of monobasic potassium phosphate in 900 ml of distilled water. Adjust the pH to 6.0 with 2 N sodium hydroxide, and make up to a volume of 1 liter with distilled water.
2. *Ether/toluene solution:* (1:1 by volume): Prepare by mixing equal volumes of the two organic solvents.
3. *TEPAH solution:* (1.5 M): Dissolve 9.2 g of triethylphenylammonium iodide (Eastman Organic Chemicals, Rochester, NY 14650) in 20 ml of absolute ethanol. Slowly add 5.8 g of silver oxide to the ethanol solution while stirring with a magnetic bar. Allow the exchange reaction to proceed with stirring for 2 hr. Separate the TEPAH solution from the precipitated silver iodide by centrifugation; collect and store the amber TEPAH solution in a glass-stoppered tube at 3°C.
4. *GLC column:* Pack a 1.83-m-long, 2-mm-i.d. glass column with 3% OV-1 on Gas Chrom Q, 100–120 mesh (a glass wool plug is necessary at the detector end of the column but not at the inlet end). Condition by heating at 300°C for 4 hr with no carrier gas flow, then at 240°C with a carrier gas flow of 40 ml/min overnight. Following conditioning the column is attached to the detector and is ready for operation; it is used exclusively for this procedure.
5. *GLC conditions:* Inlet temperature: 240°C. Column temperature: program from 165 to 230°C at 5°C/min. Flame ionization detector temperature: 250°C. Detector sensitivity: 1×10^{-9} to 3×10^{-10} A. Flow rates: air, 400 ml/min;

hydrogen, 40 ml/min; carrier (prepurified nitrogen), 40 ml/min (uncorrected); inlet pressure, 2.5 kg/cm^2.

6. *Additional equipment:* Evaporator, automatic pipettors (1 and 10 ml), mechanical shaker, 13-ml glass-stoppered extraction tubes, Concentratubes® (Laboratory Research Co., Los Angeles, CA 90036), Lang-Levy micropipettes (5, 10, 20, 30, 40, 50 μl), disposable Pasteur pipettes, vortex mixer, 10-μl microsyringe.
7. *Drug standard solution:* Weigh out and transfer to a single 50-ml volumetric flask 25 mg of mephenytoin, 25 mg of primidone, 50 mg of 5-ethyl-5-phenylhydantoin, 50 mg of phenobarbital, and 50 mg of phenytoin. Dissolve and make up to volume in absolute ethanol, and store at 3°C. (Obtain pure antiepileptic drugs from their manufacturers.)
8. *Internal standard solution:* Weigh out and transfer to a single 50-ml volumetric flask 25 mg of 5-methyl-5-phenylhydantoin (MPH), 25 mg of 5-allyl-5-phenylbarbituric acid (alphenal), and 25 mg of 5-(4-methylphenyl)-5-phenylhydantoin (MPPH). Dissolve and make up to volume in absolute ethanol, and store at 3°C. (Obtain pure internal standards from Applied Science Laboratories, State College, PA 16801, or Aldrich Chemical Co., Milwaukee, WI 53233.)

PROCEDURE

Allow 8 extraction tubes for a blank, 6 standards, and a control, as well as one tube for each patient sample. Label the tubes, and add 20 μl of internal standard solution to each one, except the blank. Add drug standard solution to the standard tubes in the following volumes: 5 μl to S-1, 10 μl to S-2, 20 μl to S-3, 30 μl to S-4, 40 μl to S-5, and 50 μl to S-6. Take each tube to dryness under a stream of air, then add 1 ml of phosphate buffer (pH 6) to each tube. Add 1 ml of blank plasma to the blank and each standard tube (using a total of 7 ml). Add 1 ml of control plasma to the control tube (the control is made up with your choice of antiepileptic drug concentrations and included in each run as a measure of precision).

Pipette 1 ml of patient serum or plasma into the remaining labeled tubes; record the patient's name and the tube number. Add 5 ml of ether/toluene solution to each tube. Stopper and seal the tubes and shake at 180 cpm for 5 min, then centrifuge at 250 $\times$ *g* for 5 min.

Set up a test tube rack of Concentratubes and label in the same order as the extraction tubes. Transfer about 4 ml of the (upper) ether/toluene layer from each extraction tube to the appropriately labeled Concentratube. Then add 50 μl of TEPAH solution to each Concentratube while mixing on a vortex mixer. Continue mixing each sample for 15 sec after the TEPAH is added. Stopper the Concentratubes and centrifuge for 5 min at 250 $\times$ *g*. Inject 1 μl of the (lower) TEPAH layer into the GLC with a 10-μl syringe, and press the temperature program start button. Rinse the syringe in absolute ethanol.

The standards, blank, and control should be run first, followed by patient samples. The blank should be devoid of peaks that would interfere at antiepileptic drug or internal standard retention times. At 1×10^{-9} A, the solvent front should return to within 10% of baseline before the MPH peak elutes. Antiepileptic drug and internal standard peaks should be well resolved and symmetrical in shape.

Calculations

Concentrations of the antiepileptic drugs in patient samples are calculated by computing the appropriate peak height ratio (PHR) and dividing by the mean slope (PHR/antiepileptic drug concentration in standards) for that antiepileptic drug, taken from the tabulated standard curve. The dimensions are PHR/[PHR/(μg/ml)] = μg/ml.

HPPH and *p*-Hydroxyphenobarbital: Determination in Urine

Robert A. Williamson and Henn Kutt

PRINCIPLE

Free *p*-hydroxyphenytoin(HPPH) and *p*-hydroxyphenobarbital (HPPB) are quantitatively determined by methylation following direct extraction from urine. Conjugated HPPH and HPPB concentrations are also determined following initial hydrolysis with concentrated hydrochloric acid to cleave the glucuronic acid conjugate. This method is also suitable for quantitation of unmetabolized phenytoin and phenobarbital.

REAGENTS AND CHEMICALS

1. Ethyl acetate, reagent grade
2. Methanol, reagent grade
3. HPPH (5-*p*-hydroxyphenyl-5-phenylhydantoin)[1]
4. *p*-OH-PB (5-*p*-hydroxyphenobarbital)[1]
5. MPPH (*p*-tolylhydantoin) (S_1)[1]
6. MPH (*p*-tolylphenobarbital) (S_2)[1]
7. TMPAI (trimethylphenylammonium iodide)[1]
8. Silver oxide, finely powdered
9. Sodium hydroxide
10. Sodium bicarbonate
11. Celite 535
12. Concentrated HCl

SOLUTIONS

1. 2.5% NaH_2CO_3 in distilled water
2. 8.5% NaOH in distilled water
3. HPPH, 10 mg/ml in methanol
4. *p*-OH-PB, 5 mg/ml in methanol
5. MPPH (S_1), 0.6 mg/ml in methanol
6. MPB (S_2), 0.3 mg/ml in methanol
7. TMPAH, 0.2 M (dissolve 526 mg of TMPAI in 10 ml of methanol, add 350 mg of silver oxide, stir for 3 hr)
8. Phosphate buffer, pH 7.7

---

[1] Aldrich Chemical Co., 940 West St. Paul Ave., Milwaukee, WI 53233.

PREPARATION OF CALIBRATION URINE SAMPLES

To 9.8 ml of drug-free urine add 0.2 ml of HPPH (solution 3) to give final concentration of 200 μg/ml. Make serial dilutions to obtain 100, 50, and 25 μg/ml. Similar action with *p*-OH-PB (solution 4) results in concentrations of 100, 50, 25, and 12.5 μg/ml. This covers the concentration ranges usually found in 1 ml of patients' urine samples. Both calibrators may be added to 9.6 ml of the same calibration urine.

HYDROLYSIS AND EXTRACTION

1. Into a pyrex digestion tube place 0.1 ml of MPPH (solution 5) and/or MPB (solution 6). Add 1.0 ml of urine and an equal volume of concentrated HCl. Heat slowly to boil in a heating block and continue slow boil for 30 min.
2. Allow to cool and pour the tube content into a small beaker; wash after with 1.0 ml of distilled water. Neutralize in beaker with 8.5% NaOH to bring the pH to around 5.
3. Transfer the mixture into 45-ml glass-stoppered centrifuge tube and add 15 ml of ethyl acetate. Shake for 10 min and centrifuge for 5 min.
4. Purification of extract

   HPPH: Transfer ethyl acetate phase (about 14 ml) to another 45-ml tube, shake with equal volume of 2.5% sodium bicarbonate solution (10 min), spin (5 min).

   p-OH-PB: Pass ethyl acetate through a small column (e.g., Pasteur pipette) filled with Celite 535. Stir Celite with phosphate buffer pH 7.7 to pack the column.
5. Place purified ethyl acetate into another 45-ml tube, evaporate to *dryness*. Reconstitute the *dry* residue with 80 μl of 0.2 M TMPAH and inject 1 to 2 μl into gas chromatograph.

CHROMATOGRAPHY CONDITIONS

Instruments: Hewlett-Packard model 402 or 7610. Column packing: 5% OV-17; oven temperature 260°C for HPPH, around 200°C for *p*-OH-PB. Port temperature 30°C above oven temperature; FID temperature 300°C

CALCULATIONS

Construct calibration curve from calibration urine samples plotting concentration against peak height or area ratios of drug over internal standard.

Read unknown sample concentration (μg/ml) from the curve.

Calculate 24-hr output (mg/24 hr) considering total 24-hr urine volume.

Antiepileptic Drug Determinations: Preparation of Internal Standards in an Aqueous Buffer and of Spiked Drug Plasma Samples for Calibration and Intralaboratory Quality Control

Kenneth H. Dudley and Daniel L. Bius

PRINCIPLE

The procedures described below were designed for a gas chromatographic on-column methylation technique in which 1 ml of an aqueous buffered internal standard solution of pH 7.6 and 1 ml of plasma are mixed prior to extraction and workup (see Chapter 4). All weighings are made to the nearest 0.01 mg on an analytical balance with a sensitivity of 0.01 mg. Class A pipettes (Fisher Scientific Co., Pittsburgh, PA) are used in the preparation of all stock and spiked solutions. MLA pipettes (Medical Laboratory Automation, Inc., Mount Vernon, NY) are used for mixing *spiked plasma I* and *spiked plasma II* (see Table 1).

TABLE 1. *Summary of final drug concentrations in calibration and intralaboratory quality control samples*

Calibration and quality control sample	Spiked plasma[a] I (ml)	Spiked plasma[b] II (ml)	Final drug concentrations (μg drug/ml plasma)				
			ES	PB	PD	DPH	CBZ
A	0.10	0.90	15	6	2	4	18
B	0.20	0.80	30	12	4	8	16
C	0.30	0.70	45	18	6	12	14
D	0.40	0.60	60	24	8	16	12
E	0.50	0.50	75	30	10	20	10
F	0.60	0.40	90	36	12	24	8
G	0.70	0.30	105	42	14	28	6
H	0.80	0.20	120	48	16	32	4
I	0.90	0.10	135	54	18	36	2

[a] Contains ES, PB, PD, and DPH.
[b] Contains CBZ only.

PREPARATION OF AN INTERNAL STANDARD SOLUTION OF 5-(P-METHYLPHENYL)-5-PHENYLHYDANTOIN (MPPH) IN AN AQUEOUS BUFFER OF PH 7.6

An internal standard solution of 5-(*p*-methylphenyl)-5-phenylhydantoin (MPPH) may be prepared with excellent accuracy by weighing out 20.00 ($\pm$ 0.02) mg of the compound and dissolving this quantity in 40.00 ($\pm$ 0.06) ml of absolute ethanol at ambient temperature. This stock solution, if stored in a Teflon-lined screw-cap tube at 4°C, is stable indefinitely; if stored in this manner, the solution is allowed to attain ambient temperature before use. An internal standard buffer solution may then be prepared on a daily basis (for daily use only) by diluting 1.00 (± 0.006) ml of the ethanol stock solution to 50.00 (± 0.05) ml with 0.25 M phosphate buffer of pH 7.6. The final concentration of the internal standard buffer solution is 10.00 (± 0.05) μg/ml of buffer, the accuracy of ±0.05 being derived by summing the maximal errors resulting from the tolerances listed at each step for the analytical equipment.

Other internal standards, with amounts given in parentheses, may be weighed and dissolved together with MPPH (20 mg) in ethanol, as follows: α,α,β-trimethylsuccinimide (100 mg); 5-ethyl-5-*p*-tolylbarbituric acid (60 mg); 5-ethyl-5-(*p*-tolyl)hexahydropyrimidine-4,6-dione (30 mg); and cyheptamide (8 mg). A buffer solution, which contains multiple internal standards, may be prepared by dilution of the ethanol stock with buffer of pH 7.6 as described above.

PREPARATION OF SPIKED PLASMA SAMPLES FOR CALIBRATION AND INTRALABORATORY QUALITY CONTROL

A solution is prepared by dissolving 30 mg of phenobarbital (PB), 10 mg of primidone (PD), 20 mg of phenytoin (DPH), and 75 mg of ethosuximide (ES) in 20 ml of absolute ethanol. This drug-stock ethanol solution is stored in a tube with a Teflon-lined cap at 4°C indefinitely. *Spiked plasma I* is prepared by diluting 1 ml of the drug stock ethanol solution to 25 ml with blank plasma.

A solution is prepared by dissolving 10 mg of carbamazepine (CBZ) in 20 ml of absolute ethanol. This drug-stock ethanol solution is stored as described above. *Spiked plasma II* is prepared by diluting 1 ml of the CBZ-stock ethanol solution to 25 ml with blank plasma.

Spiked plasma I and II are stored at 4°C and are not used after 5 days. All solutions stored at 4°C are allowed to attain ambient temperature before use or before use in the preparation of other solutions.

Calibration and intralaboratory quality control samples, which may be prepared from *spiked plasma I and II,* are summarized in Table 1. Spiked plasma samples containing only ES, PB, PD, and DPH are prepared by diluting the volumes listed under the *spiked plasma I* column to 1 ml with blank plasma. Spiked plasma samples containing ES, PB, PD, DPH, and CBZ are prepared by blending the volumes listed under *spiked plasma I* and *spiked plasma II* columns. The final drug concentrations for each calibration sample are summarized in Table 1. In this method, the final volume of the spiked plasma sample (A through I) is 1 ml. Internal standard(s) may be added as a solution in buffer prior to an extraction step.

Samples A through I may be used for calibration purposes. Two to four of these samples may be prepared on a daily basis as checks on intralaboratory control.

B. Sources

SOURCES OF COMMERCIALLY AVAILABLE ANTIEPILEPTIC DRUG CONTROLS IN A BIOLOGICAL MATRIX:

Lederle Diagnostics
American Cyanamid Company
Pearl River, NY 10965
(914/735–5000)

Ortho Diagnostics
Raritan, NJ 08869
(201/524–2444)

Syva Company[1]
3181 Porter Drive
Palo Alto, CA. 94394
(415/493–2200)

Wellcome Reagents
Burroughs Wellcome Co.
3030 Cornwallis Road
Research Triangle Park, NC 27709
(919/549–8371)

Utak Laboratories
10315 Woodley Avenue
Granada Hills, CA. 91344
(213/892–2204)

SOURCES OF COMPOUNDS FOR GAS-LIQUID CHROMATOGRAPHIC ANALYSIS OF ANTIEPILEPTIC DRUGS

Many laboratories that analyze drugs by gas-liquid chromatography do not utilize the appropriate internal standards for the various antiepileptic drugs. This is particularly true of laboratories that derivatize the barbiturates. It has been clearly established that methylation of phenobarbital results in erratic decomposition of the compound. We strongly urge laboratories to utilize *p*-tolylphenobarbital as the internal standard for phenobarbital and *p*-tolylphenytoin as the internal standard for phenytoin.

To serve as an appropriate internal standard, a drug must be as close as possible in chemical structure to the drug under analysis, so that it will have the same or similar chemical and physical properties when carried through different extraction techniques and derivatization reactions.

A number of antiepileptic drugs or compounds and metabolites are commercially available. Listed below are those available in crystalline form from the Aldrich Chemical Company, 940 West St. Paul Avenue, Milwaukee, WI 53233; telephone 414/273–3850.

Drug or Compound	*Catalog No.*
α,α-Dimethyl-β-methylsuccinimide [internal standard for ethosuximide]	16,350–3
5,5-Diphenylhydantoin [phenytoin; Dilantin]	16,192–6

[1] Only commercially available source of GLC calibrators for antiepileptic drugs.

Drug or Compound	*Catalog No.*
5-Ethyl-5-(*p*-hydroxyphenyl)barbituric acid [*p*-hydroxyphenobarbital; metabolite of phenobarbital]	19,501–4
2-Ethyl-2-phenylmalonamide [phenylethylmalonamide, PEMA; metabolite of primidone (Mysoline)]	19,502–2
5-Ethyl-5-(*p*-tolyl)barbituric acid [*p*-tolylbarbital; internal standard for phenobarbital]	17,957–4
2-Ethyl-2-(*p*-tolyl)malonamide [methyl PEMA, MPEMA; internal standard for PEMA]	19,496–4
5-(*p*-Hydroxyphenyl)-5-phenylhydantoin [major metabolite of phenytoin]	16,154–3
Iminostilbene [decomposition product of flash methylation of carbamazepine; a minor carbamazepine metabolite]	14,365–0
5-(*p*-Methylphenyl)-5-phenylhydantoin [internal standard for phenytoin]	16,145–4
α-Methyl-α-phenylsuccinimide [desmethylmethsuximide; major metabolite of methsuximide (Celontin)]	86,058–1
4-Methylprimidone [4-methylpimacolone; internal standard for primidone (Mysoline)]	19,494–8
α-Methyl-α-propylsuccinimide [proposed alternate internal standard for ethosuximide]	19,495–6

SOURCES OF COMMERCIALLY UNAVAILABLE DRUGS AND METABOLITES

The easiest way to obtain drugs that are not commercially available is to call the manufacturer of the drug, whose telephone number is listed in the *Physicians' Desk Reference* (Medical Economics Company, Oradell, NJ 07649). Ask the Medical Director's Office to refer you to the appropriate person from whom to request the compound of interest. Follow the telephone call with a letter to that individual, requesting the appropriate quantity of drug and describing its intended use. The manufacturer will send you an investigator's form in which you will again describe the intended use of the drug. Upon completion and return of the form to the manufacturer, the drug will be forwarded.

It should be noted that manufacturers do not have inexhaustible supplies of drug metabolites. They should not be requested unless you are establishing the appropriate assays, because you will be denying the drug to another investigator who could utilize the compound.

Subject Index